Electrochemical Interfaces for the Detection of Agricultural Pollutants

Online at: https://doi.org/10.1088/978-0-7503-5879-8

Electrochemical Interfaces for the Detection of Agricultural Pollutants

Edited by
Chandra Sekhar Rout
Centre for Nano and Material Sciences, Jain (Deemed-to-be University), Jain Global Campus, Kanakapura, Bangalore 562112, Karnataka, India

IOP Publishing, Bristol, UK

ISBN 978-0-7503-5879-8 (ebook)
ISBN 978-0-7503-5877-4 (print)
ISBN 978-0-7503-5880-4 (myPrint)
ISBN 978-0-7503-5878-1 (mobi)

DOI 10.1088/978-0-7503-5879-8

Version: 20240701

IOP ebooks

British Library Cataloguing-in-Publication Data: A catalogue record for this book is available from the British Library.

Published by IOP Publishing, wholly owned by The Institute of Physics, London

IOP Publishing, No.2 The Distillery, Glassfields, Avon Street, Bristol, BS2 0GR, UK

US Office: IOP Publishing, Inc., 190 North Independence Mall West, Suite 601, Philadelphia, PA 19106, USA

To everyone who pursues research in material science, electrocatalysis, and electrochemical environmental analysis for sustainable agriculture.

Contents

Preface

The ever-evolving landscape of modern agriculture and the necessity for environmental sustainability have spotlighted the imperative role of technology in addressing the challenges faced by the farming industry. Given the significant impact of agricultural pollutants on both crop yield, and the health and well-being of our ecosystem, as well as the food supply and our future, meticulous management of these pollutants is of utmost importance. It is imperative that we undertake a comprehensive approach to managing agricultural pollutants, taking into account the complex interplay between environmental, economic, and social factors. Failure to do so may lead to irreparable harm to our agricultural systems, which could have far-reaching consequences for human and environmental health. Therefore, it is incumbent upon us to prioritize the development and implementation of effective strategies for managing agricultural pollutants, to safeguard our food supply and the long-term sustainability of our planet.

Electrochemical Interfaces for the Detection of Agricultural Pollutants is an essential resource in this crucial domain. This book is a culmination of extensive research and dedication to developing and applying electrochemical sensing technology for monitoring and mitigating agricultural pollutants. In the following pages, the readers will embark on a comprehensive journey through the field of electrochemical sensors and their profound impact on detecting pollutants in the agricultural sector. We explore the fundamental principles, electrochemical methodologies, and emerging applications of electrochemical sensing, all aimed at enhancing our ability to address and combat the myriad pollutants that threaten our ecosystem. This book delves into the diverse aspects of electrochemical sensors, from their theoretical foundation to their practical implementation, from the sensing of chemical fertilizers and pesticides to monitoring heavy metals. The objective is to present state-of-the-art electrochemical sensors and inspire further attention to address the urgent environmental challenges that we face today. This book is both a compilation of knowledge and a call to action to harness the potential of electrochemical sensing technology to safeguard our ecosystem.

Chapter 1 begins with an introduction to analytical techniques, the fundamentals of voltammetry, and its related techniques. Followed by the fundamentals of electrochemical sensors, the role of electrode materials in the fabrication of electrochemical sensors, and finally the significance of electrochemical sensors for environmental analysis. Chapter 2 describes carbon and its allotropes. Chapter 3 describes the characteristics of 0D, 1D, 2D, and 3D carbon allotropes in the fabrication of electrochemical sensors for pollutant detection. Furthermore, chapter 4 substantiates the fundamentals of biosensors and the application of carbon-based nanomaterials to immobilize bioreceptors. Chapter 5 discusses the emerging agricultural pollutants and their impact on public health. Chapter 6 elaborates on carbon-based electrochemical sensors-assisted environmental analysis for fertilizer contamination. Meanwhile, chapter 7 deals with electrochemical sensing of pesticide residues from the environment. Chapter 8 narrates the detection of heavy metal ion contamination. Chapter 9 provides a description of the electrochemical biosensors that have been developed to detect various agricultural contaminants. Chapter 10 discusses carbon nanomaterial modified field-effect transistors, impedance-based, and potentiometric sensors for agricultural pollutant detection. Chapter 11 focuses on implementing electrochemical sensors for detecting agricultural pollutants and their potential prospects. Finally, this book concludes by summarizing the information presented throughout its contents.

Acknowledgements

I want to express my deep gratitude to all those who have contributed to completing this book, *Electrochemical Interfaces for the Detection of Agricultural Pollutants.* The realization of this book was made possible through the collective efforts and support of numerous individuals and my academic institution. First, and foremost, I extend my heartfelt appreciation to my dedicated research team, whose unwavering commitment and efforts played a vital role in completing this book. I thank Jain (deemed-to-be) University for providing essential resources, infrastructure, and funding. My appreciation goes to my family and friends for their patience, support, and encouragement throughout the writing process. Finally, I sincerely thank the readers and the broader community interested in electrochemical sensing technology for pollutant detection. Your dedication and curiosity in making our world a better and cleaner place have been a constant source of motivation. Finally, on behalf of all the authors, I would like to thank the anonymous reviewers who thoroughly assessed this work and added to its quality. We have also received significant assistance from the IOP's publishing team, who have contributed to the success of this book; hearty thanks!

Editor biography

Chandra Sekhar Rout

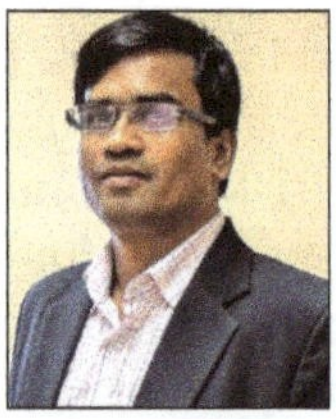

Professor Chandra Sekhar Rout is a full professor at the Centre for Nano and Material Sciences (CNMS), Jain University. Before joining CNMS, he was a DST-Ramanujan Fellow at IIT Bhubaneswar, India (2013–17). He received his BSc (2001) and MSc (2003) degrees from Utkal University and his PhD from JNCASR, Bangalore (2008) under the supervision of Prof. C N R Rao, Bharat Ratna. He did his postdoctoral research at National University of Singapore (2008–09), Purdue University, USA (2010–12) and UNIST, South Korea (2012–13). He was awarded the prestigious Ramanujan Fellowship and Young Scientist award of the Department of Science and Technology, Government of India in 2013, the Emerging Investigator Award 2017 from Elsevier, the IAAM medal 2017 from the International Association of Advanced Materials 2017, and the Young Researcher award from the Venus International Foundation in 2015. His research interests include preparing and characterizing 2D layered materials and their hybrids for chemical sensors and biosensors, supercapacitors and energy storage devices, field emitters, and electronic devices. He has authored more than 200 research papers in international journals and has edited six books. His current h-index is 57, with total citations >13 600. He was ranked in the top 2% of scientists in India by the Stanford study in 2020–22. He serves as a board member of various reputed journals. He is the associate editor of *RSC Advances*, a journal of the Royal Society of Chemistry, and *The American Journal of Engineering and Applied Sciences* of Science Publications. He has completed several sponsored projects funded by the government of India and has supervised PhD, postdocs, and MSc students. He has delivered over 50 invited talks at various national and international conferences and traveled to countries such as the USA, UK, Israel, Singapore, South Korea, Brazil, and Russia for collaboration.

List of contributors

Mr Vishwanath Ankalgi
Centre for Nano and Material Sciences, Jain (Deemed-to-be University), Jain Global Campus, Kanakapura, Bangalore 562112, Karnataka, India

Ms B R Karishma
Centre for Nano and Material Sciences, Jain (Deemed-to-be University), Jain Global Campus, Kanakapura, Bangalore 562112, Karnataka, India

Dr G Manasa
Centre for Nano and Material Sciences, Jain (Deemed-to-be University), Jain Global Campus, Kanakapura, Bangalore 562112, Karnataka, India

Ms M Monisha
Centre for Nano and Material Sciences, Jain (Deemed-to-be University), Jain Global Campus, Kanakapura, Bangalore 562112, Karnataka, India

Ms Mansi Pathak
Centre for Nano and Material Sciences, Jain (Deemed-to-be University), Jain Global Campus, Kanakapura, Bangalore 562112, Karnataka, India

Ms S Pavithra
Centre for Nano and Material Sciences, Jain (Deemed-to-be University), Jain Global Campus, Kanakapura, Bangalore 562112, Karnataka, India

Prof. Chandra Sekhar Rout
Centre for Nano and Material Sciences, Jain (Deemed-to-be University), Jain Global Campus, Kanakapura, Bangalore 562112, Karnataka, India

Chapter 1

Elementary concepts of electrochemical sensors for real-time detection

G Manasa and Chandra Sekhar Rout

Recently, electrochemical sensors have played a pivotal role in real-time detection, leveraging the principles of electrochemical reactions at electrolyte/electrode interfaces. This chapter provides a concise overview of the elementary concepts surrounding the design of electrochemical sensors. The discussion in this chapter encompasses fundamental aspects, including various electrochemical techniques, electrode classification, the need for electrode modification, and the necessity of nanomaterial catalysts. It also addresses the importance of electrochemical sensors, among other classical techniques, by exemplifying the recent trends in the sensing domain. Understanding the fundamental concepts is essential for designing and using electrochemical sensors effectively for real-time detection in various applications.

1.1 Introduction

All our sensations, thoughts, emotions, learning abilities, knowledge processing, and memory result from nerve conduction. Due to chemical and electric events, impulses are transmitted through an electron domino effect. Likewise, due to oxidoreduction reactions, various dynamic physiochemical processes occur in the body, such as the Krebs cycle, urea cycle, ornithine cycle, trans-amination catalyst, and lipid peroxidation. Electrochemistry can be used as a tool to better understand such redox reactions [1–3]. Electroanalytical chemistry is based on electrical properties that include the current, potential, and quantity of electricity produced depending on concentration when it is made part of an electrochemical cell [4, 5]. It comprises a group of quantitative and qualitative analytical methods that measure the variation of electrical parameters (current, potential) and relate this to chemical parameters (concentration). It plays a vital role in understanding the electron transfer process

doi:10.1088/978-0-7503-5879-8ch1

and the number of electrons involved in a chemical reaction. Hence, electrochemistry is a chemical and electric energy relationship that can be applied to systems that undergo redox reactions [6].

1.2 Analytical techniques of the twenty-first century

Electroanalytical techniques are robust and have a broad scope of applications due to their versatility. These techniques are most suitable for investigating the redox properties of various substances, ranging from pharmaceuticals to essential biomolecules and organic pollutants, which may be synthetic or naturally occurring [7]. The choice of several available methods depends on the type of analysis required for the sample under investigation. Each technique has a different degree of sophistication, sensitivity, and selectivity. They may also vary in cost and time of analysis.

1.2.1 Fundamentals of analytical chemistry

Foresee, a redox-active analyte, can be studied by measuring one of the four parameters, i.e., potential, current, charge, and time. Thus, the system's response depends on which parameter is applied as an excitation signal; however, a combination of these parameters can be used. The three categories are conductometry (electrical conductivity of a solution), potentiometry (measurement of the difference in electrode potentials), and voltammetry (measurement of the current in the cell while actively varying the cell potential). In brief, measurements using conductometry rely on the ability of electrolyte solutions to dissociate into ions. These measurements involve detecting changes in the electrical resistance of a solution. A conductometric cell comprises an electrolyte solution, two electrodes (anode and cathode), and a battery (current reading detection unit) to perform conductometric measurements. The concentration of electrolytes is indicated by the amount of current generated, which is determined by the number of ions present. Ohm's law describes the electrolytic properties of a conductor: $V = I \cdot R$ (where V = voltage, R = resistance, I = current), while the conductance can be calculated using the formula: $G = I/R$ (G = conductance) [8]. On the other hand, potentiometry measures the potential of a potentiometric cell. It comprises four components: a reference electrode (RE), a salt bridge, an analyte solution, and an indicator electrode. Hydrogen, calomel, or silver/silver chloride are the most commonly used REs. Indicator electrodes can either be metallic or ion-selective. A salt bridge is a barrier between the standard electrode and the analyte solution. Potentiometric methods are governed by the Nernst equation, which is used to calculate the potential (E) [8]: $E_{(cell)} = E_{(indicator)} - E_{(reference)}$.

Several instrumental analysis methods, such as mass spectrophotometry, HPLC, GC, GC–MS, and capillary electrophoresis, have been favored in detecting specific molecules, which are appealing choices for chemical analysis. Although these techniques provide accurate detection and selectivity, they are not appropriate for quickly processing numerous samples, conducting real-time detection, field studies, or in situ monitoring. In most cases, these instrumental methods, including the spectroscopic and optical techniques, require preliminary separations, limiting their use [9].

The electroanalytical technique of voltammetry has received attention because it is robust and straightforward, so an inept person can also handle it. Most importantly, it is comparatively an inexpensive and not-so-sophisticated technique. In comparison, the principal advantage of the voltammetric approach is the possibility of direct analysis, and hence convenience without the need for separation or pretreatment. Therefore, electrochemical sensors of various kinds can be an alternative. Moreover, the instrument required for voltammetric analysis is straightforward to handle and inexpensive as a reward for advances in voltammetry, kinetic information, excellent detection limits, and a wide dynamic range have been achieved. In addition, this technique favors real samples where minimal volumes of real samples are analyzed for low concentrations of molecules under investigation. For these reasons, and due to its specificity, reproducibility, and rapidity, voltammetry uniquely suits organic or inorganic substances in pharmaceutical compounds, biologically critical molecule analysis, and detecting electroactive toxic molecules for health and the environment.

This rapidly progressing sensing technology is a field of electrochemistry. This is vital because the electrochemical investigation of essential biologically active molecules elucidates biological processes and their inter-relationships in living organisms [10–12]. Monitoring redox dynamic species has been aided by electrochemical sensors, which are robust, economical, small, portable, and easily handled. Chemical sensors are miniature (but not all) electric transducers that respond to the chemical reaction through electric signals, depending on the concentration of the analyte.

Many biomolecules are designed by nature to be redox active at particular conditions, making it very difficult to elucidate the mechanistic details of the reaction. Hence, the effect of buffer, pH, and potential are studied to understand the mechanism [13, 14]. Thus, systematic examination of the electrode processes provides insight into the electrochemical mechanisms and behavior analogous to biochemical reactions. In addition, redox reactions can be mimicked at the electrode's surface, providing evidence for the involvement of hydrogen and electron atoms in the response.

1.2.2 Sensors

The advanced fundamentals and applications of interdisciplinary research span chemistry, physics, biology, materials, and nanoscience, and solve problems whose solutions are beyond the scope of a single discipline. For instance, the high sensitivity and selectivity of the developed electrochemical sensors allow the monitoring of various target analytes of interest [15–17]. This aids physicians in making rapid and accurate diagnoses, ensuring that the patient gets the proper treatment quickly. The rapid advances in the field of sensing technology have expanded the application of commercialized sensors, such as a blood glucose biosensor [18]. Sensor technologies form an interdisciplinary domain that combines several modalities of sensing, actuation, and signal processing. Electrochemical sensors are classified according to the applied electrochemical transduction mode and are mainly (i) potentiometric sensors, (ii) conductometric/impedimetric sensors, and (iii) voltammetric/amperometric sensors (figure 1.1). Ion-selective electrodes (ISEs) are often employed for potentiometric measurements. When using sensor networks for measurements that require high temporal and spatial precision, ISEs are especially appealing due to their fast reaction times, insensitivity to light, and comparatively low cost compared to alternative methods. Specific ions interact with an electrode membrane material more favorably than others, and the sensors operate based on this principle. The potential change resulting from this interaction can be used to calculate the analyte concentration using the traditional Nernst equation. On the other hand, measurement of the impedance shift caused by a change in target analyte concentration is done in the impedimetric sensors. This is in contrast to different types of sensors. For example, impedimetric measurements can potentially sense the electron transfer at high frequency and determine low analyte concentrations. Meanwhile, the concentration of the analyte is measured by amperometric sensors using the current response at a working electrode (WE) relative to the RE. Through this chapter and the subsequent chapters, I will take you through the fundamentals and application of voltammetric sensors for

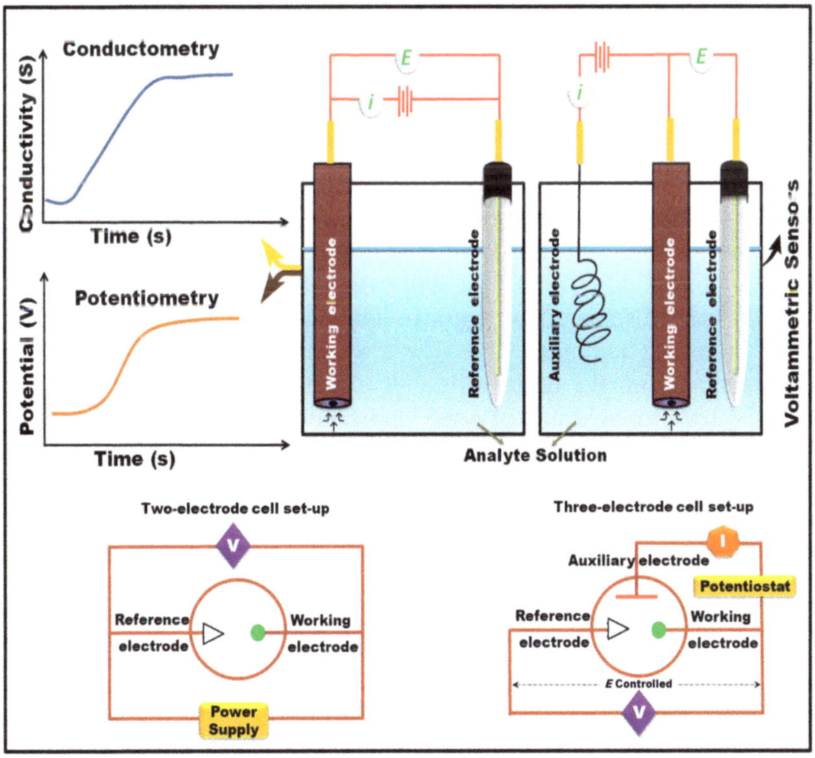

Figure 1.1. Graphical illustration of a two- and three-electrode setup and their circuits.

agro-pollutant detection. The essential advantage of this technique is its good precision and sensitivity, coupled with a more extensive linear concentration range and the ability to simultaneously determine several analytes by controlling the process through applied electrode voltage, favoring robust analysis time [19]. Ukhade *et al* have comprehensively looked at detecting, monitoring, and preventing pollutants using different forms and types, such as chemical sensors, biosensors, etc [20].

1.3 Voltammetry and its related techniques

Voltammetry, a division of electrochemistry, came into existence after Jaroslav Heyrovsky observed polarography in 1922, who was subsequently awarded the Nobel Prize for his discovery. However, voltammetry experienced several difficulties. Nevertheless, during the 1960s and 1970s, significant advances were made in voltammetric theory, methodology, and instrumentation. This enhanced the method's sensitivity and expanded into a wide range of analytical techniques. Low-cost operational amplifiers were developed around the same time. These amplifiers made it much easier to produce affordable instrumentation, which was a considerable boon for the industry. Over the past 10 years, this electroanalytical technique has significantly developed and it is now a highly adaptable and effective analytical method. The difference between these techniques is the way in which the potential is applied. The basis of these techniques is linear sweep voltammetry, wherein the current is estimated with a linear increase in the applied potential over time of the WE.

An electrochemical method called cyclic voltammetry (CV) is used to quantify the current level produced by an electrochemical cell during an oxidation or reduction reaction. To perform a CV, the voltage of a WE is cycled and the resulting current is measured. A cyclic voltammetric experiment consists of two or several linear potential sweeps. Thus, the start, switching, and end potentials must be defined. Typically, two linear units, called the half cycles, are combined, and the beginning and the end potentials are often identical. The number of possibilities for such an experiment is almost unlimited [21]. The CV curve is generated by scanning the potential starting from the initial value (E_1) (forward sweep—anode) to the final potential (E_2) (reverse sweep—cathode) that finally returns to the initial potential (E_1) (figure 1.2(a) inset). Figure 1.2(a) illustrates the CV's experimental result. When the scanning rate is constant, the voltage is increased from E_1 to E_2. An initial background current is noticed. As the potential progresses the electrochemical oxidation reaction takes place on the surface of the electrode, and the current gradually increases to a maximum and decreases. This reaction results in significant CV parameters, such as current (I_{pa} and I_{pc}) and potential (E_{pa} and E_{pc}) for the target analyte. CV is employed for qualitative analysis, including (i) determination of reversibility of the redox reaction, (ii) determination of reaction mechanism, and (iii) determination of electrochemical surface area (ECSA). However, CV has low sensitivity and is rarely used for quantitative analysis.

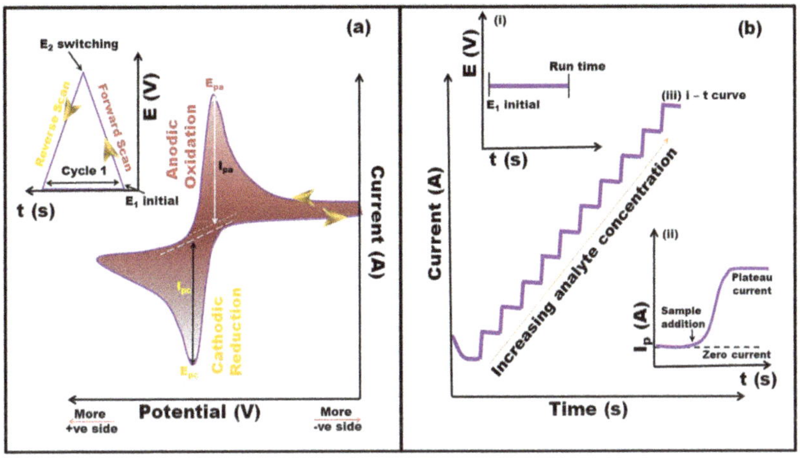

Figure 1.2. (a) Cyclic voltammogram, inset: triangular waveform: potential versus time. (b) Amperometry: inset: (i) plot of potential versus time, (ii) principle of amperometric measurement, (iii) amperogram: *i*–*t* curve.

1.3.1 Charge transfer

At the interface between the electrode and the electrolyte, an exchange of electrons occurs in any of the following three ways [22]:

(a) Reversible electron transfer: When the kinetics at the WE are faster than the mass transport, the system is electrochemically reversible. The concentration of the target species at the surface of the electrode can be expressed using the Nernstian equation:

$$C_o/C_R = \exp\left[\frac{nF(E - E^\circ)}{RT}\right]$$

Here, the concentrations of the oxidized (C_o) and reduced (C_R) species are equivalent at the electrode's surface.

(b) Irreversible electron transfer: When the electrode's kinetics are slower than the mass transport, the system is electrochemically irreversible ($k^\circ < m_{trans}$). The electrode's kinetics are expressed using the Butler–Volmer equation:

$$\text{Oxidation: } k_f = k \exp\left[\frac{-(1 - \propto)nF(E - E^\circ)}{RT}\right]$$

$$\text{Reduction: } k_f = k \exp\left[\frac{-\propto nF(E - E^\circ)}{RT}\right]$$

The rate constant for electron transfer in a redox process is denoted by k_f. This constant depends on the applied potential, which accounts for the steep rise in response peak current k, which is the standard heterogeneous rate constant.

(c) Quasi-reversible electron transfer: When mass transport and electron transfer rates are comparable, a mixed control situation is termed quasi-reversible reaction ($k^\circ \sim m_{trans}$).

Table 1.1 represents the diagnostic traits of cyclic voltammograms obtained from reversible electron transfer [23–28].

1.3.2 Electrochemical processes and transfer of electroactive material towards the electrode surface

When the WE in the electrolyte under external voltage has an excess charge on its surface, it forms an electrical double layer. Furthermore, when an electrochemical reaction occurs with the transfer of charge, the process produces a faradaic current that arises from the electron transfer across the electrolyte-WE interface. This faradaic current is proportional to the concentration of the electroactive species reduced or oxidized and is in good agreement with Faraday's law [29]:

$$Q = F\, n_e\, m$$

Here, Q is the amount of charge transferred through an electrochemical system, which is proportional to the moles of analyte (m) reacted at the WE by the total number of electrons exchanged by each species (n_e).

The sensing mechanism is based on electrochemical dynamic theory. Hence, the Nernst equation was used to describe the relationship between the electrode potential and the analyte concentrations being reduced (C_R) or oxidized (C_O) on the surface of the electrode. A typically reversible electrode reaction can be expressed as:

$$O + ne^- \leftrightarrows R$$

While the Nernst equation can unveil the quantitative relationship [30]:

$$E = E^\circ + \frac{RT}{nF} \ln \frac{C_o}{C_R}$$

Here, E° is the standard electrode potential for the reaction (V), R is the universal gas constant, T is the temperature (K), n is the transferred electron number in molecular redox, and F is Faraday's constant.

The rate of an electrochemical reaction happening at the electrode surface can be directly measured by the Faradaic current that flows at any time. Two important processes determine the current's value: (a) mass transport and (b) charge transfer kinetics.

Furthermore, as the sensing signal, the response current determines the reaction rates, as furnished by the Butler–Volmer equation [31]:

$$I = nFAk^\circ\{C_o \exp\ [-\alpha\eta] - C_R \exp[(I - \alpha)\eta]\}$$

Here, $\eta = nF(E - E^\circ)/RT$, k° is the heterogeneous electrochemical reaction rate constant, A is the WE surface area, and α is the electron transfer coefficient.

Table 1.1. Cyclic voltammograms and their diagnostic tests for reversible, irreversible, and quasi-reversible systems.

Diagnostic traits for cyclic voltammograms		
Reversible systems	Irreversible systems	Quasi-reversible systems
The Randles–Sevcik equation provides the value for peak current: $I_p = (2.69 \times 10^5)\ A.C.\sqrt{D}.\ \sqrt{v}.\ \sqrt[3]{n}$	Peak current is represented by: $I_p = (2.99 \times 10^5).n.A\ C.\sqrt{D}.\ \sqrt{v}.\ \sqrt{\alpha n}$	The square root of the scan rate is not adequately reflected in the peak. This I_p may not rise proportionately with the scan rate.
$\Delta E_p = E_{pa} - E_{pc} \simeq \frac{59}{n}$ mV	$\Delta E = E^\circ - \left(\frac{RT}{n_\alpha\ F}\right)\left[0.78 - \left(\ln\frac{k^\circ}{\sqrt{D}}\right) + \ln\sqrt{\frac{\alpha\ n_\alpha\ Fv}{RT}}\right]$	ΔE_p possibly attains $\frac{59}{n}$ mV at a low scan rate but increases with an amplifying scan rate.
	$E_p - E_{p/2} = \frac{47.7}{\alpha n}$ mV	ΔE is more significant than $\frac{59}{n}$ mV. It magnifies with an increase in the sweep rate.
$\frac{I_{pa}}{I_{pc}} = 1$	There is no peak in the reverse scan.	$\frac{I_{pa}}{I_{pc}} = 1$, not all cases are true until $\alpha = 0.5$.
	$E_p = \frac{30}{\alpha n}$ mV	E_p shifts more negatively or positively for reduction or oxidation, respectively.

Additionally, the diffusion process also influences the electrode process, as revealed by Fick's law, which describes the relationship between mass transfer and concentration gradient [32]:

$$\Phi = -D \left(\frac{\partial C_o}{\partial x}\right)$$

Here, Φ is the diffusion flux, D is the diffusion coefficient, and x is the distance from the electrode. As one can observe from the equation, the greater the concentration gradient of electroactive species, the larger the response current will be.

1.3.3 Other voltammetric techniques

The other techniques in voltammetry include [33–35]:

(i) Hydrodynamic voltammetry

(a) Rotating disk voltammetry (RDV)

The hydrodynamic techniques, crucial in environmental sensing, involve potential scanning while a solid disk electrode rotates around its axis, stirring the solution. The resulting voltammogram is a wave, which is a key indicator in this process.

(b) Amperometry (AMP)

An initial potential and run time must be selected to run this technique (figure 1.2(b) (i)). The potential is adjusted to a desired value during the AMP process, and the resulting current is then measured. Alternatively, when using a flow injection system, the potential can be kept constant while target analytes are measured at the WE. This technique is selective in detecting electroactive species from a sample solution; the resulting current is proportional to their concentration. By using a fixed potential, the charging current is minimized and the background signals are reduced, which improves the detection limit. Figure 1.2(b) (ii) indicates the electrochemical response with a weak zero current in the absence of the target analyte under detection, and the magnitude of this blank is typically attained while calibrating at a steady polarization voltage. When a target analyte is introduced, certain species become mobile across the electrolyte and undergo oxidation or reduction at the electrode. The current response to this process increases until it reaches a plateau, at which equilibrium is reached. The current at the plateau is directly proportional to the concentration of the target analyte. Thus, when a constant potential is applied during AMP measurement, the analyte response produces a Faraday response [36]. However, AMP cannot perform qualitative analysis. In addition, the hydrodynamic process of the amperometry significantly improves the mass transport at the WE surface, swirling the solution. Flow systems demonstrate superior performance in environmental monitoring compared to steady-state batch systems. This is because the flow conditions enable better transportation of solutions in multistep assay procedures, which results in online detection.

(ii) Pulse method: Different potential modulations enhance the speed and sensitivity, achieving low detection limits. This technique involves the application of a pulse voltage to produce a charging current in the electrode, which quickly decays to zero. This process causes the target analyte to generate an electrode response (Faraday current). The Faraday current is regulated by the movement of reactive species at the electrode interface. This movement slows down gradually with the reaction of the reactive species on the electrode. However, the decay rate of the redox current is much slower than that of the charging current. Hence, the current is measured later in the applied pulse voltage, and the resulting current measurement corresponds to the redox current. The three types of pulse techniques are [34]:

(a) Normal pulse voltammetry: This method uses a sequence of potential pulses with increasing amplitude. The current is measured after each pulse, and enough time is given for the charging current to decay. The measured current is displayed on the vertical axis of the generated voltammogram, while the pulse potential is plotted on the horizontal axis. The experiment is typically conducted in a solution that is not stirred.

(b) Differential pulse voltammetry (DPV): In the DPV technique, a series of periodic, constant pulses of potential is superimposed on a linear scan. To measure the current of each pulse accurately, two points are selected for sampling (i_1 and i_2). The first point is taken just before the application of the pulse, and the second point is taken at the end of the pulse. These points are selected to allow for the decay of the non-faradaic charging current. The difference between current measurements at these points for each pulse is calculated and graphed against the base potential, as depicted in figure 1.3(a).

(c) Square-wave voltammetry (SWV): SWV uses a signal to stimulate that is made up of a square-wave pulse with equal amplitude and a staircase waveform with a step height. The forward pulse of the square wave overlaps with the staircase step. The difference between the forward and reverse currents measures the current, as figure 1.3(b) shows. The concentration of the electroactive species is directly related to the height of the peak.

(iii) Stripping method: This method is commonly employed for trace analysis of metals, there are also two waveform application modes of stripping voltammetry: square wave anodic stripping voltammetry and differential pulse anodic stripping voltammetry. This technique uses controlled potential electrolysis to accumulate the analyte of interest on a WE. After a short equilibrium period (the pre-concentration step), the next step is the stripping step. During this step, the electrode is subjected to a linear ramp, which results in the dissolution of the deposit (figure 1.3(c)).

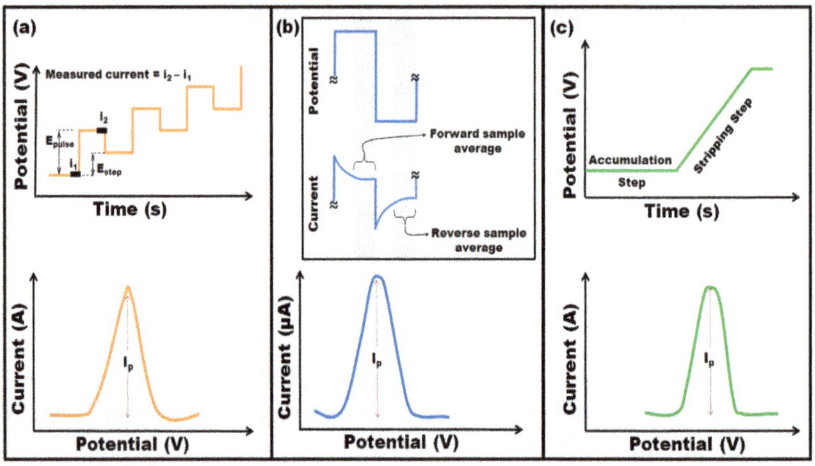

Figure 1.3. Pulse methods: (a) DPV and (b) SWV. (c) Stripping voltammetry.

As a result, a detectable current is produced at a characteristic potential and generally used for trace element analysis. The most commonly used variations are (a) anodic stripping voltammetry (ASV), (b) cathodic stripping voltammetry, and (c) adsorptive stripping voltammetry. A detailed explanation of the technique can be found in the literature [37].

1.4 Fundamentals of electrochemical sensors

One of the simplest detection motifs is direct detection, in which the measured electrochemical signal originates directly from the target analyte rather than through a label, byproduct, or mediator. Thus, various voltammetric techniques can now determine the redox-active species. A potential is applied, and the target analyte undergoes a redox reaction at a specific prospect, which produces a current signal called the Faraday current. This response current signal changes with the concentration of the target analyte. The various detection mechanisms are discussed in section 1.3. An electrochemical sensor is a device that transforms chemical data into a signal that can be used analytically, from the concentration of a single component to complete composition analysis [38]. A critical component of an electrochemical sensor is the transducer (i.e., WE substrate) that is responsible for transmitting the signal generated at the interface (nanomaterials) and analyte interaction into a readable value (figure 1.4).

1.4.1 Theoretical aspects of the electrochemical cell

A typical electrochemical cell consists of a glass round bottom flask having inlets for the electrodes and the gas purge. A three-electrode system and a sample dissolved in a supporting electrolyte are customarily used, which are the reference, counter/auxiliary, and WEs (figure 1.1). However, there are some general requirements for these electrodes [39]. First, chemical inertness over a sizeable potential region is required for high-quality electrochemical measurements. Second, the electrode

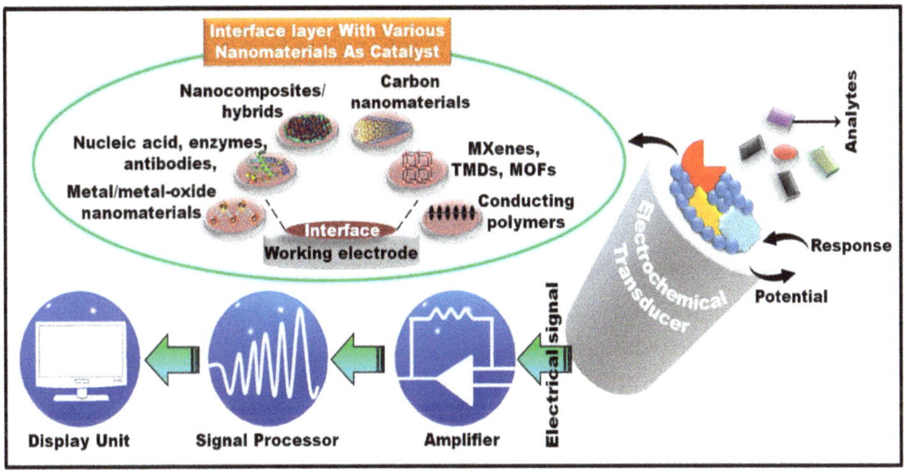

Figure 1.4. Schematic illustration of an electrochemical sensor and its processors. Various nanomaterials are employed in the fabrication of a modified electrochemical sensor.

should not interact with the supporting electrolyte. Strong adsorption, as in fouling, is instead an undesirable effect. Third, low resistance is essential for proper potential measurements. The purpose of these electrodes is described below [40]:

(i) RE: The saturated calomel (SCE) or silver-silver chloride (Ag/AgCl) electrode is commonly used in voltammetric investigations, whose potential remains constant throughout the experiment. The SCE was abandoned in favor of the more reproducible and reliable Ag/AgCl electrode. The RE provides a stable and constant reference potential against which the potential of the WE are measured. The potential is kept constant regardless of the analyte concentration or other experimental conditions. To ensure precise and accurate potential measurements, the RE acts as a reference point for the electrochemical cell. Different ways can be utilized to vary the potential. This relies on the analytical technique used and whether linear sweeps or potential steps are employed.

(ii) Auxiliary electrode (AE): In voltammetry, an additional counter or auxiliary electrode completes the electrical circuit in the electrochemical cell. It balances the current passing through the WE by acting as a source or sink of electrons. In contrast to the WE, the AE functions as a counterbalance to the redox process of the WE and is not involved in the analyte's electrochemical reaction. Carbon, platinum, and other conductive materials are frequently used as AE materials.

(iii) WE: The electron transfer usually occurs at the WE, which forms the most critical component of an electrochemical cell. The WE serves as the interface for the analyte to interact with and undergoes a redox reaction. Furthermore, the WE detects and measures the electrical current generated by the electrochemical reaction, which is proportional to the analyte concentration. Hence, to enhance the overall rate of the reaction, the catalytic effect of the electrode material concerning the charge transfer reaction has to be adequate. The bare electrode is the focal point of this setup where redox reactions occur. Among several WEs, the configuration comprises either carbon paste electrode, glassy carbon electrode, gold (Au) electrode, diamond electrode, screen-printed electrode (SPE), or platinum (Pt) electrode, which is substantiated in sections 1.3 and 1.4.2.

1.4.2 Working electrode properties

WEs are crucial components of an electrochemical sensor because they serve as the platform for the electrochemical reaction. WEs are responsible for detecting and quantifying the analyte of interest. The properties of the WE significantly impact the sensor's sensitivity and performance, including [41] surface area, conductivity, sensitivity, selectivity, stability, reversibility, and reproducibility. Thus, by optimizing these parameters, the WE can be tailored to meet the specific requirements of an electrochemical sensor.

1.4.3 Types of electrode substrates used

The different types of WE can consist of materials ranging from [42, 43]:

- Metal electrodes: Attributed to their excellent electrical conductivity, inert metals such as Pt, diamond, Au, and silver electrodes are widely used in electrochemical sensors.
- SPE: These are manufactured by employing printing techniques that allow mass production and cost-effective fabrication.
- Mercury electrodes are applicable for detection because they display a wide cathodic potential range. However, they are discontinued due to mercury's toxicity.
- Carbon electrodes, such as graphite rods, glassy carbon, carbon fibers, carbon paste electrodes, and wax-impregnated graphite, are utilized for their cost effectiveness, chemical stability, and high surface area.

Modifying an electrode typically creates sensors with specific and often predetermined properties that may not have been achievable otherwise. The ultimate goal of such modifications is to obtain sensors that are fundamentally different from their unmodified counterparts. A modified electrode exhibits improved sensing qualities, contributing to better selectivity and sensitivity against fouling and interference.

1.5 Electrode and sensor materials

The catalyst and other detection enhancers, including nanomaterial, can be easily incorporated into or coated on the electrode substrate for direct detection (figure 1.4) [44–46]. These electrode materials help avoid worries about electrode fouling by allowing them to be used only once.

1.5.1 Types

For the trace analysis of biological, environmental pollutants, industrial, and pharmaceutical species, electrochemical sensors have continued to explore new nanomaterials and design strategies to improve sensor performance. Some of the examples of nanomaterials used for electrochemical sensors include:

(i) Nanomaterials [16, 47]: Nanostructures offer advantages such as large surface area, enhanced sensitivity, and high catalytic performance (e.g., nanowires, nanoparticles, nanotubes, graphite, graphene, MXene, transition metal dichalcogenides (TMDs) and layered double hydroxides (LDHs)).

(ii) Nanocomposites [15, 48–51]: Composites combine different materials to leverage their individual properties (e.g., combining a metal with a carbon-based material).

(iii) Biomaterials [38, 52]: These include molecular recognition layers, such as antibodies, enzymes, or molecular imprints.

(iv) Conducting polymers [53]: Conducting polymers are typically organic materials that exhibit good conductivity when oxidized or doped, such as polyaniline (PANI), polypyrrole (PPy), and poly(3,4-ethylenedioxythiophene) (PEDOT).

(v) Ionic liquids [54]: Ionic liquids act as an ionic conductive medium, amplifying the electrode-analyte interface performance.

(vi) Electrodeposition and electropolymerization [55, 56]: Electrodeposition involves the controlled deposition of specific materials such as the metal coatings on the electrode surface to improve the electrocatalytic activity. Similarly, electropolymerization is the electrodeposition of monomer molecules on the electrode surface to form polymers by applying a specified potential.

Each sensor material offers specific advantages for a particular target analyte of interest. Researchers are continuously exploring various new materials and synthesis techniques to develop unique WE substrates that magnify the performance of the electrochemical sensors.

1.5.2 Significant aspects of materials and their role

Nanomaterial-based electrochemical sensors are quickly emerging as formidable analytical instruments due to their quick response, decreased over potential, good selectivity, and sensitivity. Subsequently, significant progress has been made toward synthesizing nanomaterials, their hybrids, or composites with physicochemical and electrochemical traits tailored to determine the target analyte. Nanomaterials play a substantial role in fabricating the EC sensors and have significantly contributed to advances in sensor performance. The electrode material on the WE surface works as a catalyst to catalyze the oxidation or reduction of the target analyte with the help of electricity.

The paramount characteristics include [55]: (i) functionalized and surface modification, (ii) tailored sensing traits, (iii) improved electrochemical properties, (iv) enhanced surface area, electrical conductivity, catalytic activity, adsorption capability, (v) signal amplification, (vi) durability and stability, and (vii) miniaturization and integration (e.g., into portable devices, and flexible or wearable platforms). Hence, the key takeaway from these traits is that the electrode material, with its good conductivity, must facilitate the activation of the analyte by decreasing the active energy of reactions and achieving satisfactory chemical stability in the potential window of interest.

1.5.3 Sensor engineering and state-of-the-art applications

Monitoring and mitigating environmental pollutants have become increasingly critical in the quest for a sustainable future. The health of people and ecosystems is seriously threatened by pollution, which can come from various sources, including agricultural contamination. To address this challenge, the field of environmental monitoring using electrochemical sensors has been explored in this book. The key reason behind the choice of electrochemical technique for pollutant detection is its miniaturized and portable instrumentation, which the commoner can feasibly handle. Its performance traits, such as good sensitivity, selectivity, and affordability, are also attributed to its performance traits. The efficacy of the electrochemical sensor relies heavily on the science of the nanomaterials used, as well as their surface engineering and functionalization. The electrochemical biosensors utilize the foundation of nanomaterials to detect an electric signal created by an electroactive species, either generated or drained through recognition. More importantly, the sensor's selectivity relies on the material used as a catalyst. A recent literature review demonstrates that many publications employ numerous sensing regimes in determining agricultural contaminants of (i) various classes of pesticide residues and (ii) heavy metal ions [57, 58]. Several reviews have comprehensively assessed the latest advances in electrochemical sensors and biosensors for agro-pollutants [59–63]. These reports discuss the state-of-art engineering of electrochemical sensors for agro-pollutants concerning (i) integration of nanomaterials that significantly enhanced the performance of the electrochemical sensors, (ii) selective and specific detection that enabled the detection of specific pollutants with minimal interference from other co-existing substances, (iii) simultaneous multi-analyte determination, which is essential for understanding complex pollution scenarios, (iv) increasingly more compact and portable, allowing in situ and real-time monitoring of pollutants. Hence, the upcoming chapters address agricultural pollution, which is a significant environmental and public health concern. They provide valuable insights into the electrochemical detection of these pollutants and data to support evidence-based decision-making by policymakers and regulators who often rely on well-researched, authoritative sources of information when formulating policies and regulations related to environmental issues.

1.6 Traditional methods of pollutant detection and their limitations

It is crucial to note that selecting a method depends on the specific monitoring objectives, type of pollutant, time constraints, sensitivity required, and cost. However, the most common and reliable analysis is the traditional laboratory method that involves collecting and testing environmental samples using established techniques. These methods include titration methods, atomic adsorption spectroscopy, gas chromatography, and mass spectroscopy. However, they possess shortcomings compared to electrochemical sensors, such as [61]:

(i) Electrochemical sensors provide near real-time results, making them suitable for applications where immediate data is crucial, while other techniques typically involve longer analysis time and pre-processing of samples.
(ii) Electrochemical sensors are often more compact and portable than traditional equipment, favoring on-site monitoring, while the other analytical methods are laboratory-based and do not allow on-site field testing.
(iii) Electrochemical sensors are simple to operate and cost-effective compared to other complex and expensive techniques to purchase and maintain.
(iv) Electrochemical sensors do not require the pretreatment of samples. They can easily sense significantly fewer sample volumes (which reduces the risk of sample contamination) with accuracy, while other techniques involve complex sample handling.
(v) Electrochemical sensors can analyze various sample matrices, including gases, aqueous solutions, and biological fluids, while other techniques pose limitations.

Thus, a lack of infrastructure constantly threatens field deployment in low-resource environments. According to these issues, analysis tools such as electrochemical sensors are necessary to obtain rapid and reliable information about the presence of a specific molecule/species in a sample.

1.7 Significance of electrochemical sensors in environmental analysis

Electroanalytical methods can play a crucial role in the protection of our environment. In particular, electrochemical sensors are attractive for their on-site monitoring of various priority pollutants. Various electrochemical devices, such as pH or oxygen electrodes, are commonly used in environmental analysis. The recent advances in electrochemical sensing technology will undoubtedly magnify the scope of these devices toward a broad range of inorganic and organic contaminants. Modified electrodes have been introduced as part of recent technological advances. These modifications represent a significant step forward in this field (designed with highly selective nanomaterials or biomaterial recognition layers). Another essential feature is that the electrochemical devices can respond continuously and reversibly without affecting the sample. Attributed to the expansion in the global agricultural demand due to growing population and food requirements, pesticides, heavy metal ions, and other toxins have spread through the environment through various vectors. However, with the rise of pesticide-resistant pests and weeds, the use of pesticides has markedly increased. Additionally, the consumption of heavy metal ions (HMIs) is considered toxic by the United States Environmental Protection Agency (USEPA) [59]. There is a growing concern about maintaining the quality and safety of agro-food production. Determining how soil and water are impacted by contaminants and how these pollutants affect food safety and quality is essential. Hence, detecting and determining agro-based pollutants significantly regulates their usage and minimizes their effects on health and the environment. Thus, electrochemical sensors fabricated with various nanomaterials with improved specificity, sensitivity, and selectivity are favorable.

1.8 Conclusion

Voltammetric methods are pivotal in chemical sensing applications due to their unparalleled sensitivity, selectivity, and versatility. The CV technique involves linearly sweeping the electrode potential while recording the corresponding currents. It is instrumental in studying electrode surface reactions, characterizing electroactive species, and determining redox processes and analyte concentrations. Similarly, pulse techniques use pulses that minimize noise and enhance sensitivity, making it ideal for trace analysis in complex matrices and rapid quantification in electro-analytical sensing. Amperometry, which measures current at a constant potential, provides real-time monitoring with high sensitivity, making it a vital tool for environmental pollutant sensing. EIS, a non-destructive technique, characterizes electrical properties across frequencies, enabling insights into interfacial processes and solution resistance, which are crucial for optimizing sensor performance. Potentiometry, an electroanalytical technique that measures the potential difference between two electrodes immersed in a solution, notably exploits ISEs to discern specific ions or analytes (figure 1.5). This methodology's appeal lies in its procedural

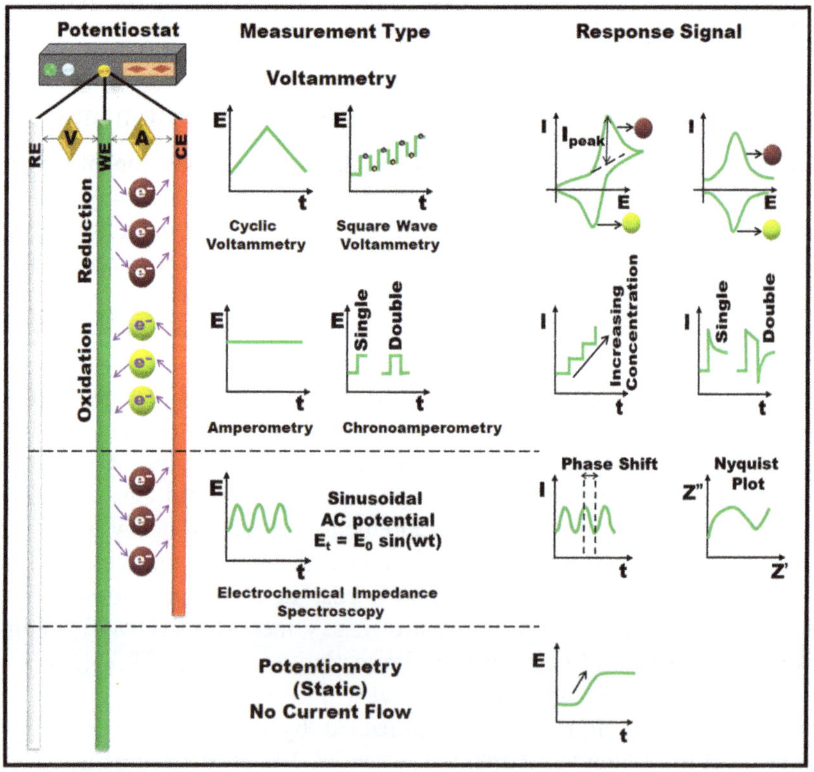

Figure 1.5. A graphical representation of an electrochemical three-electrode system, and various measurement types and response signal methods.

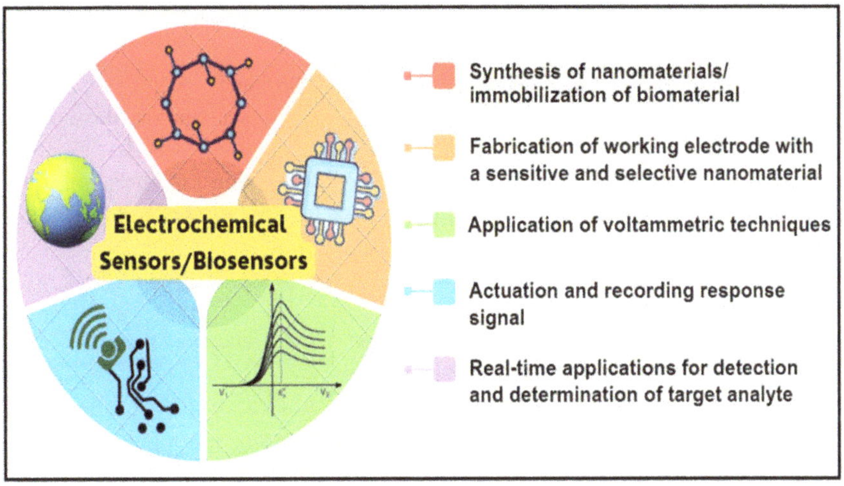

Figure 1.6. Fabrication of electrochemical sensor/biosensor for application in real samples.

simplicity. These voltammetric techniques drive advances in analytical chemistry, addressing critical societal challenges in health, the environment, and the industry. Ongoing research promises further expansion of sensing capabilities in the future.

In conclusion, voltammetry techniques represent a versatile set of electrochemical methods employed in sensor applications. These techniques have evolved significantly and have the potential to be used in various tasks. Voltammetric sensor techniques enable a robust toolbox for researchers and analytical chemists seeking to develop sensitive and selective electrochemical sensors. Their ability to provide quick, real-time data in a compact, portable format makes them indispensable for environmental monitoring (figure 1.6). Thus, the objective of the subsequent chapters is to give examples of reported works in assessing the presence of agro-pollutants and their quantification from soil/water or food samples to preserve their quality.

References

[1] Léger C and Bertrand P 2008 Direct electrochemistry of redox enzymes as a tool for mechanistic studies *Chem. Rev.* **108** 2379–438

[2] Joseph D, Rodriguez R D, Verma A, Pousaneh E, Zahn D R T, Lang H and Chandra S 2017 Electrochemistry and surface-enhanced Raman spectroscopy of CTAB modulated interactions of magnetic nanoparticles with biomolecules *RSC Adv.* **7** 3628–34

[3] Kim E, Leverage W T, Liu Y, White I M, Bentley W E and Payne G F 2014 Redox-capacitor to connect electrochemistry to redox-biology *Analyst* **139** 32–43

[4] Alberts G S and Shain I 1963 Electrochemical study of kinetics of a chemical reaction coupled between two charge transfer reactions. Potentiostatic reduction of p-nitrosophenol *Anal. Chem.* **35** 1859–66

[5] Kohen R and Nyska A 2002 Invited review: oxidation of biological systems: oxidative stress phenomena, antioxidants, redox reactions, and methods for their quantification *Toxicol. Pathol.* **30** 620–50

[6] Bard A J, Faulkner R and White H S 2022 *Electrochemical Methods: Fundamentals and Applications* 3rd edn (New York: Wiley)
[7] Scholz F *et al* 2010 *Electroanalytical Methods* (Berlin: Springer)
[8] Bhadekar R, Pote S, Tale V and Nirichan B 2011 Developments in analytical methods for detection of pesticides in environmental samples *Am. J. Anal. Chem.* **2** 1
[9] Chen H, Song Q, Tang G, Feng Q and Lin L 2013 The combined optimization of savitzky-golay smoothing and multiplicative scatter correction for FT-NIR PLS models *Int. Sch. Res. Notices* **2013** e642190
[10] Fry A 2010 *Electrochemistry in Medicine and Biomedical Applications* vol 28 no 33 (The Electrochemical Society)
[11] Zhang X, Ju H and Wang J 2011 *Electrochemical Sensors, Biosensors and their Biomedical Applications* (Amsterdam: Elsevier)
[12] Tor M W and Yitzhak 2012 *Methods for Studying Nucleic Acid/Drug Interactions* (Boca Raton, FL: CRC Press)
[13] Djokić S 2016 *Biomedical and Pharmaceutical Applications of Electrochemistry* vol **60** (Cham: Springer International Publishing)
[14] Christensen P A and Hamnet A (ed) 2007 *Techniques and Mechanisms in Electrochemistry* by P A Christensen and A Hamnet (Springer)
[15] Manasa G, Bhakta A K, Bafna J, Mascarenhas R J, Malode S J and Shetti N P 2022 An amperometric sensor composed of carbon hybrid-structure for the degradation of amino-triazole herbicide *Environ. Res.* **212** 113541
[16] Manasa G, Mascarenhas R J, Bhakta A K and Mekhalif Z 2021 Nano-graphene-platelet/Brilliant-green composite coated carbon paste electrode interface for electrocatalytic oxidation of flavanone Hesperidin *Microchem. J.* **160** 105768
[17] Rout C, Krishna S, Vivekchand S R C, Govindaraj A and Rao C N R 2006 Hydrogen and ethanol sensors based on ZnO nanorods, nanowires and nanotubes *Chem. Phys. Lett.* **418** 586–90
[18] Manasa G, Mascarenhas R J, Shetti N P, Malode S J, Mishra A, Basu S and Aminabhavi T M 2022 Skin patchable sensor surveillance for continuous glucose monitoring *ACS Appl. Bio. Mater.* **5** 945–70
[19] Stoytcheva M and Zlatev R 2014 Electrochemical sensors for environmental analysis *Encyclopedia of Applied Electrochemistry* ed G Kreysa, K Ota and R F Savinell (New York,: Springer) pp 613–6
[20] Ukhade R and Radhakrishnaiah P 2022 A comprehensive look at the detection, monitoring, and control of environmental pollution with particular focus on new and emerging solutions to address the problem *J. Mater. Sci. Eng.* **11** 1–7
[21] Skoog D A, West D M, Holler F J and Crouch S R 2004 *Fundamentals of Analytical Chemistry* (Belmont, CA: Brooks/Cole)
[22] Aristov N and Habekost A 2015 Cyclic voltammetry—a versatile electrochemical method investigating electron transfer processes *World J. Chem. Edu.* **3** 115–9
[23] Kissinger P T and Heineman W R 1996 *Laboratory Techniques in Electroanalytical Chemistry* (New York: Marcel Dekker)
[24] Savéant J-M and Costentin C 2019 Single-electron transfer at an electrode *Elements of Molecular and Biomolecular Electrochemistry* (New York: Wiley) pp 1–77
[25] Bond A M and Feldberg S W 1998 Analysis of simulated reversible cyclic voltammetric responses for a charged redox species in the absence of added electrolyte *J. Phys. Chem.* B **102** 9966–74

[26] Sun D, Xie X and Zhang H 2010 Surface effects of mesoporous silica modified electrode and application in electrochemical detection of dopamine *Colloids Surf.* B **75** 88–92

[27] Wang J and Walcarius A 1996 Zeolite-modified carbon paste electrode for selective monitoring of dopamine *J. Electroanal. Chem.* **407** 183–7

[28] Bond A M 2002 *Broadening Electrochemical Horizons: Principles and Illustration of Voltammetric and Related Techniques* (Oxford: Oxford University Press)

[29] Bamford C H, Tipper C F H, Compton R G, Bamford C H, Tipper C F H and Compton R G 1986 *Electrode Kinetics: Principles and Methodology* (Amsterdam: Elsevier Science)

[30] Compton R G and Banks C E 2011 *Understanding Voltammetry* (World Scientific)

[31] Prasad R, Kumar M and Kumar V 2018 *Nanotechnology: An Agricultural Paradigm* (Berlin: Springer)

[32] Byrnes J (ed) 2007 *Imaging for Detection and Identification* (Berlin: Springer)

[33] Simões F R and Xavier M G 2017 Electrochemical sensors *Nanoscience and Its Applications: Micro and Nanotechnologies* In: AL Da Róz, M Ferreira, ON Oliveira et al eds (Norwich: William Andrew) pp 155–78

[34] Li Z and Zhu M 2020 Detection of pollutants in water bodies: electrochemical detection or photo-electrochemical detection? *Chem. Commun.* **56** 14541–52

[35] Noviana E, McCord C P, Clark K M, Jang I and Henry C S 2019 Electrochemical paper-based devices: sensing approaches and progress toward practical applications *Lab Chip* **20** 9–34

[36] Jin W and Maduraiveeran G 2018 Nanomaterial-based environmental sensing platforms using state-of-the-art electroanalytical strategies *J. Anal. Sci. Technol.* **9** 18

[37] Singh S and Cinti S 2023 *Anodic and Cathodic Stripping Voltammetry for Metals Sensing* (Royal Society of Chemistry) pp 55–72

[38] Shanbhag M M, Manasa G, Mascarenhas R J, Mondal K and Shetti N P 2023 Fundamentals of bio-electrochemical sensing *Chem. Eng. J. Adv.* **16** 100516

[39] Inzelt G, Lewenstam A and Scholz F 2013 *Handbook of Reference Electrodes* (Springer)

[40] Grieshaber D, MacKenzie R, Vörös J and Reimhult E 2008 Electrochemical biosensors - sensor principles and architectures *Sensors (Basel)* **8** 1400–58

[41] Abraham P, Renjini S, Vijayan P, Nisha V, Sreevalsan K and Anithakumary V 2020 Review—review on the progress in electrochemical detection of morphine based on different modified electrodes *J. Electrochem. Soc.* **167** 037559

[42] Vyskočil V and Barek J 2009 Mercury electrodes–possibilities and limitations in environmental electroanalysis *Crit. Rev. Anal. Chem.* **39** 173–88

[43] Cui Y 2017 Electronic materials, devices, and signals in electrochemical sensors *IEEE Trans. Electron. Dev.* **64** 2467–77

[44] Kalcher K 1990 Chemically modified carbon paste electrodes in voltammetric analysis *Electroanalysis* **2** 419–33

[45] Zhang Y, Li F, Liu X, Lu J and Zhang G 2017 Promoting influence of activated carbon used in carbon paste electrode on platinum nanoparticles efficiency in methanol electrooxidation *Electrochim. Acta* **242** 165–72

[46] Kumar S and Adarakatti P 2018 *Modified Electrodes for Sensing* (Royal Society of Chemistry)

[47] Manasa G, Mascarenhas R J, Satpati A K, Basavaraja B M and Kumar S 2018 An electrochemical Bisphenol F sensor based on ZnO/G nano composite and CTAB surface modified carbon paste electrode architecture *Colloids Surf.* B **170** 144–51

[48] Manasa G, Bhakta A K, Mekhalif Z and Mascarenhas R J 2019 Voltammetric study and rapid quantification of resorcinol in hair dye and biological samples using ultrasensitive maghemite/MWCNT modified carbon paste electrode *Electroanalysis* **31** 1363–72

[49] Manasa G, Bhakta A K, Mekhalif Z and Mascarenhas R J 2020 Bismuth-nanoparticles decorated multi-wall-carbon-nanotubes cast-coated on carbon paste electrode; an electrochemical sensor for sensitive determination of gallic acid at neutral pH *Mater. Sci. Energy Technol.* **3** 174–82

[50] Manasa G, Mascarenhas R J, Bhakta A K and Mekhalif Z 2020 MWCNT/Nileblue heterostructured composite electrode for flavanone Naringenin quantification in fruit juices *Electroanalysis* **32** 939–48

[51] Manasa G, Raj C, Satpati A K and Mascarenhas R J 2020 S(O)MWCNT/modified carbon paste—a non-enzymatic amperometric sensor for direct determination of 6-mercaptopurine in biological fluids *Electroanalysis* **32** 2431–41

[52] Wang J 1991 Modified electrodes for electrochemical sensors *Electroanalysis* **3** 255–9

[53] Manasa G, Mascarenhas R J and Basavaraja B M 2019 Sensitively-selective determination of Propyl Paraben preservative based on synergistic effects of polyaniline-zinc-oxide nanocomposite incorporated into graphite paste electrode *Colloids Surf.,* B **184** 110529

[54] Cetinkaya A, Kaya S I, Yence M, Budak F and Ozkan S A 2023 Ionic liquid-based materials for electrochemical sensor applications in environmental samples *Trends Environ. Anal. Chem.* **37** e00188

[55] Potes-Lesoinne H A, Ramirez-Alvarez F, Perez-Gonzalez V H, Martinez-Chapa S O and Gallo-Villanueva R C 2022 Nanomaterials for electrochemical detection of pollutants in water: a review *Electrophoresis* **43** 249–62

[56] Manasa G, Mascarenhas R J, Satpati A K, D'Souza O J and Dhason A 2017 Facile preparation of poly (methylene blue) modified carbon paste electrode for the detection and quantification of catechin *Mater. Sci. Eng.* C **73** 552–61

[57] Xiang H, Cai Q, Li Y, Zhang Z, Cao L, Li K and Yang H 2020 Sensors applied for the detection of pesticides and heavy metals in freshwaters *J. Sens.* **2020** 8503491

[58] Hara T O and Singh B 2021 Electrochemical biosensors for detection of pesticides and heavy metal toxicants in water: recent trends and progress *ACS EST Water* **1** 462–78

[59] Dhamu V N, Poudyal D, Samson M, Paul A, Muthukumar S and Prasad S 2023 Review—environmental biosensors for Agro-safety based on electrochemical sensing mechanism with an emphasis on pesticide screening *ECS Sens. Plus* **2** 024601

[60] Noori J S, Mortensen J and Geto A 2020 Recent development on the electrochemical detection of selected pesticides: a focused review *Sensors* **20** 2221

[61] Umapathi R, Ghoreishian S M, Sonwal S, Rani G M and Huh Y S 2022 Portable electrochemical sensing methodologies for on-site detection of pesticide residues in fruits and vegetables *Coord. Chem. Rev.* **453** 214305

[62] Saha C, Bhushan M and Singh L R 2023 Pesticide sensing using electrochemical techniques: a comprehensive review *J. Iran. Chem. Soc.* **20** 243–56

[63] Pathiraja G, Bonner C D J and Obare S O 2023 Recent advances of enzyme-free electrochemical sensors for flexible electronics in the detection of organophosphorus compounds: a review *Sensors* **23** 1226

IOP Publishing

Chapter 2

Carbon and its allotropes for electrochemical sensing

G Manasa and Chandra Sekhar Rout

This chapter delves into the versatility of carbon and its extensive applications in chemistry, materials science, biology, and environmental science. Carbon's unique ability to form myriad organic compounds positions it as a versatile element for innovation across diverse disciplines. Carbon-based materials have emerged as critical players in sensor technology, leveraging their exceptional traits, such as high surface area, electrical conductivity, chemical stability, and biocompatibility. These traits are unique to carbon-based materials and crucial for their effectiveness in sensor technology. This chapter explores the multifaceted uses of carbon-based materials in sensor technology, underscoring their effectiveness as sensing elements for various analytes. From carbon nanotubes and graphene to carbon quantum dots and porous carbons, these materials showcase remarkable sensitivity, selectivity, and adaptability, making them prime contenders for a broad spectrum of sensing applications in material science.

2.1 Introduction

Carbon, a foundational element in material science, boasts diverse physical and chemical properties that make it indispensable across numerous applications. Its exceptional chemical stability, due to its distinctive capacity to create sturdy covalent links with other carbon atoms in various hybridization conditions (sp, sp^2, sp^3), ensures the enduring performance of carbon-based materials in diverse environmental settings [1]. This versatility of carbon, coupled with its exceptional properties, forms the basis of our exploration into its extensive applications in chemistry, materials science, biology, and environmental science.

Carbon's allotropes, including graphite, diamond, fullerenes, graphene, and carbon nanotubes (CNTs), each possess unique and fascinating properties

doi:10.1088/978-0-7503-5879-8ch2

instrumental in specific material science endeavors [2]. For instance, graphene and CNTs, two notable carbon allotropes, exhibit unparalleled electrical conductivity, a property that has revolutionized the field of electronics. Carbon materials also demonstrate a wide range of mechanical properties, from diamond's exceptional hardness, which is ideal for cutting tools, to graphite's flexibility, which makes it suitable for use in pencils. This adaptability allows the creation of materials with specific mechanical characteristics, catering to multiple structural and composite applications [3]. The high surface area of carbon-based materials, particularly porous carbons such as activated carbon and carbon aerogels, provides significant benefits in adsorption-based processes. These processes are crucial in gas storage, water purification, and catalysis, where efficient sorption of target species is essential [1–3]. CNTs and graphene exhibit inherent biocompatibility in biomedical engineering, making them suitable for drug delivery, tissue engineering, and biosensing applications [3–10]. Additionally, carbon-based materials offer exceptional tunability, allowing for precise manipulation of their atomic and molecular structures to achieve desired properties and functionalities. This feature facilitates the creation of custom materials tailored to specific applications within the material science domain.

Carbon's multifaceted properties make it an invaluable asset in material science research, which spans various disciplines, including electronics, energy, biomedical engineering, and environmental remediation [8, 11]. This chapter delves into the fascinating and diverse world of carbon allotropes, and explores their distinct properties and wide-ranging applications. Carbon materials are known for their remarkable versatility, and the various allotropes of carbon are no exception. Each allotrope possesses unique characteristics, making them suitable for different purposes. By examining their physical and chemical properties, and their applications across various industries, we can understand the significant role that carbon allotropes play in our daily lives.

2.2 Electrochemical sensor and necessity of electrocatalysis

Over the past few decades, electrochemistry has become a widely used analytical tool that has remained competitive in meeting growing demands for life analysis, environmental monitoring, and food inspection. These devices convert electrochemical data from target analytes or sensing elements into measurable analytical signals that have practical applications. However, the kinetics of electrode reactions can limit this process, especially when dealing with low analyte concentrations. Fortunately, electrocatalysis can solve this issue by promoting electron transfer between analytes and electrode surfaces, enhancing sensor sensitivity and selectivity [12]. Electrochemical detection techniques bear some resemblance to one another. However, electrochemical sensors rely significantly on different electroactive or catalytic substances placed on the electrodes [13, 14]. Therefore, developing and searching for high-quality electrode materials to improve their performance is essential. Researchers have utilized electrocatalytic materials such as carbon-based nanomaterials, metal nanoparticles, metal oxides, and molecular catalysts to customize electrode surfaces and improve sensor performance by promoting specific electrochemical reactions [15–18]. Electrocatalysis is critical in various electrochemical sensing applications, such as environmental monitoring, clinical diagnostics, food safety, and industrial process control. Carbon and carbon hybrids/composite catalysts are extensively used to detect environmental pollutants, heavy metals, and toxic gases because of their high catalytic activity and selectivity [19–21]. Electrocatalysis by carbon materials in electrochemical sensing can facilitate rapid, reliable, and cost-effective analyte detection for various applications. This chapter provides an overview of carbon and its allotropes for various electrochemical applications.

2.3 Arrangement of carbon atoms

The different configurations of C hybridization of orbitals, including sp^1, sp^2, and sp^3, offer a promising avenue for discovering and designing new C materials. The sp^3 configuration provides a strong σ bond to an adjacent atom. Four neighboring C atoms tetrahedrally surround each C atom, and the directed bond is 109.5° (figure 2.1(a)(i)). The sp^2 configuration features three-fold coordination, with three valence electrons entering trigonally directed sp^2 orbitals. This results in the formation of σ bonds in a plane style. However, the fourth electron can be found in a p-π orbital. It forms a weaker π bond with a π orbital on one or more neighboring atoms (figure 2.1(a)(ii)). In the sp^1 configuration, two out of four valence electrons occupy σ orbitals. These two electrons form a σ bond along the $\pm x$-axis (figure 2.1(a)(iii)). The remaining two electrons are located in p-π orbitals, with one occupying the y-directional orbital and the other occupying the z-directional orbital. The properties of carbon allotropes are determined by the orbital hybridization form of the carbon bond configurations, which is influenced by the microstructure organization of the carbon atoms [22, 23].

(i) sp^3 hybridization [24]: Diamond, a remarkable form of carbon allotrope, showcases sp^3 hybridization. Each carbon atom forms four single covalent bonds in a diamond with its neighboring atoms, resulting in a 3D tetrahedral network. This unique structure grants the diamond its exceptional properties, making it incredibly hard, thermally conductive, and optically efficient. In diamonds, carbon atoms form a 3D network structure. Each atom creates four strong covalent bonds in a tetrahedral configuration. These properties, in turn, make diamonds highly valuable for various industrial applications, including cutting tools, abrasives, and high-pressure anvils. The robust covalent bonds between carbon atoms in diamonds require significant energy to disrupt, contributing to their unparalleled durability and resistance to chemical degradation. This durability is a critical factor in the diamond's longevity and ability to withstand harsh conditions, making it a material of choice in various industries, including sensing applications.

(ii) sp^2 hybridization [24]: Fullerenes exhibits sp^2 hybridization of carbon atoms. This hybridization state results in each carbon atom forming three σ bonds with its neighboring carbons, while one unhybridized p orbital

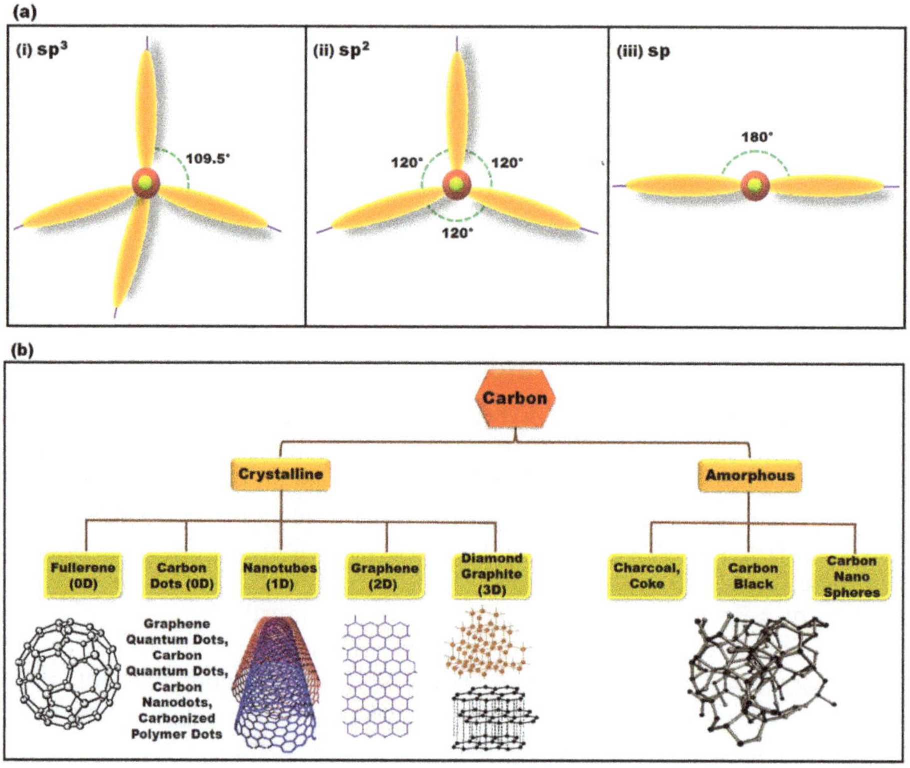

Figure 2.1. (a) Illustration of carbon configurations of (i) sp^3, (ii) sp^2, and (iii) sp. (b) Carbon allotropes.

participates in π bonding. This creates a planar hexagonal arrangement of carbon atoms, forming a closed-cage structure typically spherical and composed of interconnected hexagonal and pentagonal rings. The unique arrangement of these atoms confers significant stability and distinctive properties to fullerenes, making them highly relevant to carbon chemistry and nanomaterials research. Some notable examples of fullerenes include the iconic buckminsterfullerene (C_{60}), more extensive and smaller fullerenes such as C_{70} and C_{84}, and their higher-order derivatives. However, C_{60} is the most stable isomer with symmetry.

Graphite and graphene exemplify the sp^2 hybridization of carbon atoms, wherein each carbon atom forms three σ bonds with neighboring atoms, while the remaining p orbital participates in π bonding. Graphite is characterized by carbon atoms arranged in a hexagonal lattice, with weak van der Waals forces between layers allowing for facile sliding. This layered structure imparts lubricity and electrical conductivity, making graphite ideal for applications such as lubricants and electrodes. The arrangement of carbon atoms in graphite is a layered structure composed of stacked layers of carbon atoms arranged in a hexagonal lattice. The weak interlayer forces make it easy for the layers to slide, giving graphite unique properties such as anisotropy, lubricity, and electrical conductivity. Due to these properties, graphite is widely used in various applications such as electrochemical working electrodes, pencils, lubricants, and thermal management systems [25, 26].

Graphene, a single layer of graphite, possesses extraordinary mechanical strength, high electrical conductivity, and exceptional flexibility. These properties stem from its 2D hexagonal lattice structure and the presence of delocalized π electrons. Graphene comprises a single layer of carbon atoms arranged in a 2D hexagonal pattern. This unique structure gives graphene exceptional properties, such as high mechanical strength, electrical conductivity, and thermal conductivity. Additionally, attributed to its extensive surface area and electronic structure, it is a highly sought-after material for various applications, including flexible electronics, energy storage devices, sensors, and biomedical devices [27].

(iii) sp hybridization [28]: CNTs possess a unique sp hybridization, in which each carbon atom forms two σ bonds and possesses one unhybridized p orbital. These distinctive features, coupled with the arrangement of carbon atoms and the rolling direction of graphene sheets, enable them to exhibit either metallic or semiconducting properties. CNTs exhibit mechanical properties, a high aspect ratio, and electrical conductivity. CNTs are cylindrical structures formed by rolling up graphene sheets. A single-walled nanotube (SWCNT) consists of a single graphene layer that forms a cylinder with a diameter of approximately 1 nm and a length of up to a few millimeters. On the other hand, a multi-walled nanotube (MWCNT) comprises several concentric cylinders with a total diameter of up to 100 nm and a length of tens of microns. The properties of CNTs are significantly influenced by their atomic arrangement, diameter, and height. The exceptional properties of CNTs make them highly attractive for potential applications in nanoelectronics, sensors, and composite materials. They are also promising for advanced technologies such as field emission displays, drug delivery systems, and reinforced materials.

2.4 Allotropes of carbon and their electrochemical sensor application

Carbon is categorized into distinct allotropes based on the configuration of its atoms in distinct structures and bonding arrangements. The primary factors determining carbon's allotropes include how carbon atoms are bonded and the spatial arrangement of these atoms within the structures. Carbon is classified into its allotropes, considering the atomic structure of carbon materials (figure 2.1(b)) [29].

2.4.1 Crystalline forms of carbon

Carbon materials such as fullerene, carbon dots (CDs), CNTs, graphene, diamond, and graphite are categorized as crystalline forms due to their well-organized atomic structures. Thanks to their atomic-level organization, these materials possess remarkable properties, such as high strength, electrical conductivity, and thermal stability. The precision and regularity of their atomic arrangements, which is the foundation of their classification as crystalline forms, lay the groundwork for the diverse applications of these materials across various fields of science and technology. Meanwhile, categorizing carbon structures into 0D, 1D, 2D, and 3D forms is based on their spatial dimensionalities, which pertain to the number of spatial dimensions in which the structure extends. Each dimensional classification is explained as follows.

The molecular structure of the fullerene C_{60} is a truncated icosahedron that comprises five interlocking and six-membered carbon rings made of sp^2 hybridization [30]. This form contrasts graphite and graphene, which consists of a planar sheet of fused hexagons of sp^2 hybridization, while fullerenes are classified as a 0D closed-cage nanomaterial. The unique spherical shape of fullerene nanomaterials makes them highly desirable for sensor systems due to their large surface area. An additional advantage of fullerene nanomaterials is their carbon structure, which contains double bonds that are easily modifiable and highly responsive to chemical reactions. Nucleophilic attacks can create active sites on the fullerene sphere, allowing for chemical modifications that are necessary for surface modification or biomolecule immobilization. The spherical structure of fullerene in 60 carbons allows for the forming of 30 bonds and 30 double bonds, which can be modified using a range of chemical agents to create fullerene derivatives. The fullerene family extends beyond C_{60} and includes higher fullerenes containing five and six-membered carbon rings. C_{60}, in particular, contains 60 π electrons in its structure, which makes it susceptible to nucleophilic attack by the electron-withdrawing moieties [31]. It can also accept up to six electrons reversibly. Fullerenes can be subjected to electrophilic attacks by electron-releasing amine groups, forming immobilized C_{60} enzymes [32, 33]. The immobilization process can be harnessed to develop glucose sensors that utilize C_{60}-glucose oxidase enzymes. These enzymes are instrumental in oxidizing glucose to gluconic acid, which reacts with the C_{60} molecule. This innovative approach has immense potential in developing glucose sensors and could significantly impact healthcare [34]. Fullerenes have been utilized in different sensing applications [35, 36]. The electrical conductivity, charge transport properties, and charge separation capabilities of fullerenes make them highly sought after in sensor technology. Additionally, their photo-physical properties are also impressive and add to their desirability. However, the electrochemical sensors are highlighted in this section. The C_{60} molecules have been observed to possess excellent redox properties and can be altered to create electrodes that exhibit superior electrocatalytic activity and have a larger electroactive surface area. The electrocatalytic activity of C_{60}-modified electrodes has been improved by using a simple drop-casting method for C_{60} solution onto a supporting electrode followed by partial reduction [37]. Meanwhile, electrodes that have been modified through partially reduced C_{60} have been found to have a high electroactive surface area, as per previous research studies [37, 38]. Fullerenes with at least 60 carbon atoms have shown they can accept and donate electrons and display rich electrochemistry. These properties make them attractive for electrocatalytic applications. However, the high double-bond character of junctions of five- and six-member rings in fullerene materials can lead to addition reactions, resulting in many mono- and multiple-adducts. As a result, these addition reactions can compete with the electrocatalytic reactions, making using fullerene materials for electrocatalytic applications more challenging.

CDs are a nanocarbon crystalline family member with numerous advantages over graphene. The presence of synchronized sp^2 characterizes them and sp^3 hybridized carbon atoms make them 0D nanoparticles below 10 nm in size. One of the main advantages of CDs is their superior biocompatibility and low toxicity, as demonstrated by in vitro studies [39]. Additionally, they are suitable candidates for biosensor components thanks to their potential for use as an electron donor and acceptor [40]. As a result, CDs are one of the most widely researched members of the nanocarbon family in biosensor applications, second only to graphene and CNTs. However, CDs' inability to provide long-term stabilization, an essential feature for a biosensor design, is a significant shortcoming [41]. The stabilization techniques developed will determine the future of CDs in electrochemical sensor applications.

CNTs are categorized into two primary forms based on their number of walls: SWCNTs and MWCNTs. SWCNTs are cylindrical structures with a single graphene sheet rolled into a hollow tube, stabilized by carbon atoms linked via sp^2 bond hybridization. The chirality of CNTs, which refers to the arrangement of a hexagonal ring of sp^2 carbon atoms, determines the nanotubes' diameter, curvature, and electronic properties. Most SWCNTs are chiral ($m \neq n$), meaning they have a non-equal number of hexagonal rings along the tube's circumference. Some present armchair ($m = n$) or zigzag ($m = 0$) configurations [42]. Multi-walled carbon nanotubes (MWCNTs) are composed of numerous graphite layers held together by van der Waals forces. The interlayer spacing between these layers is measured at 3.4 Å [43]. These tubes can be visualized as concentric, closed graphite tubes with graphene sheets with multiple layers, similar to the distance between two graphene layers in graphite (~3.5 Å) [44]. CNT electrodes offer distinctive features that differentiate them from conventional electrodes, making them a compelling option for various applications. CNTs play a crucial role as molecular cables, facilitating the transfer of electrons between the transducer surface and the analyte species. They also enable direct electron transfer and mitigate the effects of surface contamination [5–7]. These unique properties have catapulted CNTs into the spotlight as a highly sought-after material for electrochemical sensors. The surfaces of as-grown pristine buckytubes possess high hydrophobicity and cannot dissolve in water or any typical solvents. Hence, incorporating functional groups onto the surface of CNTs is crucial for their solubility and to simplify their applications. The surface functionalization of CNTs may be (i) non-covalent (preserves the structural and electrical traits of CNTs) or (ii) covalent (alters the intrinsic physical properties of CNTs after chemical reactions) (figure 2.2(a)) [45]. Notably, prominent studies reveal that using electrodes modified with CNTs can markedly amplify electron transfer reactions at lower potentials and diminish the surface deterioration of sensors, as opposed to unmodified CNT electrodes. Moreover, incorporating CNTs in electrodes can lead to a marked improvement in the sensitivity of the sensors, thereby enhancing their detection performance [46–49]. The expansive surface area of CNTs allows for doping large amounts of enzymes. Using bio-functionalized CNT-modified

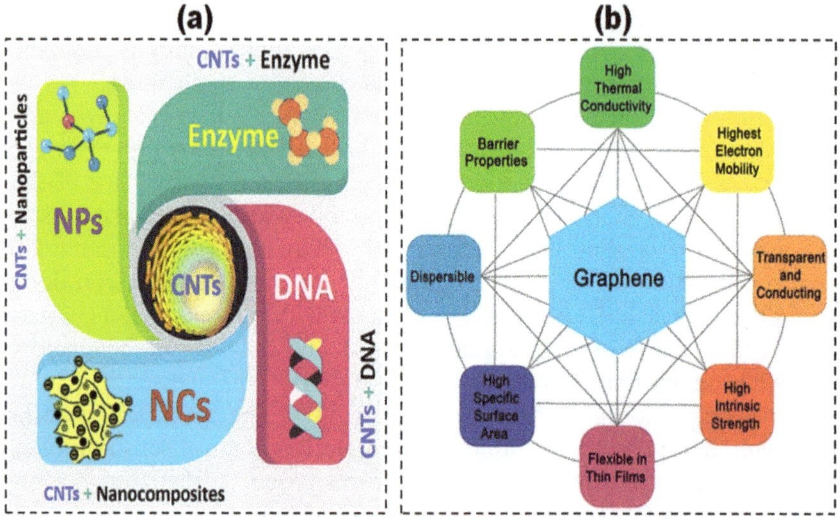

Figure 2.2. (a) Different materials, like inorganic and organic nanoparticles, nanocomposites, nanoscale polymers, hybrid materials, nucleic acids, and enzymes, are combined with CNTs to create electrochemical sensors. Reprinted from [45]. Copyright (2020), with permission from Elsevier. (b) Various characteristics of graphene for developing electrochemical sensors. Reproduced from [53]. CC BY 4.0. Copyright © 2024 by authors and Scientific Research Publishing Inc.

electrodes enables the development of sensors with superior properties, including high precision, selectivity, and rapid response. These advances pave the way for substantial improvements in sensor technology [50, 51]. The use of CNTs as mediators between enzyme components and electrodes made of glassy carbon (GC), platinum, or gold is familiar thanks to their swift electron transfer, amplified conductivity, and favorable physical and chemical properties. CNTs can be utilized to alter the surfaces of different electrodes in either an oriented or non-oriented way. Among the GCEs are the most commonly employed electrodes. Oriented electrode modifications involve depositing CNTs on the surface, which act as molecular cables, providing electrical transmission. This versatility of CNTs in electrode modification is a source of inspiration, fueling further advances in the field [52].

Graphene, a flat and hexagonal structure of carbon atoms bonded by sp^2 hybridization with a single atomic thickness, has been extensively researched for its superior physical, optical, and electrochemical properties when used in sensors. However, there are some challenges when it comes to using graphene-based sensors, including inconsistency in electrode modification methodologies, a lack of standardization in production, a high tendency for agglomeration, an inability to utilize graphene's properties fully, and concerns about physical stability. Graphene-based nanomaterials have unique properties, making them an ideal choice for developing highly efficient electrochemical sensors (figure 2.2(b)). The electrochemical activity of graphene is improved due to several key factors [54–56]: (i) Graphene sheets in 2D exhibit a vast surface area, thereby increasing the number of electroactive sites that can detect target molecules and consequently enhance sensitivity. (ii) Due to its stable nature over a wide range of temperatures, graphene serves as a reliable conductive material that can be utilized in the development of electrochemical sensors. The sp^2 hybridized p_z orbital electrons lead to faster electron transfer kinetics, which in turn result in quicker response time and lower detection limits. Graphene oxide is formed by the oxidation of graphene, which leads to the introduction of different oxygen-containing groups on the surface and edges of the graphene material. These groups could have an impact on the kinetics of electron transfer by either promoting or inhibiting the process [56, 57]. Several reports indicate that hydroxyl groups, epoxide groups, and double bonds are present in graphene oxide [58, 59]. Additional groups, including carbonyls and esters, were verified subsequently. These groups that contain oxygen showcase a reduction peak that is irreversible when subjected to electrochemical analysis. They also facilitate the mechanism of heterogeneous electron transfer by receiving protons, thereby assisting oxidation and reducing the overpotential [60–62]. During the past decade, there have been significant advances in the controlled design of graphene and its derivatives. Integrating these materials with organic polymers, biomolecules, and inorganic nanoparticles has improved their possibility for sensing applications [63–65]. Such composites show enhanced sensitivity, selectivity, and reproducibility with a wide detection range [9, 11, 27]. However, to develop novel sensing platforms, it is essential to understand the properties and changes that occur during the formation of these composites. Fine-tuning their structural features can help address stability and reproducibility issues, and improve electron transfer kinetics during electrochemical sensing. The sensitivity and selectivity of nanocomposites during sensing are significantly influenced by various factors, such as the number of defects, dopants, morphology, and size of the nanostructures [27].

Diamond embodies the pinnacle of sp^3 hybridization. Its distinctive 3D tetrahedral structure, crafted by each carbon atom's four single covalent bonds with its neighboring atoms, bestows it with extraordinary properties such as hardness, thermal conductivity, chemical inertness, optical characteristics, and biocompatibility. The robust covalent bonds between carbon atoms within the diamond structure demand substantial energy to disrupt, enhancing its durability and resistance to chemical degradation. These properties, which make it a highly coveted material in various industrial applications such as cutting tools, abrasives, and high-pressure anvils, are a testament to its unique nature. Diamond's versatility is evident in its widespread use as a sensor in various industries, including environmental monitoring and biomedical diagnostics. These sensors leverage the unique properties of diamonds to enhance safety, efficiency, and accuracy in multiple research domains and industries. Therefore, the applications of diamonds are vast and diverse, highlighting their potential for innovative and practical solutions. Using diamond-based electrochemical electrodes presents a novel approach, offering several unique advantages [66]. Optimizing the concentration of boron-atom doping in the boron doped diamond (BDD) electrode can be a valuable way to detect and measure various metal analytes accurately. Modifying the BDD electrodes with foreign materials or metallic nanoparticles makes it possible to create different structural and morphological features that allow for the specific accumulation of metal ions and anions, leading

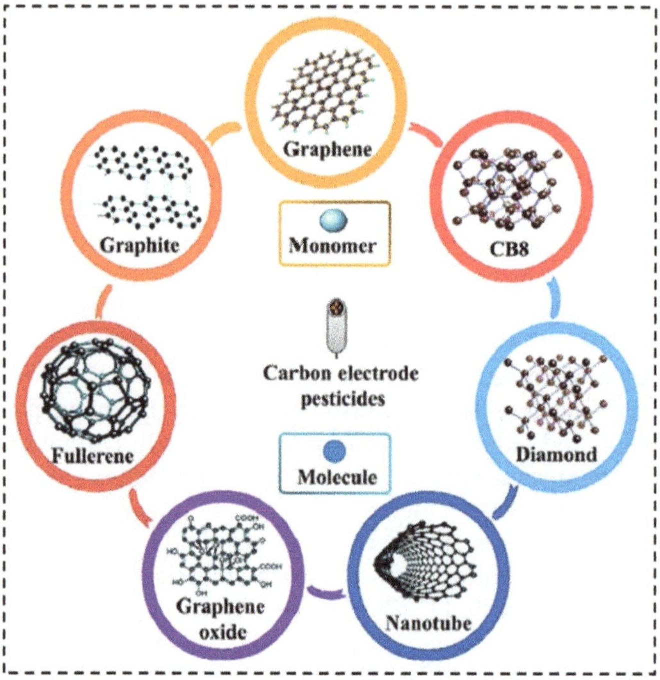

Figure 2.3. Promising carbon allotropes for electrocatalysis in fabricating electrochemical sensors. Reprinted from [45], Copyright (2020), with permission from Elsevier.

to electrochemical responses via redox reactions. For instance, introducing graphitic or nanographitic shells in the diamond-based electrodes can enhance conductivity by tuning the B/C and sp^2/sp^3 ratios. As a result, highly responsive signals can be obtained. Diamond-based electrodes possess unique structural and electrochemical resistivity features that effectively detect specific target species in aqueous media under practical operating conditions. The literature describes several examples of diamond-based electrodes that can detect target species at the picomolar level with wide linearity, providing a new way to quantify these species with specificity [66–69].

Crystalline carbon-based sensors owe much to innovations in material synthesis, functionalization, and integration techniques (figure 2.3). Researchers have developed sensors with enhanced sensitivity, selectivity, and operational stability by tailoring the carbon's surface chemistry and structural properties. These sensors have many applications, from environmental monitoring and industrial process control to health-care and wearable technology, marking a significant milestone in sensing technology.

2.4.2 Properties of amorphous carbon

Carbon is classified as amorphous due to its lack of long-range order in its atomic or molecular arrangement; unlike crystalline materials that exhibit a regular and repeating pattern, amorphous materials such as amorphous carbon exhibit a disordered structure [70]. Amorphous carbon has randomly oriented carbon atoms that are bonded together, resulting in a structure without discernible periodicity. The degree of structural disorder in amorphous carbon varies, resulting in a wide range of properties such as electrical conductivity, optical transparency, and mechanical strength [71]. Examples of amorphous carbon include charcoal, soot, coke, and activated carbon, which exhibit diverse properties depending on their synthesis methods and processing conditions.

Coke has unique electrochemical properties due to its composition and structure. Although its structure is highly disordered, it depicts good electrochemical stability, which makes it resistant to chemical reactions and oxidation, even though it generally has low electrical conductivity. Coke's high surface area and porous structure enable it to contribute to overall capacitance in composite materials or electrodes. However, its capacitance may be weaker than that of specialized carbon materials. These electrochemical properties make coke suitable for various applications, such as corrosion-resistant coatings and electrodes in specific electrochemical processes. Although not appropriate for electrochemical sensing applications, studies by researchers provide further insight into coke's electrochemical behavior and its practical implications [72, 73].

Charcoal, a carbon allotrope, has a porous structure and its surface chemistry makes it an excellent candidate for efficient adsorption and desorption of ions and molecules. Although charcoal exhibits moderate electrical conductivity due to its disordered structure, its surface can be modified to improve its conductivity and electrochemical performance. In particular, charcoal-based electrodes have demonstrated promising potential in energy storage devices, electrochemical sensors, and environmental remediation systems [74, 75]. Although there is limited literature on charcoal sensors, some examples of their potential applications have been reported [76, 77]. These examples showcase the versatility and applicability of charcoal-based sensors in future research.

Carbon black (CB), a distinctive amorphous carbon member with an average diameter of 3–100 nm, is a cost-effective and sensitive material. Its experimental simplicity, portability, and selectivity make it a compelling choice [16, 78]. Notably, CB's high conductivity sets it apart, positioning it as a promising alternative to other nanocarbon materials such as graphene and graphene-like structures, fullerenes, and CNTs. It's crucial to recognize that CB's physical properties, characterized by sp^2 and sp^3 hybridized carbon atoms, are complex. They are intricately tied to particle size, porosity, surface chemistry, aggregate morphology, and surface area. CB is often found in loosely bonded agglomerates, which presents a hurdle in obtaining consistent and rigorous data that can be standardized for biomolecular applications [79–81]. This contrasts with graphene and graphene-like structures, which are relatively more straightforward to standardize during production. Moreover, the characterization methods for these nanostructures must be developed because each structure has only a few unit cell sizes. At the same time, CB boasts good characteristics, physical properties, and the necessity for standardization during production, which present hurdles that require attention. Further research and development are needed to address these challenges and pave the way for CB's widespread adoption in biomolecular applications.

Carbon nanospheres (CNSs) are members of the amorphous nanocarbon family with a large average diameter, ranging from 50 to 350 nm. Graphitic carbon onions, with diameters ranging from 2 to 20 nm, are classified along with less graphitic carbon spheres ranging from 50 nm to 1 μm and carbon particles ranging from one to several microns [82]. The bond structure formed by matching pentagonal and heptagonal carbon rings causes CNSs to possess similar structural, physical, and electrical properties as fullerene. This is due to the rearrangement of graphene structures [82]. CNSs exhibit unique properties, making them highly versatile and valuable for many applications. CNSs can be effective support materials for drug delivery, catalysts, lubricants, and heterogeneous catalysis. The high surface area-to-volume ratio of CNSs makes them ideal for use in energy storage, capacitors, and as reinforcement agents in rubber. Encapsulation of support and electrode materials within CNSs has shown promise in several fields, including materials science and biomedical engineering. The diverse range of applications for CNSs highlights their potential as a multifunctional material for use in various industries and research fields [81, 83, 84]. However, CNSs have yet to be extensively studied for biosensor applications in comparison to other forms of nanocarbon. This is mainly due to the economic challenges of producing many CNSs under reasonable experimental conditions.

2.5 Crystalline carbon-based biosensors

Biosensors have become increasingly important in modern life and are the backbone of our ability to diagnose diseases and detect targeted biological agents in the environment. These analytical devices detect a chemical analyte by converting a biological reaction into a measurable physicochemical signal. They typically consist of a bioreceptor (i.e., antibodies, enzymes, DNAs, aptamers, microorganisms, or cells), a transducer modifying element (i.e., nanomaterial), and an electronic system with a signal amplifier, processor, and display. The target analyte is recognized explicitly by the bioreceptor, and the transducer then transforms this reaction into a distinct form of energy. This energy is subsequently amplified, processed, and converted into the desired signal [27, 85].

The development and performance of biosensors rely on the materials used to construct them and the physicochemical properties of the transducer and matrices used for enzyme immobilization, stabilizers, and mediators. Unfortunately, the large-scale use of biosensors is often hindered due to low reproducibility and poor signal stability caused by the inability to control the material used in their construction. However, nanomaterials have become an effective solution to this problem. Thanks to significant progress in synthetic methodologies, it has become feasible to create nanomaterials with precise physicochemical characteristics, surface load, and controlled shape and size. This has led to the production of a diverse range of nanomaterials. Biosensors incorporating nanomaterials offer advantages over traditional biosensors, including improved physical, chemical, and biological properties. Carbon nanomaterials, when used as a support matrix, are particularly beneficial. Biosensor design has been greatly influenced by them, providing uncomplicated techniques such as minimal background flow, surface renewal ability, and economical production [86]. Over the last few decades, carbon nanomaterials have emerged as a beacon of hope in biosensor design thanks to their unique features. These include a high surface-to-volume ratio, biocompatibility, robust mechanical strength, high electrical conductivity, and chemical stability. Carbon nanomaterials, such as fullerenes, diamonds, CNTs, and graphenes, are not just catalysts or immobilizing elements in a biosensor but potential game-changers in the field (figure 2.4). The functionalization of carbon nanomaterials presents a promising avenue for developing biosensors with unique properties, including thermal and electrical conductivity, high mechanical strength, and specificity to identify target analytes even at deficient concentrations (figure 2.2(a)) [45]. Carbon nanomaterials in biosensors have been employed as [87]: (i) the sensor system comprises a recognition element, which contains specific binding sites for the target molecules; (ii) a transducer component that transforms molecular interaction detected at the electrode surface into a quantifiable signal; and (iii) a label for target molecules for signal amplification.

Carbon allotropes, such as CNTs, graphene, fullerenes, CDs, CB, and nanodiamonds, have provided specific properties and desired biosensor features. CDs are a type of nanocarbon material with synchronized sp^2 and sp^3 hybridized carbon atoms expressed as 0D nanoparticles below 10 nm. As a result, they show biocompatibility and low toxicity. Due to their ability to act as electron donors and receivers, CDs have been explored as biosensor components. However, they lack long-term stabilization, which is a crucial requirement in biosensor design [88]. Despite this issue, CDs have received significant attention in biosensor applications and are the second-most studied member of the nanocarbon family after graphene

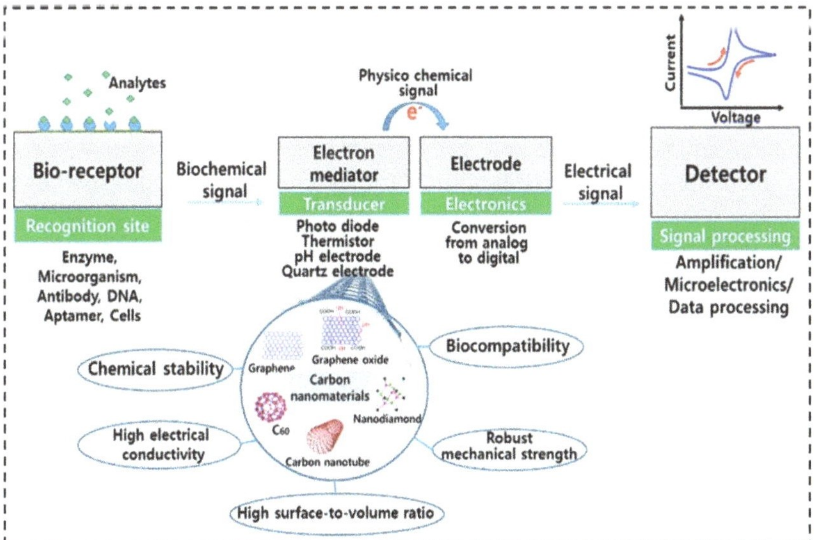

Figure 2.4. A schematic illustration of a conventional biosensor and its components with carbon nanomaterial as a transducer. Reproduced from [87]. CC BY 4.0.

and CNTs. The stabilization of CDs is crucial for their future use in electrochemical biosensor applications. This will determine whether CDs can be a viable option for these applications.

Voltammetric biosensors are widely used in various applications, but they need more stable surface architectures, which poses a challenge in achieving high sensitivity with desired biochemical and physiological events. To address this issue, researchers are exploring the use of graphene and CNTs to reduce the dimensions of biosensor elements and increase the signal-to-noise ratio for processes occurring at the device's interface. Additionally, researchers are experimenting with using multiple enzymatic labels to enhance the signal per event. Meanwhile, 1D SWCNTs and MWCNTs, and 2D graphene (e.g., graphene oxide (GO), graphene nanoribbon, and reduced graphene oxide (rGO)) possess electrical and mechanical properties that make them ideal for various biosensor applications [89, 90]. By modifying their surface, the physicochemical properties of graphene and CNTs can be adjusted to extend their scope of application. While other carbon nanomaterials such as 0D fullerenes and carbon quantum dots (CQDs) have been used as biosensors, they are less frequently used than 1D and 2D carbon nanomaterials in voltammetric biosensing applications. Incorporating polymers, nanoparticles, ionic liquids, enzymes, and DNA with 1D and 2D carbon-based nanomaterials offers multiple ways to create various sensing methods. These techniques will be discussed in the next section.

Graphene has gained considerable interest due to its extraordinary mechanical strength, optical characteristics, and extensive surface area, demonstrating high electrical conductivity. It comprises a single layer of carbon atoms arranged in a honeycomb structure. Graphene derivatives, such as graphene nanoribbons, few-layered graphene, and GO, have also been studied extensively. GO is a highly oxygenated form of graphene that is produced through the harsh oxidation of graphite, while rGO is a product of GO reduction by thermal or chemical methods [91]. The reduction method can significantly affect the functional groups and conductivity of rGO. GO and rGO are suitable for biosensor fabrication because they offer numerous sites for easy surface modification with tunable conductivity (figure 2.5) [27, 92]. However, there are some challenges when it comes to using graphene-based biosensors, including inconsistency in electrode modification methodologies, a lack of standardization in production, a high tendency for aggregation, an inability to utilize graphene's properties fully, and concerns about the physical stability of graphene in real and biological environments.

Carbon nanotubes are formed by rolling up a sheet of graphene nanoribbon, with a diameter ranging from ~0.4 to 2 nm. On the other hand, MWCNTs consist of multiple rolled-up sheets of graphene nanoribbon and have a diameter that varies from ~2 to 100 nm [93–95]. CNTs can be modified chemically, like graphene, which can alter their conductance, mechanical strength, and optical properties. These modifications can cause changes in the intrinsic properties of CNTs, which can enhance the electrical or catalytic properties of materials containing these carbon nanomaterials. Although several theories backed up by experimental evidence offer a comprehensive understanding of the complex physicochemical processes occurring

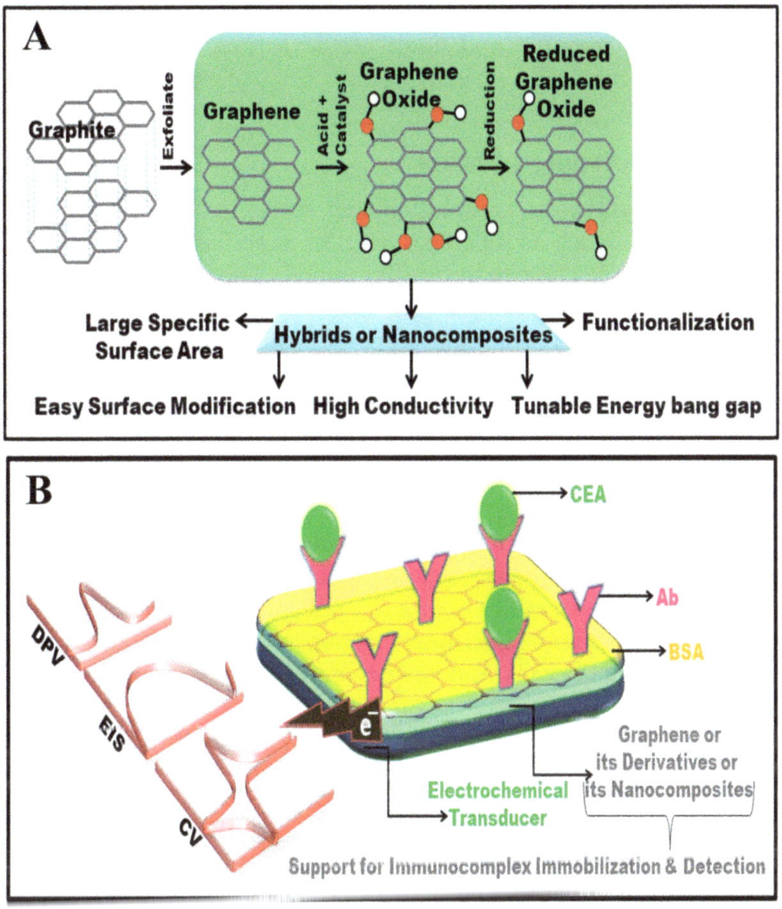

Figure 2.5. Graphene application in fabricating a biosensor: (A) graphene and its derivatives with their critical properties, and (B) graphene-based electrochemical sensor for cancer marker detection carcinoembryonic antigen. Reprinted from [27], Copyright (2022), with permission from Elsevier.

at the CNTs interface, considerable research is still needed to fully comprehend the role of CNTs in enhancing the efficiency of electrochemical sensors. This is especially true in semi-reversible electrochemical systems involving enzymes that allow biosensing without H_2O_2 [96].

While carbon nanomaterials-based biosensors hold immense promise, they are not without their share of challenges in biological applications. The fabrication of biosensors, for instance, often requires a specific size and helicity of carbon nanomaterials, a task that proves to be quite challenging during synthesis. Moreover, their fabrication is not cost-effective in large-scale production, leading to high market prices that hinder realistic commercial applications. In carbon-based biosensors, the need to immobilize an enzyme onto the surface of carbon nanomaterial-coated electrodes can potentially damage the biological receptors, posing a threat to their biological activity, biocompatibility, and structural stability.

Therefore, developing reversible, reusable, and long-lasting systems to replace current irreversible, disposable, and single-use devices remains a pressing challenge that calls for further research and innovation.

2.6 Advanced allotropic hybrids

Carbon allotropic hybrids are revolutionizing sensor technologies by combining carbon nanostructures such as fullerenes, CQDs, nanodiamonds, CNTs, graphene, and graphite (figure 2.6). These hybrids offer unprecedented opportunities for sensor innovation by leveraging the unique properties of each constituent. For instance, graphene and CNT hybrids combine graphene's high electrical conductivity and exceptional mechanical strength, while incorporating CQDs, enhancing optical properties for optoelectronic sensors [97–99]. Including fullerenes and nanodiamonds further expands the design space, enabling the creation of hybrids with tailored functionalities [100–102]. This diverse array of carbon nanostructures empowers the development of sensors with heightened sensitivity, selectivity, and stability across various applications, from environmental monitoring to healthcare diagnostics [101–103]. Researchers need to refine synthesis techniques and explore novel hybrid architectures to fully realize the potential of carbon allotropic hybrids and catalyze their integration into practical sensor devices. By doing so, we can address pressing societal needs and create more efficient, reliable, and accurate sensor devices.

These advances in allotropic forms of carbon underscore the transformative potential across various domains. Different forms of carbon material for electrochemical sensing have shown great potential in electrochemical sensing. Further research must focus on overcoming the challenges related to scalability,

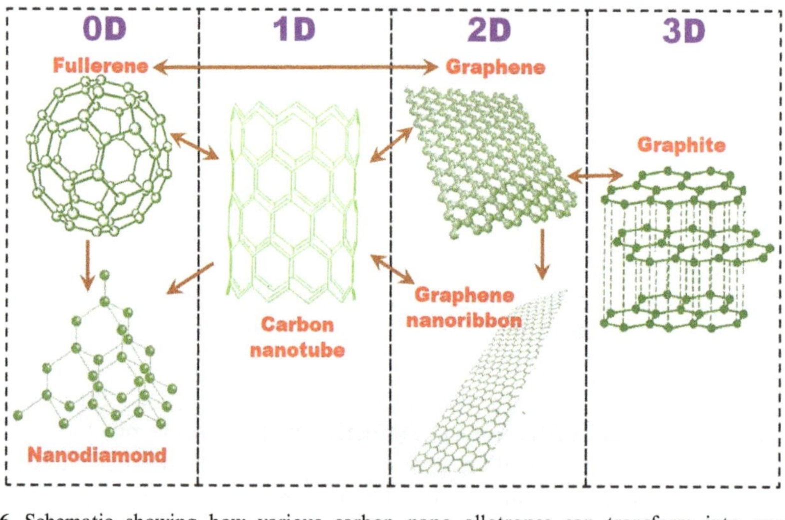

Figure 2.6. Schematic showing how various carbon nano allotropes can transform into one another, highlighting changes in dimensionality. One-sided arrows represent one-way transformations, while two-way arrows denote both-sided transformations.

reproducibility, and integration with existing technologies, which will open up additional opportunities for its applications and societal impacts. The evolution of these materials and their fabrication techniques is continuous, and carbon-based electrochemical sensors are expected to play a crucial role in enhancing our capabilities in monitoring and environmental stewardship [104].

2.7 Conclusion

This chapter delves into the use of electrochemical sensors that are crafted from nanostructured carbon allotropes (figure 2.7). Carbon materials are becoming increasingly popular as potential solutions to the challenges of constructing sensors: (i) the optical properties of these can be customized as per requirement, (ii) they possess a significantly large specific surface area, (iii) high surface free energy characterizes them, (iv) they are biocompatible in nature. These characteristics make them suitable for various roles in various types of sensors. Carbon materials exhibit highly selective and efficient sensing behaviors, which favors the signal transduction pathway. Furthermore, the suitability of carbon materials for use in electrochemical sensor construction is widely accepted. These sensors, with their sensitivity, specificity, stability, and consistency, are poised to impact environmental science and engineering significantly. Their good electrical properties, wide potential

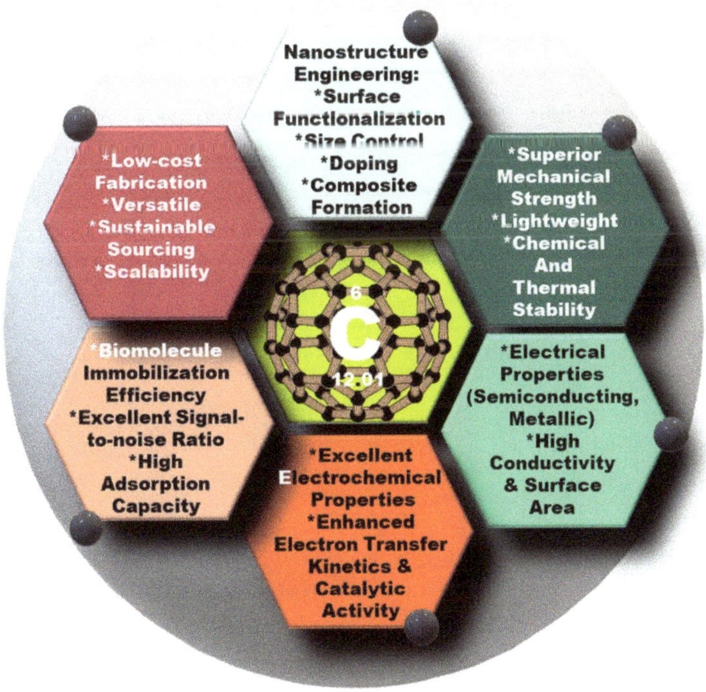

Figure 2.7. Promising traits of carbon in the fabrication of electrochemical sensors and biosensors.

window, and ease of chemical modification contribute to their effectiveness. Recent studies have demonstrated that electrochemical sensors based on carbon nanomaterials have a broad linear response spectrum and a low detection limit for various environmental pollutants. Creating new nanomaterials with suitable chemical properties and morphologies is essential to improve the electroanalytical redox mechanism.

Integrating carbon materials with different biological recognition elements such as enzymes, antibodies, and aptamers has led to remarkable advancements in sensor selectivity. However, there is still a need for significant improvements in the stability, affordability, and ease of preparation of novel or modified bio-recognition elements. Furthermore, challenges such as portability and miniaturization must be addressed.

Carbon nanotubes are highly efficient in electrochemical sensing for detecting pesticides alone or combined with various modifiers. MWCNTs have proven particularly effective because they increase the electrode surface area and enhance electron transmission between the electrode and electrolyte. Recently, 3D graphene nanomaterials/nanocomposites have emerged as a promising technique for the on-site detection of pesticides or herbicides, offering excellent performance. However, while carbon-based nanomaterials are rapidly advancing, a comprehensive evaluation of various nanomaterials under different analytical conditions of the nano-engineered sensor is still a significant area of research. The upcoming chapters highlight the application of carbon-based catalysis for electrochemical sensing of various agro-pollutants, such as pesticides, fertilizers, and heavy metal ions (figure 2.8).

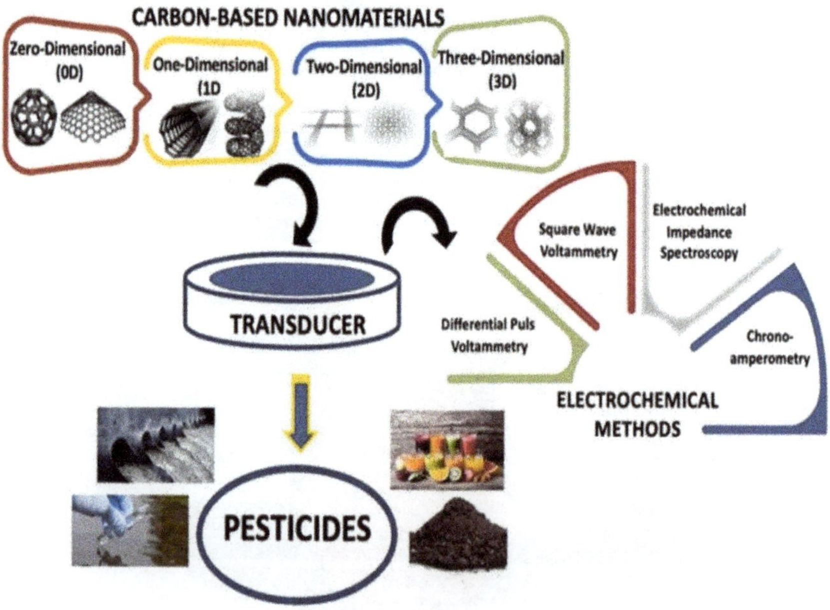

Figure 2.8. Application of various carbon allotropes in the development of electrochemical sensors for agro-pollutants such as pesticides, fertilizers, and heavy metal ions. Reprinted from [105], Copyright (2022), with permission from Elsevier.

References

[1] Zhang L, Lei Y, He P, Wu H, Guo L and Wei G 2022 Carbon material-based aerogels for gas adsorption: fabrication, structure design, functional tailoring, and applications *Nanomaterials* **12** 3172

[2] Yang I, Kwon D, Kim M-S and Jung J C 2018 A comparative study of activated carbon aerogel and commercial activated carbons as electrode materials for organic electric double-layer capacitors *Carbon* **132** 503–11

[3] Muhammad S, Yahya E B, Abdul Khalil H P S, Marwan M and Albadn Y M 2023 Recent advances in carbon and activated carbon nanostructured aerogels prepared from agricultural wastes for wastewater treatment applications *Agriculture* **13** 208

[4] Debnath S K and Srivastava R 2021 Drug delivery with carbon-based nanomaterials as versatile nanocarriers: progress and prospects *Front. Nanotechnol.* **3** 644564

[5] Manasa G, Bhakta A K, Bafna J, Mascarenhas R J, Malode S J and Shetti N P 2022 An amperometric sensor composed of carbon hybrid-structure for the degradation of amino-triazole herbicide *Environ. Res.* **212** 113541

[6] Manasa G, Bhakta A K, Mekhalif Z and Mascarenhas R J 2020 Bismuth-nanoparticles decorated multi-wall-carbon-nanotubes cast-coated on carbon paste electrode; an electrochemical sensor for sensitive determination of gallic acid at neutral pH *Mater. Sci. Energy Technol.* **3** 174–82

[7] Manasa G, Mascarenhas R J, Bhakta A K and Mekhalif Z 2020 MWCNT/Nileblue heterostructured composite electrode for flavanone Naringenin quantification in fruit juices *Electroanalysis* **32** 939–48

[8] Manasa G, Mascarenhas R J, Bhakta A K and Mekhalif Z 2021 Nano-graphene-platelet/Brilliant-green composite coated carbon paste electrode interface for electrocatalytic oxidation of flavanone Hesperidin *Microchem. J.* **160** 105768

[9] Manasa G, Mascarenhas R J, Satpati A K, Basavaraja B M and Kumar S 2018 An electrochemical bisphenol F sensor based on ZnO/G nano composite and CTAB surface modified carbon paste electrode architecture *Colloids Surf.* **B 170** 144–51

[10] Govindarajan D, Saravanan S, Sudhakar S and Vimalraj S 2024 Graphene: a multifaceted carbon-based material for bone tissue engineering applications *ACS Omega* **9** 67–80

[11] Manasa G, Shetti N, Mascarenhas R J and Reddy K R 2022 Graphene-based electrochemicals and biosensors for multifaceted applications in healthcare *Smart Nanodevices for Point-of-Care Applications* (Boca Raton, FL: CRC Press) p 1–16

[12] Sridharan G, Atchudan R, Magesh V, Arya S, Ganapathy D, Nallaswamy D and Sundramoorthy A K 2023 Advanced electrocatalytic materials based biosensors for cancer cell detection—a review *Electroanalysis* **35** e202300093

[13] Cox J A, Rutkowska I A and Kulesza P J 2020 Critical review—electrocatalytic sensors for arsenic oxo species *J. Electrochem. Soc.* **167** 037565

[14] Riaz M A and Chen Y 2022 Electrodes and electrocatalysts for electrochemical hydrogen peroxide sensors: a review of design strategies *Nanoscale Horiz* **7** 463–79

[15] Wang X, Feng Y, Dong P and Huang J 2019 A mini review on carbon quantum dots: preparation, properties, and electrocatalytic application *Front. Chem.* **7** 671

[16] Silva T A, Moraes F C, Janegitz B C and Fatibello-Filho O 2017 Electrochemical biosensors based on nanostructured carbon black: a review *J. Nanomater.* **2017** e4571614

[17] Liu X, Huang L and Qian K 2021 Nanomaterial-based electrochemical sensors: mechanism, preparation, and application in biomedicine *Adv. NanoBiomed Res.* **1** 2000104

[18] Zhu C, Yang G, Li H, Du D and Lin Y 2015 Electrochemical sensors and biosensors based on nanomaterials and nanostructures *Anal. Chem.* **87** 230–49
[19] Gibi C, Liu C-H, Barton S C, Anandan S and Wu J J 2024 Carbon materials for electrochemical sensing application—a mini review *J. Taiwan Inst. Chem. Eng.* **154** 105071
[20] Jiwanti P K, Wardhana B Y, Sutanto L G and Chanif M F 2022 A review on carbon-based electrodes for electrochemical sensor of quinolone antibiotics *ChemistrySelect* **7** e202103997
[21] Michalkiewicz S, Skorupa A and Jakubczyk M 2021 Carbon materials in electroanalysis of preservatives: a review *Materials (Basel)* **14** 7630
[22] Robertson J 1986 Amorphous carbon *Adv. Phys.* **35** 317–74
[23] Robertson J 2002 Diamond-like amorphous carbon *Mater. Sci. Eng.: R: Rep.* **37** 129–281
[24] Ye X, Qi M, Chen M, Zhang L and Zhang J 2023 Zero to three dimension structure evolution from carbon allotropes to phosphorus allotropes *Adv. Mater. Interfaces* **10** 2201941
[25] Manasa G, Mascarenhas R J, Satpati A K, D'Souza O J and Dhason A 2017 Facile preparation of poly(methylene blue) modified carbon paste electrode for the detection and quantification of catechin *Mater. Sci. Eng.* C **73** 552–61
[26] Manasa G, Mascarenhas R J and Basavaraja B M 2019 Sensitively-selective determination of Propyl Paraben preservative based on synergistic effects of polyaniline-zinc-oxide nano-composite incorporated into graphite paste electrode *Colloids Surf.* B **184** 110529
[27] Manasa G, Mascarenhas R J, Malode S J and Shetti N P 2022 Graphene-based electro-chemical immunosensors for early detection of oncomarker carcinoembryonic antigen *Biosens. Bioelectron.: X* **11** 100189
[28] Giubileo F, Di Bartolomeo A, Iemmo L, Luongo G and Urban F 2018 Field emission from carbon nanostructures *Appl. Sci.* **8** 526
[29] Li J, Yin D and Qin Y 2023 Carbon materials: structures, properties, synthesis and applications *Manuf. Rev.* **10** 13
[30] Sokolov V I 1999 Chemistry of fullerenes, novel allotropic modifications of carbon *Russ. Chem. Bull.* **48** 1197–205
[31] Zhou M, Guo J, Guo L and Bai J 2008 Electrochemical sensing platform based on the highly ordered mesoporous carbon-fullerene system *Anal. Chem.* **80** 4642–50
[32] Li R, Zhen M, Guan M, Chen D, Zhang G, Ge J, Gong P, Wang C and Shu C 2013 A novel glucose colorimetric sensor based on intrinsic peroxidase-like activity of C_{60}-carboxyfullerenes *Biosens. Bioelectron.* **47** 502–7
[33] Markovic Z and Trajkovic V 2008 Biomedical potential of the reactive oxygen species generation and quenching by fullerenes (C_{60}) *Biomaterials* **29** 3561–73
[34] Chuang C-W and Shih J-S 2001 Preparation and application of immobilized C_{60}-glucose oxidase enzyme in fullerene C_{60}-coated piezoelectric quartz crystal glucose sensor *Sens. Actuators* B **81** 1–8
[35] Keshtkar S, Rashidi A, Kooti M, Askarieh M, Pourhashem S, Ghasemy E and Izadi N 2018 A novel highly sensitive and selective H_2S gas sensor at low temperatures based on SnO_2 quantum dots-C_{60} nanohybrid: experimental and theory study *Talanta* **188** 531–9
[36] Pan S, Pei Z, Jing Z, Song J, Zhang W, Zhang Q and Sang S 2020 A highly stretchable strain sensor based on CNT/graphene/fullerene-SEBS *RSC Adv.* **10** 11225–32
[37] Wei L, Lei Y, Fu H and Yao J 2012 Fullerene hollow microspheres prepared by bubble-templates as sensitive and selective electrocatalytic sensor for biomolecules *ACS Appl. Mater. Interfaces* **4** 1594–600

[38] Li Y, Fang L, Cheng P, Deng J, Jiang L, Huang H and Zheng J 2013 An electrochemical immunosensor for sensitive detection of *Escherichia coli* O157:H7 using C_{60} based biocompatible platform and enzyme functionalized Pt nanochains tracing tag *Biosens. Bioelectron.* **49** 485–91
[39] Tuerhong M, Xu Y and Yin X-B 2017 Review on carbon dots and their applications *Chin. J. Anal. Chem.* **45** 139–50
[40] Wang J and Qiu J 2016 A review of carbon dots in biological applications *J. Mater. Sci.* **51** 4728–38
[41] Mishra V, Patil A, Thakur S and Kesharwani P 2018 Carbon dots: emerging theranostic nanoarchitectures *Drug Discov. Today* **23** 1219–32
[42] Tîlmaciu C-M and Morris M C 2015 Carbon nanotube biosensors *Front. Chem.* **3** 59
[43] Crescenzo A D, Ettorre V and Fontana A 2014 Non-covalent and reversible functionalization of carbon nanotubes *Beilstein J. Nanotechnol.* **5** 1675–90
[44] Balasubramanian K and Burghard M 2005 Chemically functionalized carbon nanotubes *Small* **1** 180–92
[45] Abd-Elsalam K A, Ramadan M M and Hassanien M K 2020 Nanocarbon-based sensors for pesticide detection: recent trends *Carbon Nanomaterials for Agri-Food and Environmental Applications* Micro and Nano Technologies K A Abd-Elsalam (Amsterdam: Elsevier) ch 18 pp 401–28
[46] Merkoçi A, Pumera M, Llopis X, Pérez B, del Valle M and Alegret S 2005 New materials for electrochemical sensing VI: carbon nanotubes *TrAC, Trends Anal. Chem.* **24** 826–38
[47] Manasa G, Raj C, Satpati A K and Mascarenhas R J 2020 S(O)MWCNT/modified carbon paste—a non-enzymatic amperometric sensor for direct determination of 6 mercaptopurine in biological fluids *Electroanalysis* **32** 2431–41
[48] Manasa G, Bhakta A K, Mekhalif Z and Mascarenhas R J 2019 Voltammetric study and rapid quantification of resorcinol in hair dye and biological samples using ultrasensitive maghemite/MWCNT modified carbon paste electrode *Electroanalysis* **31** 1363–72
[49] Manasa G, Bhakta A K, Mascarenhas R J and Shetti N P 2023 BaO-MWCNT composite material-based electrocatalytic amperometric sensor for the detection of environmentally hazardous Diuron *Microchem. J.* **191** 108778
[50] Putzbach W and Ronkainen N J 2013 Immobilization techniques in the fabrication of nanomaterial-based electrochemical biosensors: a review *Sensors* **13** 4811–40
[51] Gooding J J 2005 Nanostructuring electrodes with carbon nanotubes: a review on electrochemistry and applications for sensing *Electrochim. Acta* **50** 3049–60
[52] Deo R P and Wang J 2004 Electrochemical detection of carbohydrates at carbon-nanotube modified glassy-carbon electrodes *Electrochem. Commun.* **6** 284–7
[53] Rout D R, Senapati P, Sutar H, Sau D C and Murmu R 2020 Graphene oxide (GO) supported palladium (Pd) nanocomposites for enhanced hydrogenation *Graphene* **8** 33–51
[54] Adhikari B-R, Govindhan M and Chen A 2015 Carbon nanomaterials based electrochemical sensors/biosensors for the sensitive detection of pharmaceutical and biological compounds *Sensors* **15** 22490–508
[55] Li W, Tan C, Lowe M A, Abruña H D and Ralph D C 2011 Electrochemistry of individual monolayer graphene sheets *ACS Nano* **5** 2264–70
[56] McCreery R L 2008 Advanced carbon electrode materials for molecular electrochemistry *Chem. Rev.* **108** 2646–87

[57] Davies T J, Hyde M E and Compton R G 2005 Nanotrench arrays reveal insight into graphite electrochemistry *Angew. Chem.* **117** 5251–6

[58] He H, Klinowski J, Forster M and Lerf A 1998 A new structural model for graphite oxide *Chem. Phys. Lett.* **287** 53–6

[59] Lerf A, He H, Forster M and Klinowski J 1998 Structure of graphite oxide revisited *J. Phys. Chem.* B **102** 4477–82

[60] Ambrosi A, Bonanni A, Sofer Z, Cross J S and Pumera M 2011 Electrochemistry at chemically modified graphenes *Chem. Eur. J.* **17** 10763–70

[61] Chen D, Tang L and Li J 2010 Graphene-based materials in electrochemistry *Chem. Soc. Rev.* **39** 3157–80

[62] Gao W, Alemany L B, Ci L and Ajayan P M 2009 New insights into the structure and reduction of graphite oxide *Nat. Chem.* **1** 403–8

[63] Cuara E, Sierra U, Mercado A, Barriga-Castro E D, Cortés A, Gallardo-Vega C, Valle-Orta M and Fernández S 2021 Synthesis of copper oxides-graphene composites for glucose sensing *Carbon Trends* **4** 100050

[64] Machado M, Oliveira A M L, Silva G A, Bitoque D B, Tavares Ferreira J, Pinto L A and Ferreira Q 2022 Graphene biosensors—a molecular approach *Nanomaterials* **12** 1624

[65] Toto E, Laurenzi S and Santonicola M G 2022 Recent trends in graphene/polymer nanocomposites for sensing devices: synthesis and applications in environmental and human health monitoring *Polymers* **14** 1030

[66] Shellaiah M and Sun K W 2021 Diamond-based electrodes for detection of metal ions and anions *Nanomaterials (Basel)* **12** 64

[67] Culková E, Lukáčová-Chomisteková Z, Bellová R, Melicherčíková D, Durdiak J, Rievaj M, Vojs M and Tomčík P 2020 Voltammetric detection of silver in commercial products on boron doped diamond electrode: stripping at lowered potential in the presence of thiosulfate ions *Monatsh. Chem.* **151** 1009–17

[68] Guo Y, Huang N, Yang B, Wang C, Zhuang H, Tian Q, Zhai Z, Liu L and Jiang X 2016 Hybrid diamond/graphite films as electrodes for anodic stripping voltammetry of trace Ag^+ and Cu^{2+} *Sensors Actuators* B **231** 194–202

[69] Pei J, Yu X, Wei S, Boukherroub R and Zhang Y 2021 Double-side effect of B/C ratio on BDD electrode detection for heavy metal ion in water *Sci. Total Environ.* **771** 145430

[70] Ho M P and Lau A K-T 2015 Amorphous carbon nanocomposites *Fillers and Reinforcements for Advanced Nanocomposites* (Woodhead Publishing Series in Composites Science and Engineering) Y Dong, R Umer and A K-T Lau (Woodhead Publishing) ch 12 pp 309–28

[71] Moseenkov S I, Kuznetsov V L, Zolotarev N A, Kolesov B A, Prosvirin I P, Ishchenko A V and Zavorin A V 2023 Investigation of amorphous carbon in nanostructured carbon materials (a comparative study by TEM, XPS, Raman spectroscopy and XRD) *Materials* **16** 1112

[72] Li S *et al* 2022 Non-destructive characterisation of coke deposit on FCC catalyst and its transient evolution upon air-firing and oxy-fuel regeneration *Chem. Eng. J.* **430** 132998

[73] Bayraktar O and Kugler E L 2003 Coke content of spent commercial fluid catalytic cracking (FCC) catalysts *J. Therm. Anal. Calorim.* **71** 867–74

[74] Lu H and Zhao X S 2017 Biomass-derived carbon electrode materials for supercapacitors *Sustain. Energy Fuels* **1** 1265–81

[75] Olabi A G, Abbas Q, Abdelkareem M A, Alami A H, Mirzaeian M and Sayed E T 2023 Carbon-based materials for supercapacitors: recent progress, challenges and barriers *Batteries* **9** 19

[76] Ahmed A S, Alsultan M, Hameed R T, Assim Y F and Swiegers G F 2022 High surface area activated charcoal for water purification *J. Compos. Sci.* **6** 311
[77] Zareh M M, Ahmed R M, Saleem N O and Abd-ElSattar A 2023 Graphene oxide versus activated charcoal for La-electrochemical sensor *Mater. Sci. Eng.* B **292** 116389
[78] Lounasvuori M M, Kelly D and Foord J S 2018 Carbon black as low-cost alternative for electrochemical sensing of phenolic compounds *Carbon* **129** 252–7
[79] Bokobza L, Bruneel J-L and Couzi M 2015 Raman spectra of carbon-based materials (from graphite to carbon black) and of some silicone composites *C* **1** 77–94
[80] Marinho B, Ghislandi M, Tkalya E, Koning C E and de With G 2012 Electrical conductivity of compacts of graphene, multi-wall carbon nanotubes, carbon black, and graphite powder *Powder Technol.* **221** 351–8
[81] Mathur R B, Singh B P and Pande S 2016 *Carbon Nanomaterials: Synthesis, Structure, Properties and Applications* (New York: Taylor and Francis)
[82] Nieto-Márquez A, Romero R, Romero A and Valverde J L 2011 Carbon nanospheres: synthesis, physicochemical properties and applications *J. Mater. Chem.* **21** 1664–72
[83] Miao J-Y, Hwang D W, Narasimhulu K V, Lin P-I, Chen Y-T, Lin S-H and Hwang L-P 2004 Synthesis and properties of carbon nanospheres grown by CVD using Kaolin supported transition metal catalysts *Carbon* **42** 813–22
[84] Zhang P, Qiao Z-A and Dai S 2015 Recent advances in carbon nanospheres: synthetic routes and applications *Chem. Commun.* **51** 9246–56
[85] Kumar S, Sharma R, Bhawna , Gupta A, Singh P, Kalia S, Thakur P and Kumar V 2022 Prospects of biosensors based on functionalized and nanostructured solitary materials: detection of viral infections and other risks *ACS Omega* **7** 22073–88
[86] Malik S, Singh J, Goyat R, Saharan Y, Chaudhry V, Umar A, Ibrahim A A, Akbar S, Ameen S and Baskoutas S 2023 Nanomaterials-based biosensor and their applications: a review *Heliyon* **9** e19929
[87] Hwang H S, Jeong J W, Kim Y A and Chang M 2020 Carbon nanomaterials as versatile platforms for biosensing applications *Micromachines* **11** 814
[88] Pourmadadi M, Rahmani E, Rajabzadeh-Khosroshahi M, Samadi A, Behzadmehr R, Rahdar A and Ferreira L F R 2023 Properties and application of carbon quantum dots (CQDs) in biosensors for disease detection: a comprehensive review *J. Drug Delivery Sci. Technol.* **80** 104156
[89] Ambrosi A, Chua C K, Bonanni A and Pumera M 2014 Electrochemistry of graphene and related materials *Chem. Rev.* **114** 7150–88
[90] Zheng D, Vashist S K, Dykas M M, Saha S, Al-Rubeaan K, Lam E, Luong J H T and Sheu F-S 2013 Graphene versus multi-walled carbon nanotubes for electrochemical glucose biosensing *Materials* **6** 1011–27
[91] Dimiev A M and Tour J M 2014 Mechanism of graphene oxide formation *ACS Nano* **8** 3060–8
[92] Yin P T, Shah S, Chhowalla M and Lee K-B 2015 Design, synthesis, and characterization of graphene–nanoparticle hybrid materials for bioapplications *Chem. Rev.* **115** 2483–531
[93] Datsyuk V, Kalyva M, Papagelis K, Parthenios J, Tasis D, Siokou A, Kallitsis I and Galiotis C 2008 Chemical oxidation of multiwalled carbon nanotubes *Carbon* **46** 833–40
[94] Lota G, Fic K and Frackowiak E 2011 Carbon nanotubes and their composites in electrochemical applications *Energy Environ. Sci.* **4** 1592–605

[95] Karousis N, Tagmatarchis N and Tasis D 2010 Current progress on the chemical modification of carbon nanotubes *Chem. Rev.* **110** 5366–97
[96] Carrara S, Baj-Rossi C, Boero C and De Micheli G 2014 Do carbon nanotubes contribute to electrochemical biosensing? *Electrochim. Acta* **128** 102–12
[97] Ahmed Y M, Eldin M A, Galal A and Atta N F 2024 Electrochemical sensor based on PEDOT/CNTs-graphene oxide for simultaneous determination of hazardous hydroquinone, catechol, and nitrite in real water samples *Sci. Rep.* **14** 5654
[98] Huang Q, Lin X, Tong L and Tong Q-X 2020 Graphene quantum dots/multiwalled carbon nanotubes composite-based electrochemical sensor for detecting dopamine release from living cells *ACS Sustain. Chem. Eng.* **8** 1644–50
[99] Ghosh D, Sarkar K, Devi P, Kim K-H and Kumar P 2021 Current and future perspectives of carbon and graphene quantum dots: from synthesis to strategy for building optoelectronic and energy devices *Renew. Sustain. Energy Rev.* **135** 110391
[100] Mazloum-Ardakani M and Khoshroo A 2014 High performance electrochemical sensor based on fullerene-functionalized carbon nanotubes/ionic liquid: determination of some catecholamines *Electrochem. Commun.* **42** 9–12
[101] Elugoke S E, Fayemi O E, Adekunle A S, Nkambule T T I, Mamba B B and Ebenso E E 2021 Conductive nanodiamond-based detection of neurotransmitters: one decade, few sensors *ACS Omega* **6** 18548–58
[102] Lee S-K, Song M-J, Kim J-H, Kan T-S, Lim Y-K, Ahn J-P and Lim D-S 2014 3D-networked carbon nanotube/diamond core–shell nanowires for enhanced electrochemical performance *NPG Asia Mater.* **6** e115 e115
[103] Koo D, Sung J, Suh H, Bae S and So H 2023 Comprehensive analysis of CNT/NS/GO composites: dispersion effect of graphene oxide for environmental sensor application *Compos. A: Appl. Sci. Manuf.* **173** 107639
[104] Georgakilas V, Perman J A, Tucek J and Zboril R 2015 Broad family of carbon nanoallotropes: classification, chemistry, and applications of fullerenes, carbon dots, nanotubes, graphene, nanodiamonds, and combined superstructures *Chem. Rev.* **115** 4744–822
[105] Karadurmus L, Cetinkaya A, Kaya S I and Ozkan S A 2022 Recent trends on electrochemical carbon-based nanosensors for sensitive assay of pesticides *Trends Environ. Anal. Chem.* **34** e00158

Chapter 3

Application of carbon allotropes in the fabrication of electrochemical sensors

G Manasa, Pavithra Siddu and Chandra Sekhar Rout

The global population explosion has created an immense demand for increased food supply, compelling scientists and engineers to devise novel methods for enhancing agricultural production. Given the limited land and water resources, the only viable means of increasing agricultural productivity involve sound agronomy and robust technological support. However, modern agricultural practices have raised significant environmental concerns regarding the global pollution crisis, escalating due to anthropogenic factors such as industrialization and urbanization. The contamination of the biosphere by toxic agro-environmental pollutants, including pesticides, dyes, polycyclic aromatic hydrocarbons, heavy metals, and others, poses a significant threat. Electrochemical sensors have emerged as a promising sensing technology to address this challenge, offering rapid detection, affordability, selectivity, and sensitivity in identifying hazardous agricultural pollutants. The allotropes of carbon, such as quantum dots, carbon nanotube, carbon nanofiber, graphene, and its derivatives, are widely used to improve electrochemical sensor performance attributed to their greater specific area, porosity, and catalytic effects. This chapter gives an overview of the determination of agricultural pollutants utilizing various carbon allotrope-based electrochemical sensors.

3.1 Introduction

Significant advances have been made in detecting agricultural pollutants through electrochemical sensors [1]. Carbon-based electrochemical sensors are extensively employed to detect a diverse range of target species due to their affordability, efficient electron transfer kinetics, chemical stability, and biocompatibility. These sensors offer several advantages over other sensing techniques, such as high sensitivity and selectivity, rapid response time, and low detection limits.

doi:10.1088/978-0-7503-5879-8ch3

Additionally, they can be easily integrated with various electronic devices, making them an ideal choice for applications across several industries, including healthcare, food, and environmental monitoring. Conventional carbon-based electrode substrates, such as carbon fibers, pyrolytic graphite, and glassy carbon electrodes (GCE), are frequently employed [2].

Due to their small size (ranging from 1 to 100 nm), nanomaterials have unique properties that enable enhanced reactivity, selectivity, and sensitivity. They have found widespread applications in various fields, such as biotechnology, electronics, energy, and materials science. The high surface area of nanomaterials enables them to have a remarkable surface-to-volume ratio and specific surface area, making them attractive for many industrial and academic pursuits. In particular, carbon nanomaterials (CNMs) possess exceptional interfacial adsorption properties, improved electrocatalytic activity, remarkable biocompatibility, and rapid electron transfer kinetics, making them superior to many conventional materials used in electrochemical sensors [3]. Notably, for a considerable period, carbon was only known to exist in two natural crystalline allotropic forms, namely graphite and diamond.

The discovery of fullerene by Kroto and colleagues in 1985 opened a new era for studying synthetic carbon allotropes. Allotropes are materials with the same chemical composition but different physical properties. Carbon has the most allotropes of any element, including 0D nanoparticles, such as quantum dots [4]; 1D structures, such as carbon nanotubes (CNTs) and carbon nanofibers (CNFs) [5]; and 2D layered materials, such as graphene [6]. Graphene–CNT hybrids are 3D structures that combine both materials [7]. These allotropes have distinct crystal structures and properties, as illustrated in table 3.1 and figure 3.1. The hybridization and its structure have a great significant impact on the electrochemical activity of the individual allotropes with multiple favorable features, such as wide potential window, cost-effectiveness, high chemical stability, relativity innocuous electrochemistry along the substantial surface area to volume geometry, and rich surface chemistry that facilitates a variety of redox processes. These outstanding characteristics make CNMs highly sought after for an array of electrochemical applications, predominantly in the realm of sensors. Several carbon-based sensors have been

Table 3.1. Comparative properties of carbon nanomaterial hybridization.

Carbon nanomaterials	Dimensions	Hybridization	Electrical conductivity (S cm^{-1})	Thermal conductivity (W m^{-1} K^{-1})	Experimental specific surface area (m^2 g^{-1})	Hardness	Tenacity
Fullerene	0	Mostly sp^2	10^{-10}	0.4	80–90	High	Elastic
CNT	1	Mostly sp^2	Structure-dependent	3500	~1300	High	Flexible, elastic
Graphene	2	sp^2	~2000	4840–5300	~1500	—	Flexible, elastic
Graphite	3	sp^2	Anisotropic: $2–3 \times 10^4$	Anisotropic: 1500–2000, 5–10	~10–20	High	Flexible, non-elastic

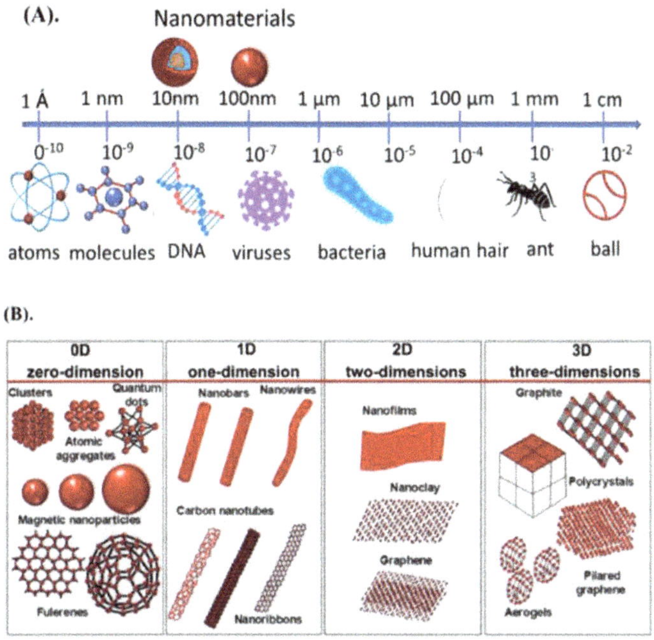

Figure 3.1. (A) Comparative nanomaterial size with standard materials, and (B) schematic illustrations of low-dimensional nanostructures in 0D, 1D, 2D, and 3D. Reproduced from [8]. CC BY 4.0.

validated in literature to have the ability to detect and quantify toxins, pharmaceutical ingredients, antioxidants, pathogens, heavy metals, pesticides, and various other small organic molecules. The critical agricultural pollutants have severely threatened human health (figure 3.2). Therefore, they urgently eed to be detected and monitored.

Anthropogenic activities have led to water and soil pollution in ecosystems. The three most significant contributors to this pollution are human settlements, industries, and agriculture. Pesticides and over 100 000 other chemicals are registered and used in our daily lives, and they inevitably contaminate the fresh water and soil. The quality of water, soil fertility, and purity of fruits and vegetables are declining, which can harm aquatic organisms and humans. This poses a significant threat to waterbodies and can have far-reaching consequences for aquatic ecosystems, from individuals to entire watersheds. If access to nutritious food and clean drinking water is limited, this can endanger human health. More than one-third of the global population lacks safe drinking water. Streams, rivers, lakes, and ponds, collectively known as freshwaters, are exposed to pollutants such as pesticides, heavy metals, and nutrients. These pollutants can have a negative impact on the quality of fresh water. Excessive amounts of nitrogen and phosphorus in freshwater bodies often result in eutrophication, a common cause of water quality degradation. Numerous attempts have been made to enhance fresh water quality, both directly and indirectly. Monitoring food and water quality remains crucial in numerous

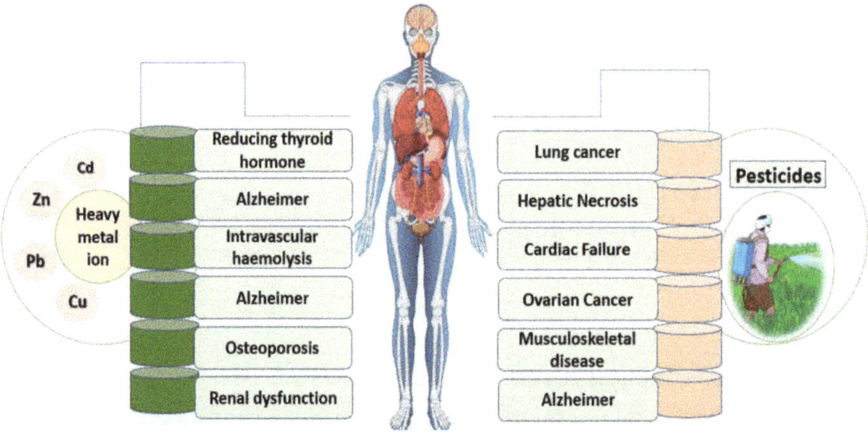

Figure 3.2. The effect of pesticides and heavy metals on human health.

ecological studies because it is vital for safeguarding ecosystems and ensuring human health.

Carbon-based materials are inexpensive and environmentally beneficial. Despite being one of the most fundamental nanomaterials, carbon still attracts considerable interest because of its exceptional electrical conductivity, quick charge transfer, excellent stability, and simplicity of adjustment. In addition to changing carbon's morphological structure, attempts have also been made to change the elements that make up its chemical structure.

Even though the material's morphology can be readily changed to have a larger surface area and more pores, the end product is typically an amorphous carbon material. Both chemical and physical techniques can be used to change the chemical structure of carbon. Functional groups have been shown to dramatically enhance the electrochemical characteristics of sensors in detecting pesticides and heavy metals in agriculture, which cause diseases and are toxic to humankind and the environment. This chapter reviews recent advances in carbon materials under sensors.

3.1.1 Synthesis of carbon allotropes

Carbon allotropes are a subject of intense study in materials science and nanotechnology. The formation of these allotropes involves the reorganization of carbon atoms from various carbon precursors, which can be achieved using multiple synthetic methods. Of particular interest are the techniques that allow for energy-saving reactions and the use of low-cost starting materials. In this paper, we will provide an overview of the synthesis of carbon allotropes, including the various methods and techniques used to achieve this. We aim to understand this complex and rapidly evolving field comprehensively.

(a) **Carbon dots (CDs):** The two methods that are most frequently used for creating CDs are top-down and bottom-up. These synthesis approaches can be carried out using optical, chemical, and thermal techniques. In optical synthesis, a carbon target is frequently ablated using a laser in a solvent or water [9]. The carbon precursor usually undergoes several steps before creating CDs, including carbonization, polymerization, and dehydration. The precursor is subjected to direct heat treatment at a temperature to induce the carbonization process. However, this pyrolysis method appears less attractive because of its time-consuming heating durations, which can last from a few hours to many days. Because it is rapid and reliable, microwave-assisted synthesis thus becomes a practical choice [10].

(b) **Graphite:** In 1896, American scientist Edward Acheson invented the first synthetic graphite made up of carbon atoms, which are connected in flat, stacked layers. This type of carbon is an excellent choice for electrode materials in electrical arc lamps due to its exceptional electrical conductivity. Under normal circumstances, graphite is the most stable form of carbon. The delocalization of the pi-electrons in the carbon atoms allows graphite to conduct electricity. This substance has a glossy black appearance. It possesses excellent electrical and thermal conductivity, is chemically inert, greyish-black, visually opaque, and exhibits properties of both metals and non-metals. The crystal structure of this material is likely responsible for its exceptional qualities. Another fascinating aspect is graphite's hexagonal arrangement of carbon atoms in a planar condensed ring structure.

(c) **Carbon nanotube:** There are three fundamental methods for creating CNTs: laser ablation, chemical vapor deposition (CVD), and arc discharge techniques [11]. In contrast, laser ablation employs intense laser pulses and a catalyst to target carbon within an inert air-filled furnace. Despite being able to produce high-quality CNTs, laser beam bombardment will cause the carbon precursor to evaporate and a graphene coating to grow on the substrate. Both procedures demand a high synthesis temperature to evaporate the carbon precursor [12]. The process of arc discharge requires a vacuum chamber and two carbon electrodes. These electrodes are used as the predecessors to carry out the process. The chamber is filled with inert gas to spread carbon deposition and create multi-walled carbon nanotubes (MWCNTs) with near-perfect shapes. A comparable set of circumstances must include catalysts such as Ni, Fe, Co, Pt, and Rh to produce single-walled carbon nanotubes (SWCNTs). The CVD process is also utilized to make CNTs at significantly low temperatures.

(d) **Graphene:** The most common method for preparing graphene is mechanical exfoliation, which creates microscopic graphene flakes by repeatedly peeling with Scotch tape [13]. The solvent-graphene interaction controls the exfoliation mechanism, which balances the energy required to exfoliate graphite into single-layer graphene. Nevertheless, the number of graphene layers, defects, and challenges in eliminating the remaining solvents are outside the control of this liquid exfoliation approach, which can be detrimental when used as a sensing material on an optical fiber sensor [14]. Another chemical process that can be used to produce graphene is the reduction of GO. This approach has a significant drawback: it cannot completely reduce the GO through the reduction procedure. Additionally, this method yields defects that are often of lower quality than pure graphene, which cannot be eliminated by annealing. The final product is a reduced graphene oxide.

3.2 0D nanomaterials for sensing applications

In November 1985, Harry Kroto (University of Sussex) and Richard Smalley (Rice University) published a report in Nature that led to the discovery of C_{60}. This discovery enabled the production of carbon nanotubes that are linked to fullerenes. Buckyballs, also known as fullerenes, are made up of carbon molecules and come in various sizes and shapes. Since the introduction of graphene in 2004, fullerenes have been extensively researched as carbon nanotubes. This research has created a new area of nanoscale material science and technology study. Although fullerenes [15] and CNTs have an indistinguishable range of diameters, the materials are anticipated to have various size effects on their structures and properties. Fullerenes are well-recognized as 0D materials. This has multiple implications for their characteristics and structures [16].

3.2.1 Introduction and sensor performance enhancing properties of 0D materials

Carbon allotropes with 0D, such as carbon quantum dots and graphene quantum dots (GQDs), have attracted considerable attention from researchers. Semiconductor nanocrystals such as GQDs have found widespread application in various fields. Several GQDs, such as MOSs GQDs, metal dichalcogenide GQDs, and carbon-based GQDs, have been reported to form composites, enhancing their sensing performance. GQDs in sensing layers motivate electron transfer and provide active adsorption sites. Due to their exceptional advantages, superior and universal fluorophores have been identified as fullerenes with enhanced quantum confinement effects. These advantages include highly adjustable photoluminescence and electrochemiluminescence, biocompatibility, exceptional photostability, ultra-small size, and 0D structures [17]. Nodes of innovative electrochemical sensing applications of 0D carbon nanomaterials can be found near recently developed properties. These nanomaterials are abundant in edge sites, have a large specific surface area, and are conductivity good. As a result, GQDs exhibit excellent electrochemical properties, making them ideal for use in numerous technological applications. Moreover, their structures can be modified through specific doping or surface and edge modification, which can still enhance or tune some of their properties [18]. Factors such as area, structure, crystallinity, and chemical composition can significantly improve the electrochemical properties of the sensor.

3.2.2 Application of 0D materials as electrochemical transducers for agricultural pollutants

0D carbon material properties are good candidates for sensors; hence, Prasad *et al* [19] have fabricated CDs (C-dots)/ZrO_2 electrochemical sensors to detect nitroaromatic organophosphorus pesticides. Electrochemical deposition created the C-dots/ZrO_2 nanocomposite on a GCE. The developed material has been characterized by scanning electron microscope (SEM), transmission electron microscope (TEM), x-ray diffraction (XRD), and x-ray photoelectron spectroscopy (XPS). Cyclic voltammetry was employed for the electrochemical analysis. This study focused on examining the ideal parameters, including the influence of factors such as pH, accumulation time, accumulation potential, scan rate, quantity of multiple C-dots, and ZrO_2. By using adsorptive stripping voltammetry, the C-dots/ZrO_2 modified GCE enabled the quick and precise measurement of methyl parathion in rice samples. With a detection limit of 0.056 ng ml^{-1}, the stripping response was substantially linear over the range of methyl parathion concentrations from 0.2 to 48 ng ml^{-1}. This innovative electrochemical nanocomposite-based electrochemical sensor successfully found methyl parathion in rice samples. Furthermore, Selvakumar and co-workers [20] reported the electrochemical synthesis of AuNPs decorated AC60 modified SPCE, which was used for hydrazine amperometric detection. The developed material has been subjected to SEM analysis, which demonstrates that AuNPs (average size of 75 ± 8 nm) were uniformly adorned on the surface of AC60. For the detection of hydrazine, the AC60-AuNPs modified SPCE showed low oxidation potential and good electrocatalytic activity. The fabricated modified electrode shows a more comprehensive linear response range of 0.13 μM to 1.21 mM (response time of 1.3 s), and lower limit of detection (LOD) of 0.038 μM with a sensitivity of 0.583 μA μM^{-1} cm^{-2} for hydrazine detection. The good selectivity and practicality of AC60-AuNPs modified SPCE confirm its applicability in real-world scenarios. In another study, Akeem [21] created an electrochemical sensor to detect glyphosate (Glyp). Glyp is a common herbicide and a significant environmental pollutant that can harm human health. The authors developed Cu0-doped graphitic carbon quantum dots (CuO-OGQ) to detect trace amounts of Glyp in agricultural produce, vegetables, water, and fruits. DPV, CV, and EIS techniques were used to examine the electrochemical behavior of the synthesized material. The electroactive area of CuO-OGQ is 0.428 cm^2, which is 1.35 times greater than OGQ's (0.318 cm^2) and approximately seven times larger than a bare glassy carbon electrode (0.0612 cm^2). The developed Glyp sensor demonstrated a LOD of 2.02 ng ml^{-1} (S/N=10) and a high sensitivity of 179.7 μA ng ml^{-1} over a wide concentration range of 0.01 to 40.0 μM under optimal testing conditions. The sensor's ability to detect Glyp is not affected by competing substances such as ascorbic acid, glucose, or other metal ions, as indicated by its selectivity tests. In samples, the CuO-OGQ sensor demonstrated a recovery rate of 90%–102% for accurate detection of Glyp. It functioned 95% of the time, even after 30 days, making it a dependable, constant, and selective tool for environmental analysis.

3.3 1D nanomaterials-based sensors

Carbon-based nanomaterials such as CNTs and CNFs have demonstrated tremendous promise as electrocatalysts for agricultural sensing applications. These materials have unique qualities that enable them to effectively detect a range of agriculturally relevant analytes, including nutrients, insecticides, and soil components. Since they have large surface areas, they offer active sites for catalytic reactions. This characteristic increases the sensitivity of electrochemical sensors, enabling the detection of traces of analytes.

They are corrosion-resistant, chemically inert, and biocompatible. They have high electrical conductivity, guaranteeing effective electron transfer during electrochemical reactions. This conductivity is essential for quick and precise sensor responses. To improve selectivity and sensitivity, the surface of 1D CNMs can be functionalized with particular chemical groups or biomolecules [21]. Amperometric, potentiostatic, and impedance-based sensors are just a few of the many sensor types that can use these functionalized CNMs, making them adaptable.

3.3.1 Sensor performance enhancing properties of 1D materials

1D nanomaterials, which include nanorods, nanowires, nanobelts, nanofibers, and nanotubes, have appealing topologies and morphologies. Various complex shapes, such as core–shell, firetube, multichannel, and quasi-1D hierarchical structures, have been designed and fabricated to improve sensing capabilities. These intricate morphologies are aimed at further enhancing sensing performance. One of the main causes is that the shell's thickness and hollowness are easily adjustable, allowing one to use synthesis processes by adjusting these 1D structure factors. The depletion layer's surface area and width are largely affected, which will enhance the sensor's properties. Several researchers have developed a 1D-carbon-based hybrid electrode material that efficiently detects heavy metal ions. For example, Matlou *et al* [22] reported the detection of Hg^{2+}. In their work, drop coating, electrodeposition, electropolymerization, and self-assembled monolayers (SAMs) have all been used to modify the electrode. The SAM method was used to attach SWCNT-PABS (single-walled carbon nanotubes-poly (m-amino benzene sulfonic acid)) to the surface of a gold electrode. This process is facilitated by a thiol moiety (dimethyl amino ethane thiol). The resulting product detects Hg^{2+} in water using SWASV as an analytical tool. The material developed, characterized by AFM, was used to study the surface topography. The sensor exhibited high sensitivity and could detect concentrations as low as 0.06 μM. Under ideal conditions, the sensor's linear concentration range was between 20 and 250 ppb. The estimated limit of LOD of the sensor was below the maximum limit the World Health Organization allowed for inorganic mercury in drinking water, which is 6.0 μM. The analytical applicability of the proposed method with the sensor electrode was tested with a real water sample. In another study, Liu *et al* fabricated a CNT-NEA (nanoelectrode array) to detect Pb^{2+} and Cd^{2+} ions. The CNTs-NEAs have been developed by enclosing the CNTs' side walls with a passive epoxy layer. This layer decreases the current leakage and removes the electrode capacitance, leading to a low background current and a high signal-to-noise ratio. Coating the prepared CNTs-NEAs with a bismuth film can efficiently detect Pb^{2+} and Cd^{2+} ions using voltammetry analysis, with a detection limit of 0.04 $\mu g\ l^{-1}$. It is indicated that the efficient side wall sealing on the CNT is responsible for the low background contributions surrounding the stripping signal for the specified target metals. The detection limit of the CNT-NEAs is much lower than the previous reports with a GCE (0.8 $\mu g\ l^{-1}$). The CNT-NEAs have a high signal-to-noise ratio, which improves the stripping signal and low detection limit. Deng *et al* [23] fabricated 2,2′-azinobis (3-ethylbenzothiazoline-6-sulfonate) diammonium salt (ABTS)-MWCNTs nanocomposite/Bi film modified GCE for the DPV detection and quantification of Cd^{2+} and Pb^{2+}. Optimal sensitivity was achieved by optimizing the concentration of bismuth, preconcentration potential, preconcentration time, and solution pH. The Bi/ABTS-MWCNTs electrode exhibited superior performance due to the chelating agent of ABTS adsorbed on MWCNTs. Linear responses were obtained for the determination of Cd^{2+} and Pb^{2+} separately and at the same time. The linear range obtained for Cd^{2+} was from 0.5 to 35 $\mu g\ l^{-1}$, while for Pb^{2+} it was from 0.2 to 50 $\mu g\ l^{-1}$. The detection limits for Cd^{2+} and Pb^{2+} were 0.2 and 0.1 $\mu g\ l^{-1}$, respectively. Therefore, it would be possible to successfully identify trace heavy metal ions in actual samples using the Bi/ABTS-MWCNTs/GC electrode, which has a well-defined stripping response. Niu *et al* [24] have reported the simplified fabrication of bismuth-carbon-based screen-printed electrodes (Bi-C SPEs) for Pb^{2+} and Cd^{2+}. An ink formulation for screen printing required a nanocomposite of bismuth nanoparticles and amorphous carbon, which was synthesized by sol–gel and pyrolysis. The material was then milled down to achieve a specific particle size distribution. The carbon's porous structure and the high surface area of the bismuth nanoparticles allow metal ions to be detected at concentration levels below 4 ppb. The electrochemical detection of Pb^{2+} and Cd^{2+} ions of metals was carried out by the SWASV method with a detection limit of 99.0 and 157.0 ngl^{-1} and liner range of 0.1–120.0 μgl^{-1} and 0.16–120.0 μgl^{-1}, respectively. Furthermore, tap water and wastewater collected from an influent of an urban wastewater treatment plant were utilized to carry out real sample analysis with good recoveries. Similarly, Deshmukh *et al* [25] reported the simultaneous detection of three metal ions, namely Cu^{2+}, Pb^{2+}, and Hg^{2+} ions. Their work employed the DPV-based determination of metal ion concentrations by polyaniline (PANI), SWCNTs, and ethylenediaminetetraacetic acid (EDTA) modified stainless steel electrode. The process of SS surface modification by PANI/SWCNTs nanocomposite is visually represented in figure 3.3(a). The same picture also shows the additional modification of PANI/SWCNTs nanocomposite using EDTA chelating ligand. AFM, SEM, and Fourier-transform infrared spectroscopy (FT-IR) analysis have been carried out for morphological and structural compositional analysis of EDTA_PANI/SWCNTs nanocomposite. This work demonstrated well-resolved voltammetric peak potentials for each metal ion without significant mutual interference through DPV, and the individual determination individually determined LODs were Cu^{2+} 0.08 mM, Pb^{2+} 1.65 mM, and Hg^{2+} 0.68 mM. More interestingly, as illustrated in figure 3.3(b). This determination promotes the presence of one metal over the other. Hence, when they co-exist in real samples, the EDTA chelation ability and PANI/SWCNTs nanocomposite structure increase the sensitivity of EDTA_PANI/SWCNTs/SS-based electrodes for individual detection of the targeted metal ions.

Tarley *et al* [26] prepared a specialized material called ion imprinted poly (methacrylic acid), which was loaded with 1-(2-pyridylazo)-2-naphthol, a chelating agent that is selective towards lead ions (Pb^{2+}). They tested its effectiveness as a modifier element for a GCE and MWCNT, which will detect Pb^{2+} using differential pulse anodic stripping voltammetry (DPASV). Poly (methacrylic acid) was chosen as the functional monomer for the material because of its ability to form metal ion complexes with cations, making it an ideal candidate for this application. Meanwhile, azo compounds, such as the 1-(2-pyridylazo)-2-naphthol, can form

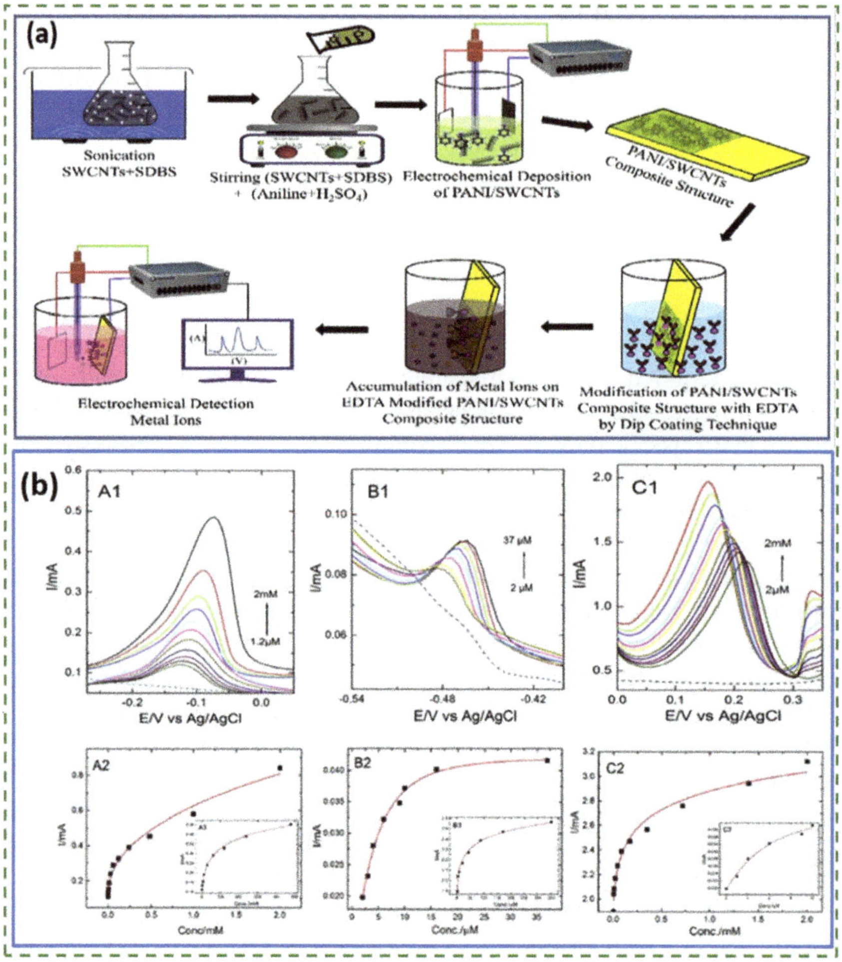

Figure 3.3. (a) Schematic of the EDTA_PANI/SWCNTs. (b) The nanocomposite of EDTA_PANI/SWCNTs was tested for individual analysis of Cu^{2+} (A1), Pb^{2+} (B1), and Hg^{2+} (C1) using DPV response. A2, B2, and C2 are peak currents plotted against Cu^{2+}, Pb^{2+}, and Hg^{2+} concentrations, respectively. Reprinted from [25], Copyright (2018), with permission from Elsevier.

stable and colored complexes with metals. SEM and thermal gravimetric analysis (TGA) have characterized the material. They demonstrated voltammetric peak potentials for Pb^{2+} without significant mutual interference through DPASV. The sensor provided two linear ranges from 0.50 to 12.0 $\mu g\ l^{-1}$ and 15.0–22.0 $\mu g\ l^{-1}$ of Pb^{2+}, and LOD and limit of quantification were calculated to be 0.16 $\mu g\ l^{-1}$ and 0.50 $\mu g\ l^{-1}$, respectively. At the same time, the sensor's reproducibility and relative standard deviation (RSD) values were satisfactory. To check the practical feasibility of the developed sensor, the compositions were analyzed with actual samples, such as tap and mineral water, physiological serum, and synthetic urine, with satisfactory recovery values (95%–103%). Table 3.2 presents the comparative performance of 1D-carbon allotropes sensors on various heavy metal ions and pesticides.

Table 3.2. Different 1D-carbon allotropes for detecting various heavy metal ions and pesticides.

Electrochemical sensors	Method	Analyte	Detection limit	Linear range	References
DMAET-SWCNT-PABSA/Au electrode	SWASV	Hg^{2+}	0.0634 μM	20.0–250.0 ppb	[22]
CNTs-epoxy-Bi electrode	SWV	Cd^{2+}	0.04 μg l^{-1}	0.5–8.0 μg l^{-1}	[27]
ABTSMWCNTs-Bi-GC	DPSV	Pb^{2+}	0.1 μg l^{-1}	0.2–50.0 μg l^{-1}	[23]
		Cd^{2+}	0.2 μg l^{-1}	0.5–35.0 μg l^{-1}	
B-PMWCNTs electrode	CV, EIS	Pb^{2+}	99 ng l^{-1}	0.1–120.0 μg l^{-1}	[24]
	SWASV	Cd^{2+}	157 ng l^{-1}	0.16–120.0 μg l^{-1}	
EDTA-PANI/SWCNTs/stainless steel	DPV	Cu^{2+}	0.08±0.01 μM	2 mM–1.2 μM	[25]
		Pb^{2+}	1.65±0.01 μM	1.8 mM–4.0 μM	
		Hg^{2+}	0.68±0.01 μM	2.0 mM–2.0 μM	
IIP/PAN/MWCNT/GCE	DPASV	Pb^{2+}	0.16 μg l^{-1}	0.50–22.0 μg l^{-1}	[26]
GCE-MWCNT/poly (PCV)/Bi	DPASV	Cd^{2+}	0.20 μg l^{-1}	1.0–300.0 μg l–1	[28]
		Pb^{2+}	0.40 μg l^{-1}	1.0–200.0 μg l^{-1}	
HCNT/CNH/GCE	DPV	Nitenpyram	4.0 nM	20.0–2000.0 nM	[29]
CNT/GCE	CV	Fenitrothion	0.090 μM	0.54–6.84 μM	[30]
FT@CNT/GCE	DPV	Chlorantraniliprole	8.1 nmol l^{-1}	0.01–7.0 μmol l^{-1}	[31]
$ZnFe_2O_4$/SWCNTs	CV	Carbendazim	0.09 and 0.05 μM	0.5–100.0 μM	[32]
AuNPs-PANABA-MWCNT	CV	2,4-Dichlorophenoxy acetic acid	0.3 ppb	1.0–100.0 ppb	[33]
MWCNT-IL/RGO/SiC/CILE	CV	Bentazone	0.25 nM	1.0–150.0 nM	[34]
GO-MWCNTs	SWV	Isoproturon	0.1 μmol l^{-1}	0.30–15.0 μmol l^{-1}	[35]

3.3.2 Application of 1D materials as electrochemical transducers for agricultural pollutants

The strong adsorption capabilities of CNTs are utilized by two extraction techniques—solid-phase extraction (SPE) and solid-phase micro-extraction (SPME). SPE technology is one of the most used extraction techniques for pre-treating biological, food, and environmental materials. Several research investigations have demonstrated SWCNTs and MWCNTs to be effective adsorbents for the preconcentration of lead, nickel, and cobalt ions. Pesticides containing organophosphate (OP) and chlorophenols. CNTs/SiO_2 nanohybrids were created by Saraji *et al* for SPME coating. They assessed the effectiveness of these hybrids in extracting some organophosphorus pesticides (OPPs) from water samples, vegetables, and fruits [36]. The OPPs were found using gas chromatography and corona discharge ion mobility spectrometry. When CNTs/SiO_2-coated SPME was compared to commercial SPME fibers, the adsorption capacity and mass transfer rate were considerably higher, indicating greater extraction efficiency. Excellent linearity was observed from 0.01 to 3.0 $\mu g\ l^{-1}$ for the samples, and the LOD range for water samples was 0.005–0.020 $\mu g\ l^{-1}$, while the limits of quantification (LOQ) were 0.010 and 0.050 $\mu g\ l^{-1}$. The range of spiked recoveries was between 79±9 and 99±8. As a result, the created materials have potential and can be used for OPP analysis in actual sample data. Feria and colleagues [37] have employed MWCNTs and carboxylated c-SWCNTs to identify several pesticide kinds in virgin olive oils. It was interesting to observe that the carboxyl functional groups in the structure of c-SWCNTs allowed for improved interactions between pesticides and CNTs, as evidenced by their superior sorbent properties compared to MWCNTs. The low LODs achieved were between 1.5 and 3.0 $\mu g\ l^{-1}$. For the accurate detection of fenuron (FU) and diuron (DIU), Mani *et al* [38] designed amperometric sensors using a composite composed of GO-MWCNT. A straightforward solution-based method was used to manufacture the GO-MWCNT composite. The GO-MWCNT films modified GCE showed promising electrocatalytic activity in the oxidation of DIU and FU. The modified electrode exhibited reduced overpotential and significantly increased peak currents. GO-MWCNTs have demonstrated electrocatalytic efficiency that is noticeably better than DMF-dispersed MWCNTs. A GO-MWCNT-based amperometric sensor with a wide linear range between 9.0 μM and 0.38 mM and a sensitivity of 0.645 $A\ M^{-1}\ cm^{-2}$ has been developed. The amperometric sensor can detect FU with a 1.20 $\mu A\ \mu M^{-1}\ cm^{-2}$ sensitivity over a wide linear range of 0.9 and 47.0 μM. Additionally, the sensor has respectable repeatability with RSD values of 3.87% and 3.25%, 3.96%, and 2.70% for reproducibility, and stability results were examined using GO-MWCNT coated on GCE rotating disk in the presence of DIU and FU. Amperometric tests have been conducted at the GO-MWCNTs/GCE with a speed of rotation of 2500 rpm and 1.0 mM DIU. Even after 3600 s continuous use, just 8% of the initial Ip was reduced, demonstrating the electrode's strong operational stability in determining DIU. Additionally, the electrode has good operational stability to detect FU—even after 3600 s of nonstop operation, only 7% of the initial Ip was reduced. Various water samples from agricultural areas have been used to evaluate the practicability of the constructed amperometric sensor. Duran *et al* [39] proved the practicality of the solid-phase extraction technique by adsorbing nickel, copper, lead ions, and cobalt as their o-cresolphthalein complex onto MWCNTs before conducting atomic absorption spectrometric measurements. A study was carried out to examine how different variables affect the retrieval rates of analyte ions. These variables comprised the acidity of the solutions, the quantities of the complexing agent, the kind of solvent, the volume of the sample, the rates of flow of the solution, and the existence of matrix ions. The investigated metals were observed to have a detection ranging from 1.64 to 5.68 $\mu g\ l^{-1}$. Analyzing certified reference material HR 1 (Humber River sediment) confirmed the method's validity; the findings concurred with verified values. Trace element concentrations in environmental samples have been successfully determined with acceptable findings by examining and implementing the best experimental conditions that guarantee the procedure's performance. Manasa *et al* [32] fabricated BaO-MWCNT/MCPE (Barium oxide-MWCNT/carbon paste electrode) via one-step bulk modification in another work. FE-SEM, EDS, and EIS characterized the structural morphology of the modified composite. The MCPE-based sensor exhibited good electrocatalytic activity and the lowest charge transfer resistance for the detection of DIU (the target analyte). By increasing the effective surface area on MCPE, the devised sensor enhanced the electrocatalytic performance and sensitivity, resulting in reduced activation energy. The electrochemical analysis is carried out through CV with a low detection limit value of 0.31×10^{-6} mol l^{-1}, a limit of quantification of 1.06×10^{-6} mol l^{-1}, and good reproducibility. The developed sensor portrays good selectivity, sensitivity, and reliability for DIU determinations and also displays quick response with portable and cost-effective potentiostats. Du *et al* [40] developed MWCNT as a new sorbent for SPE of OP. A rapid, precise, and discriminative electrochemical technique for detecting OP pesticide using methyl parathion (MP) as a representative was obtained by combining SPE with SWV analysis. MWCNT has a strong affinity for phosphoric groups, and nitroaromatic OP compounds can easily bind to the surface of MWCNT. The stripping response had a high degree of linearity within the MP range of 0.05–2.0 $\mu g\ ml^{-1}$, with a LOD of 0.005 $\mu g\ ml^{-1}$ Garlic samples' MP content could be determined with a reasonable degree of precision. MWCNT is a promising sorbent for various solid-phase extractions due to its quick extraction speed. Yuanyuan Dong *et al* [32] fabricated $ZnFe_2O_4$/SWCNTs nanohybrid through a facile one-step hydrothermal method for detecting CBZ and TBZ. The electrochemical behaviors of the prepared composite were investigated using CV DPV. The developed sensors exhibit good performance, such as excellent sensitivity, an appreciable LOD of 0.09 and 0.05 μM, and a comprehensive linear range of 0.5–100.0 μM, with good stability and repeatability. CBZ and TBZ in various real samples have been investigated, and the results were satisfactory.

3.4 2D nanomaterials as electrocatalysts for sensing

Graphene sheets are hexagonal lattice structures, monolayers of sp^2 hybridized carbon atoms covalently bound together. The lattice constant of a single sheet of graphene is almost 1.42 Å. By mechanically exfoliating bulk graphite, Andre Geim and Konstatin Novoselov produced monolayer graphene in 2004 [41]. Because of its incredible physical and chemical characteristics, graphene has emerged as a wonder material with many applications in the material sciences. Graphene is considered the most desirable 2D nanomaterial due to its direct and zero bandgaps. The conductivity and bandgap of graphene are determined by the way its layers are stacked, and it has a specific surface area of 2630 m^2g^{-1}. Scotch tape, solution-phase exfoliation, CVD, and organic synthesis techniques prepare graphene. GO is created during the solution-phase exfoliation process by oxidizing graphite in a highly acidic environment. Graphene on GO can be treated chemically, electrically, or thermally to reverse its shape. Graphene is an excellent material for sensing applications because of its high tensile strength, high conductivity, and ease of production [42].

3.4.1 Sensor performance enhancing properties of 2D materials

In comparison to conventional bulk materials, the design process of 2D materials is more malleable owing to their nanoscale thickness and atomically thin layered structure. This flexibility in design allows for the creation of unique materials with desirable properties, such as increased strength or enhanced conductivity. The utilization of 2D materials in various fields, including electronics, energy storage, and biomedical applications, has shown great potential due to their exceptional properties. This offers improved processability for electronic devices because of its greater flexibility. Large accessible specific surface areas, room-temperature stability, high electron mobility, and other physical, chemical, and structural characteristics are advantageous for sensing performances. Graphene and its derivatives, such as GO and reduced graphene oxide (rGO), have been extensively reported as sensors in recent decades for sensing and detecting sensors in various fields. Hence, several researchers have developed 2D carbon electrochemical sensors to determine agricultural pollutants simultaneously. Yinxiu Zuo [43] reported the detection of Hg^{2+}. Their research suggested a PEDOT/GO composite through liquid/liquid interfacial polymerization. EDOT monomer and GO were dispersed separately in the organic and water phases. The PEDOT/GO nanocomposite obtained showed remarkable catalytic activity towards Hg^{2+} ions. SEM and TEM were used to examine the surface morphology of the material. The findings indicated that the PEDOT had a composition resembling that of miniature rods that were bound to the exterior of GO nanosheets. This composition had the potential to enhance the quantity of electroactive locations within the nanocomposite. DPSV was applied to determine Hg^{2+}, and the calculated detection limit was 2.78 nM with a linear range of 10.0 nM to 3.0 μM. It was demonstrated that Hg^{2+} determination in tap water samples can be successfully applied. In another work, Dai [44] reported an electrochemical metal ions sensor based on a phytic acid functionalized PPy/GO nanocomposite-modified electrode shown in figure 3.4(a). The PPy/GO nanocomposite was prepared using ferric chloride in situ polymerization. Adsorption by electrostatic attraction was used to attach Phytic acid onto the surface of the PPy/GO nanocomposite. The nanocomposites were further characterized using TEM, ATR-IR, and Raman spectroscopy. A sensor was developed using the DPV technique for

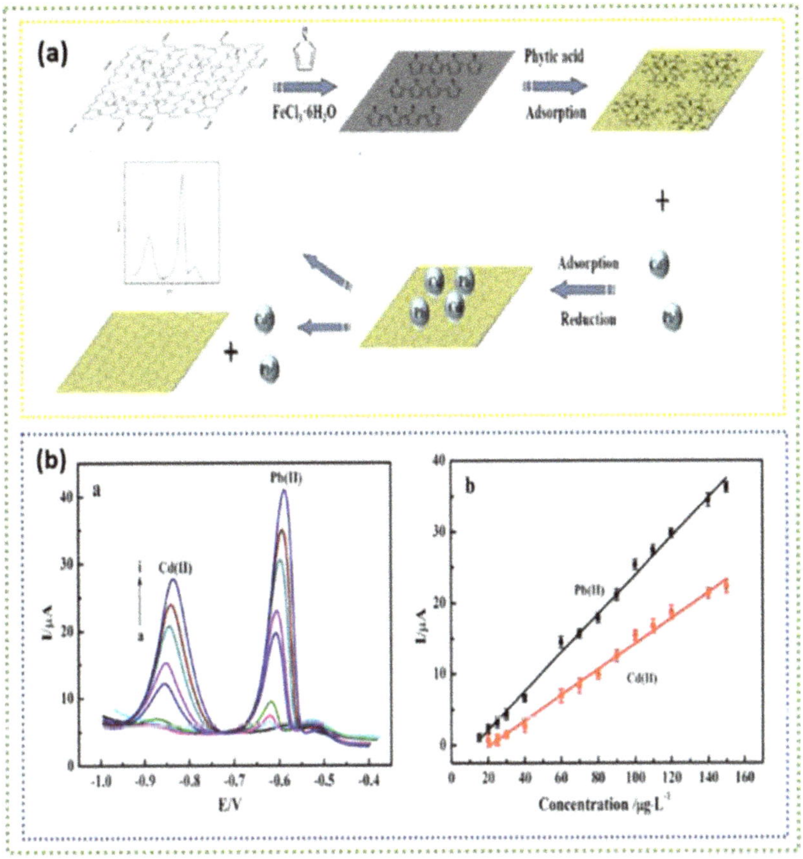

Figure 3.4. (a) Schematic diagram for synthesizing the PA/PPy/GO nanocomposites. (b) a. Electrochemical performance and b. the matching calibration plots of the PA/PPy/GO modified electrode with respect to the concentrations of Pb(II) and Cd(II). Reprinted from [44], copyright (2016), with permission from Elsevier.

electrochemical analysis of trace metal ions. The modified electrode was able to quantify Cd(II) and Pb(II) in an acetic acid-sodium acetate buffer solution with high reproducibility and stability, and a linear working range of 5.0–150.0 $\mu g\ l^{-1}$ was observed, as shown in figure 3.4(b). To evaluate the practical application of the PA/PPy/GO electrode, it was used to determine in the real tap water samples and analyzed. The prepared electrode has the potential for practical application in determining metal ions in real samples, as demonstrated by the standard deviation (SD) and RSD values falling within the range of 0.5–1.2 $\mu g\ l^{-1}$ and 5.1%–11.0%, respectively. Yinxiu Zuoa [45] has synthesized a nanocomposite to modify GCE by in situ growth of Co_3O_4 nanoparticles on GO and subsequent hydrazine reduction process. The nanocomposite is composed of Co_3O_4, rGO and chitosan (Co_3O_4/rGO/chitosan) and has been developed in-house. The fabricated material has been characterized by SEM, TEM, XPS, and XRD to analyze the surface morphology, crystalline structure, and elemental composition, and its electrochemical properties were investigated using DPASV techniques (linear dynamic range: 1.0–200.0 nM). The nanocomposite comprising rGO with high conductivity and surface area, cobalt oxide nanoparticles (Co_3O_4 NPs) A sensitive Pb(II) sensor with a detection limit of 0.35 nM has been developed by combining two materials—one with strong Pb(II) adsorption ability and the other with excellent Pb(II) complex-forming ability, namely chitosan. The study also revealed satisfactory results with regard to reproducibility and stability. The positive charge of chitosan enables its interaction with the negatively charged rGO, thus increasing the strength of the Co_3O_4/rGO nanocomposite. A new opportunity for vegetable analysis is presented by the hybrid nanocomposite Pb(II) sensor.

Hussein and co-workers [46] have fabricated poly(aniline-co-o-toluidine)/graphene oxide nanocomposite by in situ oxidative polymerization method with ultrasonic assistance. The material has been subjected to FE-SEM, TEM, FT-IR, XRD, and TGA for chemical structure analysis. In addition, electrical conductivity has been conducted. They demonstrated the SWV technique to study the electrochemical analysis and showed the LOD and quantification limit (LOQ) of 5–500 μM, with 0.0215 μM and 0.0719 μM, along with RSD of 0.12%, respectively. The invented sensor displayed good stability, selectivity, and sensitivity and has exhibited potential for detecting Cr(VI) in real samples. Table 3.3 presents the comparative performance of 2D carbon allotrope sensors on various heavy metal ions and pesticides.

3.4.2 Application of 2D materials as electrochemical transducers for agricultural pollutants

Agricultural pollution and ecological contamination have emerged as significant side effects of modern development, contributing to worldwide concerns. Pesticide contamination, in particular, poses a serious threat to both human and animal health. The accumulation of pesticides on vegetable and fruit leaves has raised concerns among consumers, as these chemicals can impair the body's normal functions. As such, the use of electrochemical sensors for pesticide detection has become increasingly popular, especially those employing low-dimensional materials and device configurations. These sensors have shown promising results, providing effective detection of harmful pesticides, and could play a valuable role in addressing the issue of pesticide contamination. AChE on gold nanoparticles and graphene oxides, a nanosheet (AChE/AuNPs/cr-Gs) was synthesized by Lin and co-workers to sense the presence of organophosphate pesticide [51]. In recent years, there has been an increasing interest in the development of electrochemical sensors for the detection of various pesticides in food products. Several research groups have reported the use of 2D nanomaterials for the fabrication of electrochemical sensors, which have demonstrated improved detection limits and comparable results. Notably, these sensors have the potential to assist organizations in regulating the use of pesticides in food goods to prevent adverse health effects. For instance, Moga and colleagues utilized a graphene-based nanocomposite to detect paraoxon-ethyl, while an rGO and zirconium oxide nanohybrid was used to immobilize AChE for detecting

Table 3.3. Different 2D nanomaterials catalyst sensors for various heavy metal ions and pesticides.

Electrochemical sensors	Method	Analyte	Detection limit	Linear range	References
PEDOT/GO/GCE	DPSV	Hg^{2+}	2.78 nM	10.0 nM–3.0 mM	[43]
Co_3O_4/RGO/CHIT/GCE	DPASV	Pb^{2+}	0.35 nM	1.0–200.0 nM	[45]
Au NPs/PANI-co-PoT/GO/Au	SWV	Cr^{4+}	0.0215 μM	5.0–500.0 μM	[46]
PA/PPy/GO/GCE	DPV	Cd^2+	2.13 $\mu g\ l^{-1}$	5.0–150.0 $\mu g\ l^{-1}$	[44]
	DPV	Pb^{2+}	0.41 $\mu g\ l^{-1}$	5.0–150.0 μg l	
GO-Fe_3O_4-PAMAM/GCE	SWASV	Cd^{2+}	130 $ng\ l^{-1}$	0.4–120.0 $\mu g\ l^{-1}$	[47]
		Pb^{2+}	70.0 $ng\ l^{-1}$	0.2–140.0 $\mu g\ l^{-1}$	
MWCNT-IL/RGO/SiC/CILE	CV	Bentazone	0.25 nM	1.0–150.0 nM	[34]
HCP5 @AuNPs-ERGO/GCE	DPV	Methyl parathion	0.001 μM	0.005–30.0 μM	[48]
AChE/CS@TiO2m-CSm/rGO/GC	DPV	Dichlorvos	29.0 nM	0.036–22.6 μM	[49]
rGO/Cu/CuO–Ag/GCE	DPV	Carbaryl	0.005–0.003 μM	0.05–20.0 μM	[50]

chlorpyrifos. Similarly, Wang *et al* developed a non-enzymatic electrochemical sensor for carbofuran (CBF) and carbaryl (CBR) detection using an (rGO/CoO) nanocomposite to diminish the negative impact of Ache. The non-enzymatic AChE-based electrochemical sensor was highly sensitive, selective, and stable, enabling the detection of CBF and CBR. Moreover, electrochemical sensors have been employed to discriminate between a number of pesticides, including carbofuran, dichlorvos, methyl parathion, and triazophos. The use of 2D nanomaterials has enhanced the detection limits of these sensors, making them reliable tools for detecting poisonous and dangerous pesticides in food products. Given the serious health problems associated with the use of pesticides, these sensors have the potential to contribute to the ongoing efforts to minimize their usage on plants and food goods.

In another work, Hashemi *et al* [50] synthesized ternary nanocomposite Cu/CuO–Ag modified glassy carbon electrode (rGO/Cu/CuO–Ag/GCE) electrochemical sensors in their study based on carbaryl (CA) and Fenamiphos (FEN) detection in fruit and vegetable sample. The characterization of the proposed sensor was studied through TEM, XRD, and FT-IR analyses. The electrochemical properties of the sensor were investigated using CV and DPV techniques. The rGO/Cu/CuO–Ag/GCE was used in conjunction with a cost-effective for detecting low levels of CA and FEN. The modified electrode displayed two separated oxidation signals with excellent sensitivity to determine carbaryl and fenamiphos simultaneously. The broad linear ranges of 0.05–20.0 and 0.01–30.0 μM and the detection limits were found as 0.005 and 0.003 μM for CA and FEN, respectively. Nevin *et al* [52] utilized an electroanalytical approach to detect a synthetic fungicide called propamocarb (PM), which belongs to the carbamic acid class of fungicides. They produced rGO through an environmentally friendly ultrasonic microwave-assisted technique and studied non-enzymatic electrochemical sensors based on rGO. The modified non-enzymatic electrochemical sensor demonstrated high sensitivity, selectivity, reproducibility, and a rapid response time within 1 min. It also exhibited an LOD of 0.6 μM and a dynamic range of 1.1–5.0 μM, with a high sensitivity of 101.1 $\mu A\ \mu M^{-1} cm^{-2}$ for PM. The researchers then successfully applied high-sensitivity sensors on an actual cucumber sample.

3.5 3D nanomaterials for electrochemical sensor fabrication

3D carbon nanomaterials are materials consisting of carbon in the form of nanostructures, such as graphene aerogels and carbon nanohorns (CNHs). Graphene aerogels are three-dimensional structures composed of interconnected graphene sheets. They are lightweight, highly porous, and have a large surface area that exhibits exceptional mechanical strength, low density, and high electrical conductivity. CNHs are carbon nanoparticles with a unique horn-shaped structure composed of conical graphene sheets. These nanoparticles possess high chemical reactivity and surface area and can be functionalized to suit specific applications. Due to their nanoscale dimensions, they exhibit unique properties and can be used in various applications, such as energy storage, electronics, biomedical devices, and sensing. The 3D graphene has an interconnected structured framework, ample gaps, substantial specific surface area, and free binder, making it a promising electrode material for electrochemical sensors. However, the 3D graphene-based electrochemical sensor has limited repeatability, poor selectivity, low sensitivities, and an extended dynamic response. To address these issues, the preparation methods have undergone continuous improvement. Furthermore, various nanomaterials, including carbon-based materials, metal–organic frameworks, metal and metal compounds, and polymers, have been gradually incorporated into the 3D graphene-based electrode Through proper material design and preparation, electrochemical sensors can offer advantages such as affordability, convenience, effectiveness, selectivity, and sensitivity when detecting analytes. Consequently, the use of these materials has increased in agricultural applications and environmental pollution, including pathogenic bacteria, pesticide residues, heavy metal ions, etc. The unique properties of 3D nanomaterials, including their large specific surface area and quantum size effect, have made them a subject of considerable research interest. These materials strongly depend on their sizes, forms, dimensionality, and morphologies, all of which determine their ultimate performance and applications in diverse areas such as catalysis, magnetic material, and electrode material for sensors. Higher surface areas provided by nanostructures allow for more molecules to be absorbed in a smaller space, and 3D porosity in such materials could result in better molecule transport, thereby enhancing sensor performance. Consequently, the synthesis of 3D carbon materials with a controlled structure and morphology is an intriguing prospect that has captured the attention of researchers.

3.5.1 Sensor performance enhancing properties of 3D materials

In recent years, electrochemical sensor detection has become an efficient approach to detecting agriculture pollutants by converting changes into an electrical signal with quick response, sensitivity, selectivity, miniaturization facile operation, and low cost. 3D carbon nanomaterial plays a vital role in enhancing the electrochemical sensor performance. These materials have an ordered and interconnected framework in 3D, which gives them unique advantages such as more significant surface area, sufficient spaces, and a free binder. This makes them ideal for many challenging applications. Their network has the ability to provide excellent anchoring as a supporting substrate for chemical functionalities or nanomaterials. This particular feature makes them ideal for loading catalysts and enzymes to create an electrochemical sensor. This sensor is capable of detecting analytes quantitatively with high sensitivity and selectivity. By using a novel 3D carbon material and composites, we can efficiently enhance the electrochemical sensing property and achieve trace-level detection of analytes with improved reproducibility. Carefully controlling 3D sensing materials can optimize sensing's functional features. Preparing homogeneous 3D materials remains challenging, particularly for multicomponent materials containing carbon nanomaterials with hierarchical structures. Furthermore, due to the complexity of the structure, it is difficult to conduct a systematic investigation into how shape, size, structure, and morphology affect sensing performances. More research on nanoparticle creation mechanisms is required to develop the morphology.

3.5.2 Application of 3D materials as electrochemical transducers for agricultural pollutants

Rahmani *et al* [53] fabricated an electrochemical sensor to determine 1-naphthyl methylcarbamate (carbaryl). An efficient nanocomposite has been synthesized by functionalizing 3D graphene and incorporating Au NPs (3DG-Au), which have a high surface area and catalytic capabilities. Thiourea was used as a crosslinking agent to impregnate the graphene with sulfur and nitrogen functional groups. Gold nanoparticles modified graphene doped with sulfur and nitrogen atoms. An analysis was conducted using the 3DG-Au nanocomposite that had been modified to detect carbaryl through the DPV method. Optimization of various experimental parameters, including pH, type of electrolyte, accumulation time, and accumulation potential, was carried out. Using these optimized parameters, the linear response of the sensor was achieved within the range of 0.004–0.3 μM of carbaryl, with a detection limit of 0.0012 μM (S/N=3). The obtained results showed a 3.1% RSD value. The sensor's stability, selectivity, and reproducibility were appropriate, and it was successfully used to detect carbaryl in water samples, vegetables, and fruit with good recoveries. Lakshmi and co-workers proposed a simple electrochemical sensing mechanism developed to detect urea in water using nanocomposites of CuO/ZnO and Fe_2O_3/ZnO modified on a pencil graphite electrode. The sensing platform can detect urea at the soil's surface and diagnose diseases related to urea cycle disorders. Cu and Fe-based ZnO nanocomposites are used to enhance the electrochemical sensing performance of urea. The increased oxidation current concerning urea concentration confirmed the sensing responses. The results show that Fe_2O_3/ZnO coated graphite electrode responds more against urea than ZnO and CuO/ZnO. The CV studies also validate urea determination at the Fe–ZnO in the dynamic range of 0.8–4.0 μg ml^{-1}, with an LOD of 2.5 μg ml^{-1}. This shows that the inexpensive Fe_2O_3/ZnO modified pencil graphite electrode may be a useful analytical instrument for urea sensing. Annu *et al* [54] fabricated a modified pencil graphite electrode (CLs/PGE) to detect atrazine in BR buffer at pH 4.3. The electrochemical experiments were carried out using SWV and CV. The modified sensor exhibited a linear calibration curve over a 5.0 ng ml^{-1} concentration range to 320 ng ml^{-1} with a LOD of 0.008 ng ml^{-1}. It demonstrated a strong catalytic reaction to the ATZ reduction, with a distinct reduction peak at 880 mV. The constructed sensor performed exceptionally well, measuring ATZ with a 3.0% relative standard deviation precision. The created sensor could effectively detect ATZ without being hampered by common metabolites. With its high sensitivity, good selectivity, and reproducibility, the voltammetric approach was successfully applied to real sample analysis. This makes it appropriate for additional environmental sample analyses. The recommended method has been successfully used to detect ATZ in drinking water, recovering 98.8%–99.1%. Jaqueline Santos *et al* [55]. An electroanalytical method has been developed that is affordable, simple, and effective. This method uses a graphite oxide paste electrode (GrO-PE), as shown in figure 3.5, to directly detect traces of glyphosate (GLY) herbicide in groundwater samples, soybean extracts, and lettuce extracts. The interactions between the GLY and the sensor surface were

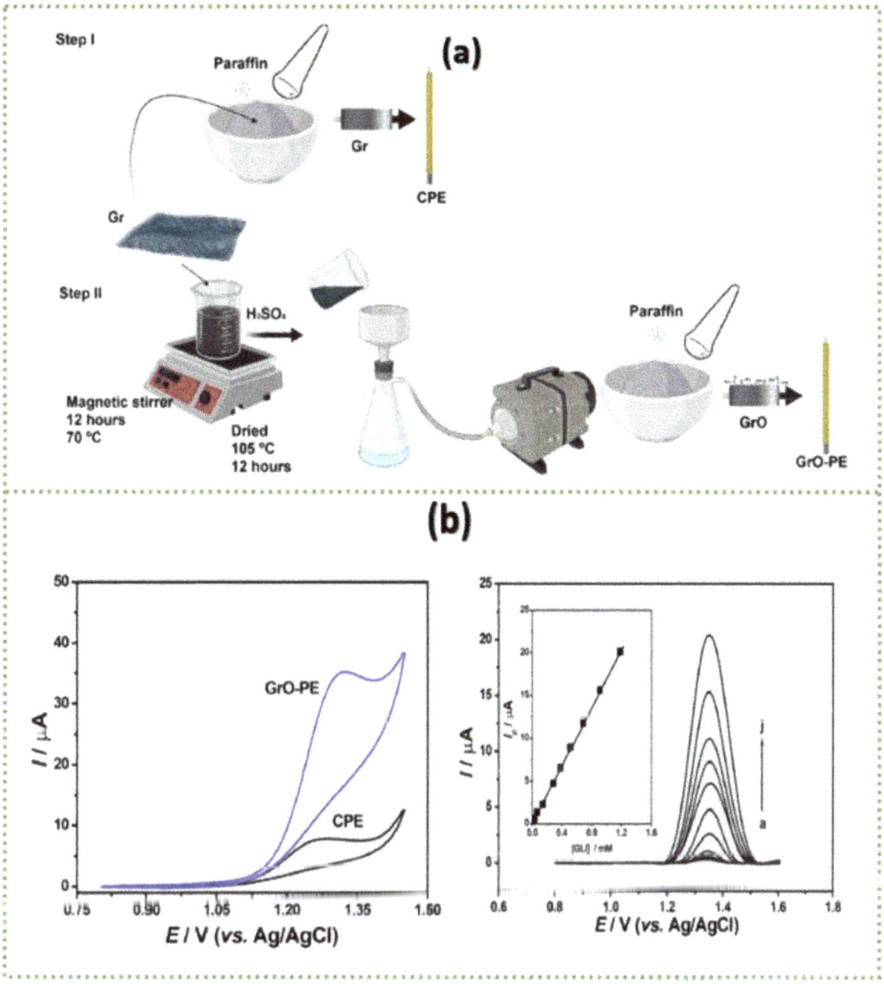

Figure 3.5. (a) Schematic illustration of sensor fabrication: Step 1—CPE, Step 2—GrO-PE. (b) Cyclic voltammograms and square wave analytical curve for GLY. Reprinted from [55], copyright (2020) with permission from Elsevier

investigated using both CV and SWV, and the transport properties on the sensor surface were studied using electrochemical impedance spectroscopy (EIS). The proposed sensor demonstrated a linear response regarding peak current intensity against the concentration range for GLY, which was between 1.8×10^{-5} and 1.2×10^{-3} mol l^{-1}. 1.7×10^{-8} mol l^{-1} and 5.6×10^{-8} mol l^{-1} are the limits of detection and quantification, respectively. This methodology's strong analytical performance was demonstrated with excellent repeatability, precision, and reproducibility. Furthermore, it shows remarkable selectivity by effectively avoiding interference from other compounds. GLY traces in real samples were successfully found using the GrO-PE sensor, with recovery percentages varying from 98% to 102%. The obtained values demonstrate that the GrO-PE is a valuable and practical tool for

GLY detection. Its lack of sophisticated handling or lengthy modifications makes it an attractive option for environmental study.

3.6 Conclusion

Carbon and its allotrope materials have shown great potential in agricultural applications because they can enhance the quality of life and environment. This chapter discusses the latest progress in producing and creating electrochemical sensors that utilize carbon nanomaterials to identify various agropollutants. The distinctive chemical and physical characteristics of nanostructured materials must be noted to distinguish them from bulk and micro-sized materials. This chapter provides a comprehensive overview of the factors that can be modified to improve the exceptional characteristics of these nanomaterials. (figure 3.6). However, employing such a nanocomposite to provide highly effective catalysis for electrochemical sensors still presents difficulties. To overcome the limitations affecting the performance of these sensors, the nanomaterial's manufacturing processes, morphologies, and selective catalysts need to be optimized. Therefore, there is still a high demand for intelligent surface structure designs to achieve durability and efficiency. Consequently, the ongoing investigation must be dedicated to developing active carbon allotrope materials for sensor applications. Although nanostructure aspects such as 0D, 1D, 2D, and 3D nanomaterials have received considerable attention, a more comprehensive understanding of how synthesis methods, content, size, and shape affect the catalytic activity of 0D, 1D, 2D, and 3D-based nanomaterials will be necessary for future development. In electrochemical sensor applications, the performance of nanomaterials based on 0D, 1D, 2D, and 3D structures can be improved by developing new synthesis and fabrication processes that are simple, effective, and offer precise control over the size and morphology of the resulting

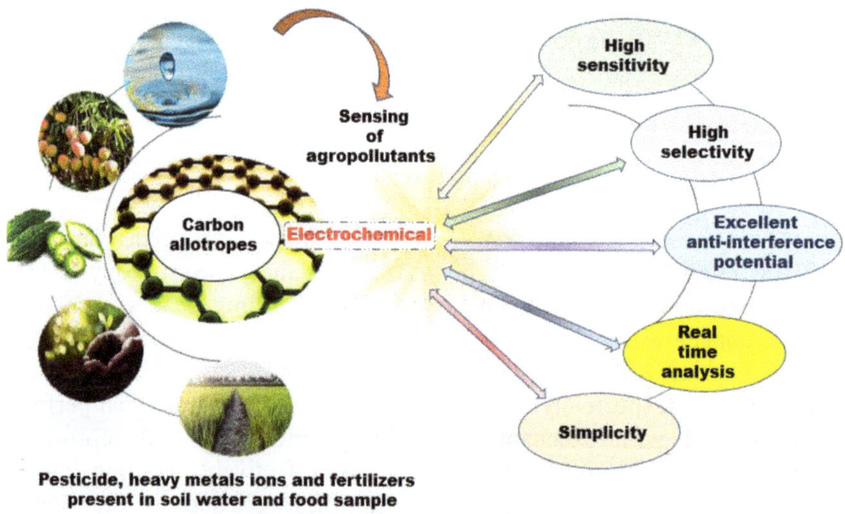

Figure 3.6. Carbon nanomaterial-based electrochemical sensors for agropollutant detection from environmental samples.

products. Additionally, when the chemical and physical characteristics of 0D, 1D, 2D, and 3D-based nanomaterials are better understood, more opportunities will arise to use these qualities in magnetic, electric, and optical-based applications. Creating 0D, 1D, 2D, and 3D-based nanomaterials can help to advance current technologies, and more studies will produce even more incredible outcomes that will benefit society and industry.

References

[1] Tang L, Zeng G-M, Shen G-L, Li Y-P, Zhang Y and Huang D-L 2008 Rapid detection of picloram in agricultural field samples using a disposable immunomembrane-based electrochemical sensor *Environ. Sci. Technol.* **42** 1207–12

[2] Karthik P S, Himaja A L and Singh S P 2014 Carbon-allotropes: synthesis methods, applications and future perspectives *Carbon Lett.* **5** 219–37

[3] Li J and Han Y 2023 Artificial carbon allotrope γ-graphyne: synthesis, properties, and applications *Giant* **13** 100140

[4] Yang T, Liu Y, Wang H, Duo Y, Zhang B, Ge Y, Zhang H and Chen W 2020 Recent advances in 0D nanostructure-functionalized low-dimensional nanomaterials for chemiresistive gas sensors *J. Mater. Chem.* C **8** 7272–99

[5] Xu Q, Li W, Ding L, Yang W, Xiao H and Ong W-J 2019 Function-driven engineering of 1D carbon nanotubes and 0D carbon dots: mechanism, properties and applications *Nanoscale* **11** 1475–504

[6] Anichini C, Czepa W, Pakulski D, Aliprandi A, Ciesielski A and Samorì P 2018 Chemical sensing with 2D materials *Chem. Soc. Rev.* **47** 4860–908

[7] Dong X, Wang X, Wang L, Song H, Zhang H, Huang W and Chen P 2012 3D graphene foam as a monolithic and macroporous carbon electrode for electrochemical sensing *ACS Appl. Mater. Interfaces* **4** 3129–33

[8] Asghar N, Hussain A, Nguyen D A, Ali S, Hussain I, Junejo A and Ali A 2024 Advancement in nanomaterials for environmental pollutants remediation: a systematic review on bibliometrics analysis, material types, synthesis pathways, and related mechanisms *J. Nanobiotechnol.* **22** 26

[9] Cayuela A, Soriano M L and Valcárcel M 2015 Photoluminescent carbon dot sensor for carboxylated multiwalled carbon nanotube detection in river water *Sensors Actuators* B **207** 596–601

[10] Zulfajri M, Sudewi S, Ismulyati S, Rasool A, Adlim M and Huang G G 2021 Carbon dot/polymer composites with various precursors and their sensing applications: a review *Coatings* **11** 1100

[11] Sinha N, Ma J and Yeow J T W 2006 Carbon nanotube-based sensors *J. Nanosci. Nanotechnol.* **6** 573–90

[12] Zaporotskova I V, Boroznina N P, Parkhomenko Y N and Kozhitov L V 2016 Carbon nanotubes: sensor properties. a review *Mod. Electron. Mater.* **2** 95–105

[13] Nag A, Mitra A and Mukhopadhyay S C 2018 Graphene and its sensor-based applications: a review *Sensors Actuators* A **270** 177–94

[14] Cho B *et al* 2014 Graphene-based gas sensor: metal decoration effect and application to a flexible device *J. Mater. Chem.* C **2** 5280–5

[15] Shetti N P, Mishra A, Basu S and Aminabhavi T M 2021 Versatile fullerenes as sensor materials *Mater. Today Chem.* **20** 100454

[16] Shi X, Liu S, Sun Y, Liang J and Chen Y 2018 Lowering internal friction of 0D–1D–2D ternary nanocomposite-based strain sensor by Fullerene to boost the sensing performance *Adv. Funct. Mater.* **28** 1800850

[17] Ramya M, Senthil Kumar P, Rangasamy G, Uma Shankar V, Rajesh G, Nirmala K, Saravanan A and Krishnapandi A 2022 A recent advancement on the applications of nanomaterials in electrochemical sensors and biosensors *Chemosphere* **308** 136416

[18] Brainina K, Stozhko N, Bukharinova M and Vikulova E 2018 Nanomaterials: electrochemical properties and application in sensors *Phys. Sci. Rev.* **3** 20188050

[19] ReddyPrasad P, Naidoo E B and Sreedhar N Y 2019 Electrochemical preparation of a novel type of C-dots/ZrO_2 nanocomposite onto glassy carbon electrode for detection of organophosphorus pesticide *Arab J. Chem.* **12** 2300–9

[20] Palanisamy S, Thirumalraj B and Chen S-M 2015 Electrochemical fabrication of gold nanoparticles decorated on activated fullerene C60: an enhanced sensing platform for trace level detection of toxic hydrazine in water samples *RSC Adv.* **5** 94591–8

[21] Chen C, Fan Y, Gu J, Wu L, Passerini S and Mai L 2018 One-dimensional nanomaterials for energy storage *J. Phys. D: Appl. Phys.* **51** 113002

[22] Matlou G G, Nkosi D, Pillay K and Arotiba O 2016 Electrochemical detection of Hg(II) in water using self-assembled single walled carbon nanotube-poly(m-amino benzene sulfonic acid) on gold electrode *Sens. Bio-Sens. Res.* **10** 27–33

[23] Deng W, Tan Y, Fang Z, Xie Q, Li Y, Liang X and Yao S 2009 ABTS-multiwalled carbon nanotubes nanocomposite/Bi film electrode for sensitive determination of Cd and Pb by differential pulse stripping voltammetry *Electroanalysis* **21** 2477–85

[24] Niu P, Fernández-Sánchez C, Gich M, Navarro-Hernández C, Fanjul-Bolado P and Roig A 2016 Screen-printed electrodes made of a bismuth nanoparticle porous carbon nanocomposite applied to the determination of heavy metal ions *Microchim. Acta* **183** 617–23

[25] Deshmukh M A, Celiesiute R, Ramanaviciene A, Shirsat M D and Ramanavicius A 2018 EDTA_PANI/SWCNTs nanocomposite modified electrode for electrochemical determination of copper (II), lead (II) and mercury (II) ions *Electrochim. Acta* **259** 930–8

[26] Tarley C R T, Basaglia A M, Segatelli M G, Prete M C, Suquila F A C and De Oliveira L L G 2017 Preparation and application of nanocomposite based on imprinted poly(methacrylic acid)-PAN/MWCNT as a new electrochemical selective sensing platform of Pb^{2+} in water samples *J. Electroanal. Chem.* **801** 114–21

[27] Liu G, Lin Y, Tu Y and Ren Z 2005 Ultrasensitive voltammetric detection of trace heavy metal ions using carbon nanotube nanoelectrode array *Analyst* **130** 1098

[28] Chamjangali M A, Kouhestani H, Masdarolomoor F and Daneshinejad H 2015 A voltammetric sensor based on the glassy carbon electrode modified with multi-walled carbon nanotube/poly(pyrocatechol violet)/bismuth film for determination of cadmium and lead as environmental pollutants *Sensors Actuators* B **216** 384–93

[29] Wang H, Pan L, Liu Y, Ye Y and Yao S 2020 Electrochemical sensing of nitenpyram based on the binary nanohybrid of hydroxylated multiwall carbon nanotubes/single-wall carbon nanohorns *J. Electroanal. Chem.* **862** 113955

[30] Soltani-Sarvestani M, Shamspur T, Mostafavi A, Falahati-Pour S K, Mohamadi M and Saljooqi A 2020 A novel preconcentration/extraction method for fenitrothion residues and its electrochemical sensing in pistachio kernels *J. Mater. Sci. Mater. Electron.* **31** 11268–75

[31] Tümay S O, Şenocak A, Sarı E, Şanko V, Durmuş M and Demirbas E 2021 A new perspective for electrochemical determination of parathion and chlorantraniliprole pesticides

via carbon nanotube-based thiophene-ferrocene appended hybrid nanosensor *Sensors Actuators* B **345** 130344

[32] Dong Y, Yang L and Zhang L 2017 Simultaneous electrochemical detection of benzimidazole fungicides carbendazim and thiabendazole using a novel nanohybrid material-modified electrode *J. Agric. Food Chem.* **65** 727–36

[33] Fusco G, Gallo F, Tortolini C, Bollella P, Ietto F, De Mico A, D'Annibale A, Antiochia R, Favero G and Mazzei F 2017 AuNPs-functionalized PANABA-MWCNTs nanocomposite-based impedimetric immunosensor for 2,4-dichlorophenoxy acetic acid detection *Biosens. Bioelectron.* **93** 52–6

[34] Norouzi P, Larijani B, Faridbod F and Ganjali M R 2014 A novel method for ultra trace measurement of bentazon based on nanocomposite electrode and continuous coulometric FFT cyclic voltammetry *Int. J. Environ. Res.* **9** 101–8

[35] Zhou Y, Cheng F, Hong Y, Huang J, Zhang X and Liao X 2020 Rapid and sensitive detection of isoproturon Via an electrochemical sensor based on highly water-dispersed carbon hybrid material *Food Anal. Methods* **13** 839–49

[36] Saraji M, Jafari M T and Mossaddegh M 2016 Carbon nanotubes@silicon dioxide nanohybrids coating for solid-phase microextraction of organophosphorus pesticides followed by gas chromatography–corona discharge ion mobility spectrometric detection *J. Chromatogr.* A **1429** 30–9

[37] López-Feria S, Cárdenas S and Valcárcel M 2009 One step carbon nanotubes-based solid-phase extraction for the gas chromatographic–mass spectrometric multiclass pesticide control in virgin olive oils *J. Chromatogr.* A **1216** 7346–50

[38] Mani V, Devasenathipathy R, Chen S-M, Wu T-Y and Kohilarani K 2015 High-performance electrochemical amperometric sensors for the sensitive determination of phenyl urea herbicides diuron and fenuron *Ionics* **21** 2675–83

[39] Duran A, Tuzen M and Soylak M 2009 Preconcentration of some trace elements via using multiwalled carbon nanotubes as solid phase extraction adsorbent *J. Hazard. Mater.* **169** 466–71

[40] Du D, Wang M, Zhang J, Cai J, Tu H and Zhang A 2008 Application of multiwalled carbon nanotubes for solid-phase extraction of organophosphate pesticide *Electrochem. Commun.* **10** 85–9

[41] Ashraf N, Isa Khan M, Majid A, Rafique M and Tahir M B 2020 A review of the interfacial properties of 2-D materials for energy storage and sensor applications *Chin. J. Phys.* **66** 246–57

[42] Tyagi D, Wang H, Huang W, Hu L, Tang Y, Guo Z, Ouyang Z and Zhang H 2020 Recent advances in two-dimensional-material-based sensing technology toward health and environmental monitoring applications *Nanoscale* **12** 3535–59

[43] Zuo Y, Xu J, Zhu X, Duan X, Lu L, Gao Y, Xing H, Yang T, Ye G and Yu Y 2016 Poly (3,4-ethylenedioxythiophene) nanorods/graphene oxide nanocomposite as a new electrode material for the selective electrochemical detection of mercury (II) *Synth. Met.* **220** 14–9

[44] Dai H, Wang N, Wang D, Ma H and Lin M 2016 An electrochemical sensor based on phytic acid functionalized polypyrrole/graphene oxide nanocomposites for simultaneous determination of Cd(II) and Pb(II) *Chem. Eng. J.* **299** 150–5

[45] Zuo Y, Xu J, Jiang F, Duan X, Lu L, Xing H, Yang T, Zhang Y, Ye G and Yu Y 2017 Voltammetric sensing of Pb(II) using a glassy carbon electrode modified with composites

consisting of Co_3O_4 nanoparticles, reduced graphene oxide and chitosan *J. Electroanal. Chem.* **801** 146–52

[46] Hussein M A, Ganash A A and Alqarni S A 2019 Electrochemical sensor-based gold nanoparticle/poly(aniline-co-o-toluidine)/graphene oxide nanocomposite modified electrode for hexavalent chromium detection: a real test sample *Polym. Plast. Technol. Mater.* **58** 1423–36

[47] Baghayeri M, Alinezhad H, Fayazi M, Tarahomi M, Ghanei-Motlagh R and Maleki B 2019 A novel electrochemical sensor based on a glassy carbon electrode modified with dendrimer functionalized magnetic graphene oxide for simultaneous determination of trace Pb(II) and Cd(II) *Electrochim. Acta* **312** 80–8

[48] Hou X, Liu X, Li Z, Zhang J, Du G, Ran X and Yang L 2019 Electrochemical determination of methyl parathion based on pillar[5]arene@AuNPs@reduced graphene oxide hybrid nanomaterials *New J. Chem.* **43** 13048–57

[49] Cui H-F, Wu W-W, Li M-M, Song X, Lv Y and Zhang T-T 2018 A highly stable acetylcholinesterase biosensor based on chitosan–TiO_2–graphene nanocomposites for detection of organophosphate pesticides *Biosens. Bioelectron.* **99** 223–9

[50] Hashemi P, Karimian N, Khoshsafar H, Arduini F, Mesri M, Afkhami A and Bagheri H 2019 Reduced graphene oxide decorated on Cu/CuO–Ag nanocomposite as a high-performance material for the construction of a non-enzymatic sensor: application to the determination of carbaryl and fenamiphos pesticides *Mater. Sci. Eng.* C **102** 764–72

[51] Wang Y, Zhang S, Du D, Shao Y, Li Z, Wang J, Engelhard M H, Li J and Lin Y 2011 Self assembly of acetylcholinesterase on a gold nanoparticles–graphene nanosheet hybrid for organophosphate pesticide detection using polyelectrolyte as a linker *J. Mater. Chem.* **21** 5319

[52] Taşaltın N, Karakuş S, Taşaltın C and Baytemir G 2022 Highly sensitive and selective rGO based non-enzymatic electrochemical sensor for propamocarb fungicide pesticide detection *Food Chem.* **372** 131267

[53] Rahmani T, Bagheri H, Behbahani M, Hajian A and Afkhami A 2018 Modified 3D Graphene-Au as a novel sensing layer for direct and sensitive electrochemical determination of carbaryl pesticide in fruit, vegetable, and water samples *Food Anal. Methods* **11** 3005–14

[54] Annu , Sharma S, Nitin A and Jain R 2020 Cellulose fabricated pencil graphite sensor for the quantification of hazardous herbicide atrazine *Diam. Relat. Mater.* **105** 107788

[55] Santos J S, Pontes M S, Santiago E F, Fiorucci A R and Arruda G J 2020 An efficient and simple method using a graphite oxide electrochemical sensor for the determination of glyphosate in environmental samples *Sci. Total Environ.* **749** 142385

[56] Song D, Wang Y, Lu X, Gao Y, Li Y and Gao F 2018 Ag nanoparticles-decorated nitrogen-fluorine co-doped monolayer MoS_2 nanosheet for highly sensitive electrochemical sensing of organophosphorus pesticides *Sensors Actuators* B **267** 5–13

IOP Publishing

Chapter 4

Electrochemical carbon-based biosensors

G Manasa, M Monisha and Chandra Sekhar Rout

Electrochemical biosensors combine electrochemical transduction and biological detection. The biological element of the sensor identifies the substance being measured, which triggers a catalytic or binding event. This leads to an electrical signal proportional to the concentration of the substance being measured and is measured by a transducer. Working electrodes are vital in converting biological interactions into observable electrical impulses that can be subjected to various electrochemical analysis methods. These biosensors have advanced commercially and are widely used in multiple industries, including agriculture, environmental, and clinical sectors. Nanomaterials are excellent candidates for developing electrochemical sensors with improved sensitivity. Among these, carbon nanomaterials have emerged as a promising option for high-performance biosensors due to their high electrical conductivity, favorable biocompatibility, and catalytic activity. Biosensors offer a quick response, are easy to use, and are reasonably priced for real-world applications. As a result, they have been widely used in recent years. This chapter discusses the fundamentals, types of bioreceptors, immobilization techniques, and application of carbon-based nanomaterial in developing biosensors for agro-pollutant detection.

4.1 Introduction

Electrochemical biosensors combine recently developed physical and chemical sensing techniques as sensors [1]. These sensors are analytical tools that transform biochemical events such as enzyme-substrate reactions into electrical signals [2]. The first electrochemical biosensor reported by Clark was the Clark oxygen electrode for blood glucose [3]. Ideally, biosensors should be reusable, highly sensitive, and not impacted by physical parameters such as pH and temperature [4]. These biosensors are used in food industries, clinical diagnosis, and agro-industries to test for

doi:10.1088/978-0-7503-5879-8ch4

environmental contamination. The main features of biosensors are stability, expense, sensitivity, and reproducibility. The receptors in biosensors, such as nucleic acid, antibodies, enzymes, polysaccharides, and tissue, can interact with the analyte and convert it into electrical signals using a transducer (figure 4.1) [5].

The primary benefit of using biosensors compared to other standard techniques such as polymerase chain reaction (PCR), immunoassays, and biochemical analysis for analytes-based tests for identifying contaminants is that the sample can be used without prior preparation [6]. As the glucose sensor shows, electrochemical biosensors are unaffected by the disadvantages of significant sensor setup complexity and cost. Their simple interaction with regular electronic read-out and processing directly results from their close connection to advancements in low-cost microelectronic circuit manufacture. Biosensors stand out for their dependability, ease of downsizing, superior detection limits, and small analyte size [7]. Research on developing biosensors for environmental monitoring of organic pollutants and potentially dangerous compounds has contributed to society's sustainable growth by addressing ecological pollution. These biosensors are primarily utilized for detecting hazardous substances such as insecticides, including organophosphorous pesticides, parathion, and carbamates, as well as metal ions such as Hg^{2+} that can harm the environment.

Most current biosensors incorporate innovative nanomaterials and nanocomposites into their systems, which enhances analytical performance in terms of sensitivity and limit of detection (LOD) [8]. Nanomaterials, including gold nanoparticles, carbon nanotubes, metal oxide nanoparticles, and quantum dots (QDs), are utilized in biosensors with electrochemical activity as an immobilization support for recognition molecules [9]. Applying nanotechnology is envisioned as a successful idea for developing more complex multi-analyte detection systems at an affordable cost. Nanomaterials have tremendous potential for detecting chemical and biological exposure indicators. They are used as signal transducers in biosensors as a

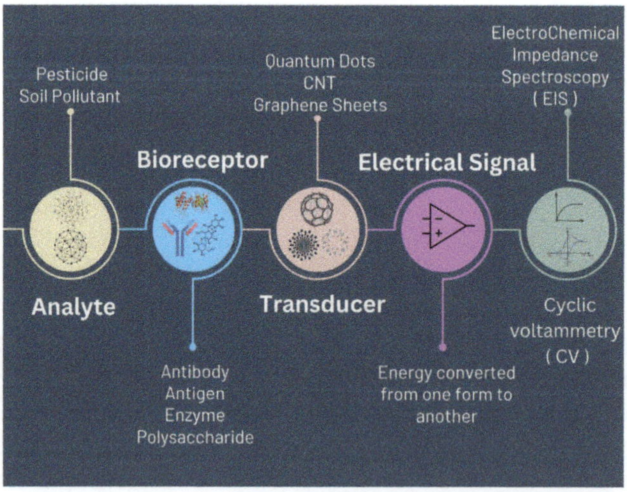

Figure 4.1. Schematic representation of an electrochemical biosensor.

recognition system, mediators of current flow, and electroactive identifiers to indicate an analyte's presence [10]. Due to their fascinating physical, chemical, and electrical capabilities, they are promising candidates for constructing the next generation of miniature biosensors [11].

4.2 Types of biosensor

Biosensors are classified based on their transducer and biorecognition components, which are crucial in biosensor fabrication. Biosensors can be categorized according to different transducers: (i) electrochemical biosensors (amperometric, potentiometric, and impedimetric biosensors), (ii) optical biosensors, (iii) calorimetric approaches, (iv) piezoelectric methods, and (v) thermoelectric method.

Based on the biorecognition components, biosensors include (i) DNA biosensors, immunosensors (antigen, antibodies, or biomarkers), (ii) whole-cell sensors, and (iii) microbial sensors [12]. In this chapter, we mainly focus on electrochemical biosensors (figure 4.2).

4.2.1 Electrochemical biosensor

(i) **Amperometric biosensor:** Amperometric biosensors have a high sensitivity level. This technique applies a potential to the working electrode relative to the reference electrode while simultaneously measuring the response current. The current is generated by electrolysis, which is enabled by electrochemical oxidation or reduction occurring at the active electrode [12]. Due to its ease of use and low LOD, amperometric detection is frequently utilized with affinity and biocatalytic sensors. A constant potential in amperometric measurements has the advantage of a small charging current coming from sensing, which reduces a background signal that impairs the detection limit [13]. Researchers have examined various electrocatalytic materials as substitutes for conventional electrodes, such as carbon-based compounds and metal and metal oxide nanoparticles. These materials exhibit domain specialist competence by acting as applicable modifiers for conventional electrodes [14].

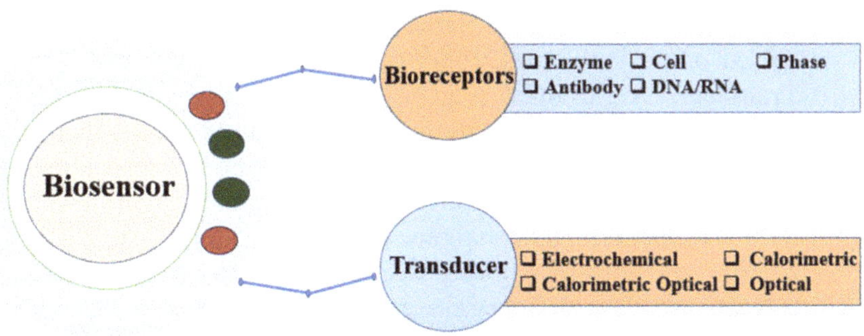

Figure 4.2. Types of biosensor.

(ii) **Potentiometric biosensor:** Potentiometric sensors work by sensing an electrochemical cell's potential while producing a low current. Ion-sensitive field transistors and ion-selective electrodes are the essential components of potentiometric biosensors. The ions accumulating at the ion-selective membrane interaction might cause the main signal output. The electrode generates an equal or almost zero current [12, 15]. The sensor detects the potential across a membrane using an electrochemical cell with two reference electrodes that only react with the charged ion of interest. A biorecognition component is held inside the membrane or immobilized on the membrane's outside surface. In light-addressable potentiometric sensors (LAPS), the photovoltaic effect optically determines the surface potential. LAPS may be the foundation for chemical imaging and multi-analyte sensing [16].

(iii) **Impedimetric biosensor:** Impedance sensing does not require a label, which is helpful for protein detection in developing third-generation biosensors. When a voltage is applied, a circuit's resistance to a current is measured by its electrical impedance [15]. This is known as the voltage-to-current ratio in a specific frequency domain. The electrical impedance induced on the electrode/electrolyte interface in the steady state of an alternating current (AC) under circumstances involving constant direct current (DC) bias is detected by the impedance biosensor [12].

4.2.2 Fundamentals of biosensor

As we know, an electrochemical biosensor contains a bioreceptor and a transducer. However, the biosensor must detect the target molecule by performing five essential functions.

(i) **Bioreceptor:** A biosensor is distinguished by the bioreceptor, also known as the biological recognition element. The bioreceptor is responsible for the sensor's recognition mechanism, which is directed towards the desired analyte. Bioreceptors are molecular species that use a biological process for identification, allowing them to attach the relevant analyte to the sensor surface for measurement. The sampling component of a biosensor has a sensitive layer that contains receptors or receptors covalently linked to the transducer. Examples of biorecognition components include enzymes, nucleic acids, antibodies, and microorganisms [17].

(ii) **Transducer:** A transducer is an element that transforms modifications in the physical or chemical properties of an electroactive species in an analyte into an observable reaction or signal. Three electrodes are required to perform this detection process: a reference electrode, an auxiliary electrode, and a working electrode. The reference electrode offers a steady potential for comparison with the working electrode, enabling electrochemical reaction transduction. The auxiliary electrode creates an electron flow channel in the working electrode by connecting it to the electrolytic solution. In contrast, the working electrode, in combination with the counter electrode, demonstrates both conductivity and chemical stability, ensuring the effectiveness of the transduction process [18].

(iii) **Signal amplifier:** A signal amplifier detects and amplifies electrical impulses before sending them to a signal processor.

(iv) **Signal processor:** The processor readies the signal for display as pictures, graphs, voltammograms, or numbers by converting it into a legible form.

(v) **Display unit:** A user interpretation system built within this device reproduces curves, graphs, voltammograms, or data that users can understand.

To be practical and effective, an electrochemical sensor must fundamentally have the following analytical characteristics:

(i) **Sensitivity:** The smallest input signal size necessary to generate an output with a given signal-to-noise ratio. The standard deviation measurement, frequently derived from the calibration curve, is the foundation for sensitivity. This curve is produced by plotting the specific analyte's concentrations on the x-axis and the observed current on the y-axis, and a more excellent value indicates increased biosensor sensitivity. The biosensor must be sensitive to even small changes in analyte concentration, such as those between ng ml^{-1} and fg ml^{-1} [19].

(ii) **Selectivity:** The biosensor device should only respond to the target analyte without reacting to other chemical entities with similar molecular structures. To determine the biosensor's selectivity, interfering chemicals are added to the measuring cell at their expected concentrations while the standard analyte concentration is already present. The assessment of selectivity is based on several factors, including the range of analyte concentrations, and the receptor and transducer choice.

(iii) **Response linearity:** The sensor's calibration parameters, such as sensitivity and linearity over the measurable analyte concentration range, must be satisfactory to calculate the lowest detection limit. The biosensor has two types of response time: transient response time and steady-state response time. Steady-state response time is determined after introducing each analyte into the measuring cell and is the duration for the biosensor to achieve a stable response. On the other hand, transient response time is the time that elapses before the first derivative of the output signal reaches its maximum value following the addition of the analyte. The activity of both the analyte and the molecular recognition system determines both response times. A higher activity level generally results in a faster response time [20].

(iv) **Reproducibility:** When the target analyte is repeatedly analyzed, the biosensor must produce the same amplitude of the analytical signal. Reproducibility is a statistic that measures the stability of a set of observations across time. Analyte concentrations are frequently measured within the biosensor's usable range, providing essential information on the device's accuracy and dependability. This measures the overall assessment of the biosensor's capacity to consistently deliver results within the prescribed range of analyte concentrations by examining drift or variation over time.

(v) **Stability:** The stability of a biosensor is greatly influenced by its preparation technique and shape. It also depends on the substrate's internal diffusion and the current environment in which it operates. To assess operational stability, analyte solutions with varying concentrations are added continuously or progressively to the biosensor. The analysis also considers differences in pH, buffer composition, and temperature [21].

(vi) **Operating life:** For bioreceptors to effectively monitor the target analyte, they must have a long operational lifetime. The biosensor gadget must be miniaturized, portable, biocompatible, and reasonably priced.

4.3 Electrochemical techniques

Voltammetry—including cycle voltammetry (CV), differential pulse voltammetry (DPV), and square wave voltammetry (SWV), along with electrochemical impedance spectroscopy (EIS)—are electrochemical techniques that are commonly employed in pesticide detection after following one of the biosensing routes illustrated in figure 4.3. In this section, we will provide a brief overview of each method's key characteristics.

(i) **Cyclic voltammetry**

CV helps study the electrochemical processes during potential scans. While a CV is not widely used for quantitative assessments due to its poor sensitivity, it provides critical insights into electroactive molecules' oxidation and reduction pathways by analyzing current peaks. This technique determines whether the process under study is reversible, irreversible, or quasi-reversible based on separating anodic and cathodic peaks. CV measures the currents at the working electrode by performing fast voltage scans in alternating directions. Typically, the scan rate is uniform in both forward and reverse directions. CV can be performed in single or multicycle modes, each providing distinct advantages. CV records essential features

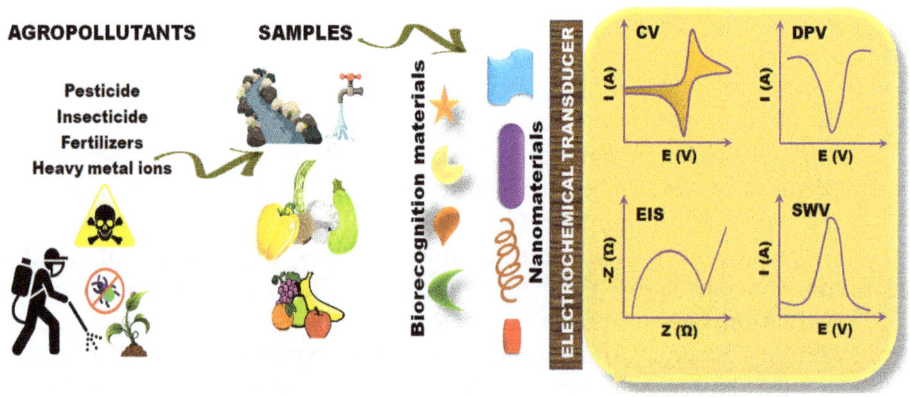

Figure 4.3. Steps to follow during electrochemical biosensing of agropollutants.

such as the anodic and cathodic peak potentials (E_{pa} and E_{pc}), corresponding peak currents (I_{pa} and I_{pc}), and half-peak potentials ($E_{p/2}$) where the cathodic and anodic currents attain half of their peak values. These factors, taken together, provide complete insights into the electrochemical behavior of the system being studied [22].

(ii) **Square wave voltammetry**

Barker pioneered the square wave-potential-time approach, which provides the working electrode with a distinct waveform with a regular square wave superimposed on top of a staircase potential foundation [23]. Here, the electrode undergoes fast potential scanning with a high-frequency square wave superimposed on each step. In SWV, the current is measured twice after each half wave. When the wave's amplitude is small and the redox system is reversible, an electroactive substance can be reduced (or oxidized) during the first half wave and then oxidized (or reduced) during the second half wave. By combining these two currents, sensitivity is increased. This technique's sensitivity can be improved by increasing the amplitude or frequency of the square wave used. Detection limits typically vary from 5.0 to 50.0 $\mu g\ l^{-1}$ [24].

(iii) **Differential pulse voltammetry**

In DPV, periodic, constant potential pulses are applied to a linear scanning process, and the resulting signal is consistently amplified. Additionally, a reading that is less susceptible to capacitive current impact can be obtained by measuring the current difference just before and after each pulse. This differential reading of the current produces a voltammogram that looks like a peak. This method allows for DPV, which is highly sensitive, with detection limits ranging from 10.0 to 100.0 $\mu g\ l^{-1}$ [22].

(iv) **Electrochemical impedance spectroscopy**

Electrochemical impedance spectroscopy is a technique for studying binding events on electrode surfaces. The Randles circuit, which functions as an equivalent electrical circuit, is used in impedance measurement by incorporating an active solution resistance (R_s) between the electrodes; R_{ct} (charge transfer resistance) explains how the redox chemical interacts with the electrode's surface through electron transport. A parallel combination of the double-layer capacitance (C_{dl}) and the capacitance between the electrode's surface and the charged species is also used in the solution of the faradaic reaction. Nyquist plot, which graphically illustrates impedance data, shows a semicircle region followed by a straight line drawn along the real axis. The Nyquist plot provides this characteristic pattern in detail regarding the electrochemical behavior of the system under study.

4.4 Types of bioreceptor

Biosensors can be classified based on their bioreceptor component or the physical–chemical transducer. The bioreceptor component may involve an enzyme, immunoaffinity recognition element, or whole-cell of microorganisms, plants, animals, or

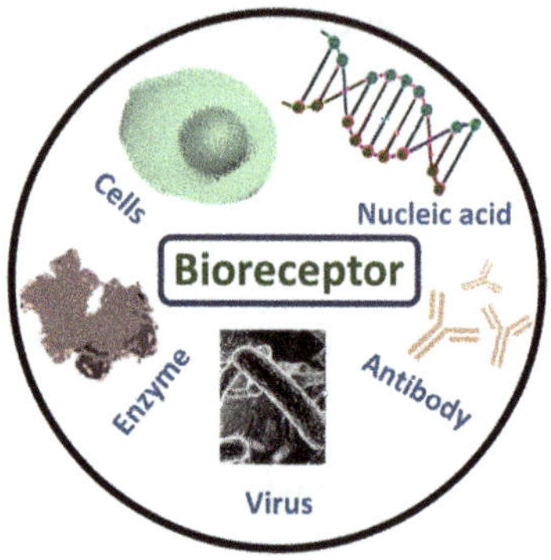

Figure 4.4. Types of bioreceptor.

DNA fragments. Physical–chemical transducers may include electrochemical, optical, piezoelectric, or thermal components. In environmental monitoring, bioreceptor elements such as whole microbial cells, enzymes, antibodies, and DNA are commonly used (figure 4.4). Analytical devices known as biosensors utilize a bioreceptor with a physicochemical detector to detect and measure chemical compounds. The bioreceptor used in a biosensor depends on the target analyte or molecule being monitored.

(i) **Enzymes:** Enzymes are widely used as bioreceptors in biosensors. They can catalyze specific processes that result in a detectable signal in the presence of their substrate. For instance, acetylcholinesterase (AChE) is used in pesticide sensors, while glucose oxidase is used in glucose sensors. However, tiny concentrations of such substances can hinder enzymatic activity. In amperometric biosensors, this inhibition is detected by a shift in the oxidation current of thiocholine at a specific voltage [25].

(ii) **Nucleic acids (DNA/RNA):** Biosensors that detect genetic material or specific sequences can use DNA or RNA molecules as bioreceptors. It is usual practice to employ DNA probes or aptamers, single-stranded DNA/RNA molecules with a strong affinity for particular targets [26].

(iii) **Whole cells:** Whole cells are designed to react to particular target molecules by sending a discernible signal. Microbial biosensors, for instance, use yeast or bacteria to find contaminants in ambient samples. A persistent organochlorine pesticide called lindane (hexachlorocyclohexane) was detected using a microbial biosensor based on polyanilines-genetically engineered *Escherichia coli* cells that express hexachlorocyclohexane [27].

(iv) **Molecularly imprinted polymers (MIPs):** MIPs, or molecularly imprinted polymers, are artificial polymers that mimic a target molecule's physical and chemical characteristics. They contain specific molecular recognition sites that enable them to be used as bioreceptors for small compounds when antibodies or enzymes are not easily accessible. Researchers have been paying close attention to MIP-based biosensing devices, which have a fundamental advantage over conventional bioassays (immunoanalytical systems). They make it possible to quickly and directly identify how the target analyte and recognition element interact [28].

(v) **Aptamers:** The bioreceptors in aptasensors are called aptamers, which are brief single-stranded RNA or DNA molecules with a high specificity and affinity for target molecules. They can either be chosen or designed to bind to various targets. Aptamers and nanomaterials have recently been coupled to boost affinity capture and the analytical signal of biosensors. For instance, electrochemical transduction-based DNA-aptamer biosensors were suggested for detecting ochratoxin A, employing DNA aptamers mounted on gold nanoparticles (AuNPs) and supermagnetic nanoparticles [29].

(vi) **Antibodies:** Proteins, hormones, and infections are just a few examples of the many target molecules that antibodies may identify because they are so highly selective. Many immunoassays, such as enzyme- linked immunosorbent assay (ELISA) and surface plasmon resonance [30], use antibodies as bioreceptors.

(vii) **Phages and viruses:** Bacteriophages and some viruses can surface-display particular peptides or proteins. These viral particles are suitable for biosensors as bioreceptors [30].

Selecting a bioreceptor for a biosensor application depends on several factors, such as the target molecule, sensitivity specifications, and ambient conditions. It is crucial to choose the right bioreceptor because each type has advantages and limitations that can impact the proper functioning of the biosensor.

4.5 Immobilization strategies

Immobilizing biomolecules, such as enzymes, antibodies, DNA, and cells, onto a transducer's surface is necessary for fabricating biosensors. This process allows the transducer to detect and react to the target analyte with high accuracy and sensitivity. Several factors must be considered to successfully attach biomolecules onto the transducer's surface, including the biomolecule type, transducer surface chemistry, and the chosen immobilization method. Therefore, it is essential to develop effective strategies for immobilization to produce biosensors with superior performance characteristics [31]. Typically, biomolecules are attached to or within a solid support. Finding an efficient immobilization technique helps to increase a biosensor's selectivity, stability, sensitivity, and reproducibility, which is crucial in fabricating the biosensor [32]. Various approaches have been reported for immobilizing desired biomolecules onto solid support materials, as illustrated in figure 4.5.

(i) **Cross-linking**

The biomaterial is covalently attached to a solid substrate, such as a polymer or glass bead, in the cross-linked immobilization technique. This technique eliminates the need for a matrix and assistance. However, enzyme molecules can become denatured or lose their catalytic properties when cross-linked with polyfunctional reagents. Polyfunctional compounds

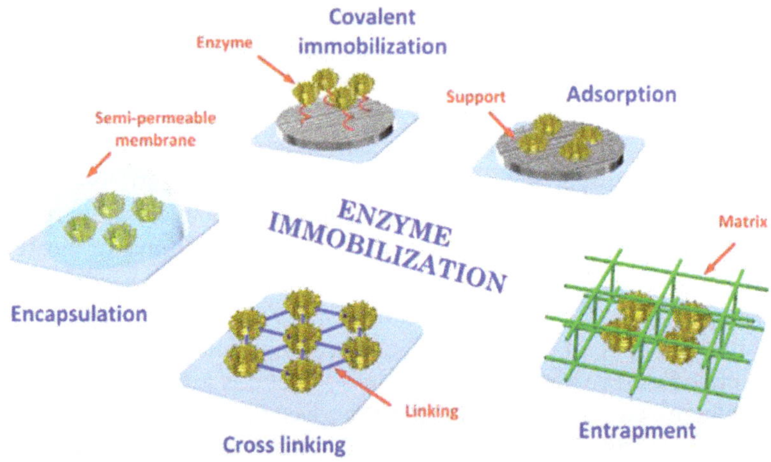

Figure 4.5. Enzyme immobilization processes. Reproduced from [39]. CC BY 4.0.

such as diazonium salt and glutaraldehyde can form covalent bonds with bioreceptors or immobilized enzymes to form a direct connection. This technology offers several advantages over traditional immobilization techniques, such as increased biorecognition material reusability, less leaching, and higher stability [33].

(ii) **Covalent bonding**

Covalent immobilization is a technique that helps to prevent leakage problems by creating a solid bond between the support and the enzyme. This method also helps to improve operational stability, especially in terms of heat, pH, and organic solvents, without affecting the transfer of reagents or products. Covalent bonds can be formed between functional groups such as $-NH_2$, alcoholic –OH, –COOH, and –SH and enzymes under appropriate conditions [34]. Enzyme immobilization requires activating supports using specific activating agents such as carbodiimides, glutaraldehyde, organic and inorganic halides, and other bifunctional agents after functionalization. This method has several advantages, including broad applicability, dependable linkage, and absence of leakage and desorption problems. However, there are also some disadvantages, such as the non-regenerative matrix, potential exposure to harsh or toxic chemicals, and loss of functional conformation of bioreceptors (enzyme and antibody). Functionalization or derivatization adds a new chemical function to a support (enzyme carrier). Meanwhile, the process of making the newly added chemical function reactive toward the enzyme is called activation. In some cases, both functionalization and activation co-occur [35].

(iii) **Adsorption**

Adsorption is the most straightforward technique for immobilizing bioreceptor molecules, including enzymes, antibodies, and DNA probes. Here, electrostatic interactions enable an enzyme or antibody to immediately adsorb onto a carrier (nanostructured materials) or transducer solid support (conducting electrodes: Pt, Au, etc). It has been demonstrated that bioreceptor molecules do not form long-lasting connections when they adsorb on solid supports. The solid substrate's bioreceptors can be stabilized by weak bonds, such as van der Waals forces, ionic interactions, and hydrogen bonds. This approach eliminates 'pore diffusion limitations' because bioreceptors are externally immobilized on the carrier or solid support. The desorption of enzymes from the carrier and decreased efficiency are drawbacks. The benefits of this approach include its simplicity, directness, affordability, lack of reagent requirements, and low activation steps [36].

(iv) **Entrapment**

Physically, bioreceptors are imprisoned within a porous matrix made of a water-soluble polymer. Bioreceptor stabilization inside the matrix may entail both covalent and noncovalent interactions. We can stop the loss of bioreceptors by regulating a matrix's pore size. Changing the polymer's concentration can adjust a matrix's pore size. Agar, carrageenan, cellulose triacetate, polyacrylamide gels, and gelatin are often used as trapping matrices. Enzymes, or bioreceptors, can be directly trapped within gels. The benefits of the entrapment method are that it is inexpensive and straightforward, there is a small risk of conformational change in the enzyme, and moderate conditions are required. The drawbacks are microbial contamination, pore diffusion limitation, and enzyme leakage [37].

(v) **Encapsulation**

Enzymes are enclosed in selectively permeable membranes. This technology is commonly used in biomedical, food, detergent, and wastewater treatment. This encapsulation method provides a simple and cost-effective immobilization method, effectively increasing enzymatic activity by increasing the contact surface area between the enzyme and the substrate [38].

4.6 Role of nanomaterials in a biosensor

The possible use of nanomaterials in biosensors is drawing increased research attention. They are employed as transducer materials, which are crucial to the fabrication of biosensors, and allow for the immobilization of more bioreceptors in an increased quantity [40]. Nanomaterials have proven to be effective in biosensing applications, producing increased sensitivities and significantly enhanced detection limits spanning several orders of magnitude. Because nanoparticles mediate current flow, their use in biosensors is extremely promising. The effective use of these nanomaterials has improved overall performance [41]. Additionally, the properties of nanoparticles, such as their large specific surface area, make it easier to immobilize a wider variety of bioreceptor cells. Electrode surface modification using a variety of new nanomaterials, including metal nanoparticles, carbon nanomaterials, nanofibers, nanowires, and nanotubes, among others, can improve analytical performance [42]. Several nanomaterials have been developed and utilized to construct biosensors through their distinct chemical and physical characteristics.

Here, the biomolecules attach to the nanoparticles by electrostatic interactions, either by dislodging the surrounding capping ions or by coming into chemical contact with ligands such as amines, thiols, etc. Nanotechnology is essential for protecting agricultural land from various threats and increasing agricultural yield. The earlier detection of the factors affecting agriculture, such as pathogens, pesticides, fungicides, and herbicides, can help prevent loss of agriculture yield and adverse environmental effects. Due to the distinctive features resulting from their quantum size effect and surface effect, low-dimensional nanomaterials are among the best candidates for producing sensor materials. The requirements for signal amplification must be met by nanomaterials used as electrodes that show excellent electron mobility, strong biocompatibility with biomolecule capture, and helpful electrocatalytic characteristics. To satisfy the demands of more precise and sensitive analysis, the enhancement of existing biosensing approaches has focused heavily on the distinctive physico-chemical features of nanomaterials.

4.6.1 Application of carbon nanomaterials in detection for electrochemical sensing

Carbon-based nanomaterials (CNMs) are one of the most frequently employed materials in biosensors. They are inexpensive, have minimal inherent toxicity, and have multifunctional surface functionalization [43]. Carbon has allotropes graphite (sp^2), diamond (sp^3), and intermittent sp^2–sp^3 hybridized macroscopic formations that are referred to as amorphous carbon [44]. CNM-based biosensors are widely used for pollution detection in the environment. Without the need for assigning or amplification procedures, good selective and sensitive analyte detection has demonstrated the exceptional physical and electrical properties of graphene and carbon nanotubes [45]. Because of their properties, CNMs went beyond their initial application as electrode materials and became essential components in electrochemical biosensing systems [46]. Biosensor sensitivity can be increased and low detection limits can be achieved using CNMs. They can function as a transduction component and immobilize many bioreceptor units in a smaller volume [47]. QDs, carbon nanotubes (CNTs), and nanoparticles are included in these nanomaterials. CNTs have multiple characteristics, including a wide surface area, strong chemical and thermal durability, electronic and optical properties, and a vital aspect ratio [48]. Owing to their high surface-to-volume ratio, they enable the transformation of the sensing signal and immobilize the bioreceptor on the atom's surface [49]. These properties make CNTs a good biosensor transducer material, which show good conductivity. They are also excellent electrode materials [50]. Numerous CNT-based electrochemical biosensors have been developed, demonstrating the effectiveness of CNTs in this field [51]. Structural and composition heterogeneity are two critical aspects of CNT electrochemistry that should be considered. Because of their structural variability, CNT walls have different characteristics from their ends. Changes in the orientation and arrangement of CNTs on the electrode's surface can affect the pace of electrode transfer, which can have a substantial impact [52, 53]. Comprehending and dealing with these heterogeneities is essential to maximizing the dependability and efficiency of CNTs-based electrochemical biosensors.

CNMs are among the nanoparticles supporting the transducer or the biorecognition component [54]. Each carbon nanomaterial has different characteristics; based on their common features, the electrochemical biosensor includes:

(i) **Electrochemical conductivity:** Because of their exceptional electrical conductivity, carbon nanomaterials can effectively manage electron transfers in electrochemical biosensors, improving sensor performance overall [55].
(ii) **Large surface area:** Carbon nanomaterials have a large surface area; more parts may be efficiently assembled inside electrochemical biosensors to maximize their performance [56].
(iii) **Electrochemical activity:** Carbon nanomaterials and their derivatives have inherent or controlled electrochemical activity, which makes them suitable for electrochemical biosensors [57].

4.6.1.1 0D carbon-based nanomaterials

0D carbon nanomaterials include fullerenes, carbon QDs, nanotoroids, diamonds, graphene clusters, onion-like carbon, and nanohorns. Carbon dots (CDs) are tiny nanoparticles with optical and electro-optical capabilities similar to QDs. They have unique features, such as quantum confinement, which make them valuable in various applications. CDs are also eco-friendly, non-toxic, and have excellent biocompatibility, which makes them ideal for use in biosensors. Two types of CDs can be identified: carbon quantum dots (CQDs) and graphene quantum dots (GRQDs). CQDs appear as hemispherical amorphous materials with diameters less than 10 nm, whereas GRQDs have lateral dimensions less than 20 nm and exhibit different structural traits and properties. These flexible carbon-based nanostructures show enormous promise in various disciplines due to their outstanding properties and functions [58].

4.6.1.2 1D carbon-based nanomaterials

Single-walled carbon nanotubes (SWCNTs), multi-walled carbon nanotubes (MWCNTs), and functionalized MWCNTs are 1D carbon nanomaterials chemically inert and biocompatible. Due to their remarkable mechanical strength, extensive surface area, and high conductivity, MWCNTs are frequently used in pesticide analysis. These properties make them ideal for enhancing the sensitivity and selectivity of pesticide-detection biosensors. Moreover, their compatibility with various recognition elements and ease of functionalization make them widely applicable in this field [59]. SWCNTs have an empty interior region typically between 0.4 and 2.0 nm in diameter. Functionalizing the surfaces of CNTs provides vital information on their electrical, optical, and physical properties, increasing their versatility and utility in various fields. CNTs are utilized as nanocarriers due to their robust electrochemical characteristics. Their aspect ratio is more significant than CDs, leading to an interconnected conductive network that increases conductivity.

Incorporating various functional groups onto the surface of CNTs through surface modification is an effective way to enhance the performance of electrochemical biosensors. By modifying the surface chemistry of CNTs, their interactions with analytes can be accurately adjusted, resulting in better sensitivity, selectivity, and overall performance of electrochemical biosensors developed for pesticide detection [60].

4.6.1.3 2D and 3D carbon-based nanomaterials

Graphene, nanoribbons, 2D networks, and Haeckelite surfaces are essential components of 2D carbon nanomaterials [61]. Dendrimers are nanometer-scale 3D macromolecules that are comparable in size to conventional proteins. Dendrimers are recognized by their hyper-branched, monodispersed, star-shaped structures and abundant surface functional groups. Dendrimers have a vast surface area because of their unique shape, making them ideal for conjugating physiologically active chemicals. Dendrimers, which comprise three distinct components—the core, the internal dendron, and the exterior surface with terminal functional groups—have become widely used in various biosensor applications. Their adjustable structure and functionalization capabilities make them valuable tools for increasing biosensor performance and adaptation across many domains (figure 4.6) [62].

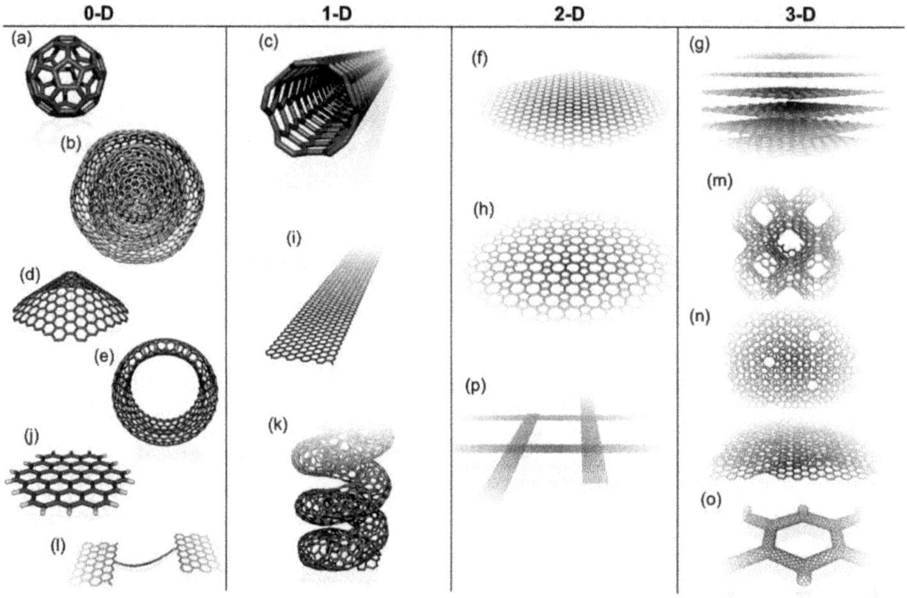

Figure 4.6. Molecular models of various sp^2-like hybridized carbon nanostructures displaying 0D, 1D, 2D, and 3D dimensionalities: (a) Buckminsterfullerene or C_{60}, (b) graphitic onions or nested giant fullerenes, (c) CNT, (d) nanohorns ors nanocones, (e) nanotoroids, (f) graphene, (g) 3D graphite, (h) Haeckelite structure, (i) graphene nanoribbons, (j) clusters of graphene, (k) helicoidal CNTs, (l) short chains of carbon, (m) Schwarzite crystals in three-dimensions, (n) carbon nanofoams, (o) 3D networks of nanotubes, and (p) 2D networks of nanoribbons. Reprinted from [63], Copyright (2022), with permission from Elsevier.

4.6.2 Electrochemical sensing of organophosphate pesticide

Organophosphate (OP) compounds are used as insecticides in modern agriculture to control various insect pests, weeds, and disease-carrying vectors [64]. These compounds can block the esterase group of hydrolytic enzymes, making them acutely toxic. Although the amount of pesticides used is relatively low, they can accumulate in the environment, soil, and crops, causing damage [65]. Pesticides are also difficult to break down, potentially threatening the environment and agricultural lands. It is essential to rapidly detect pesticide residues using carbon-based electrochemical sensors, which we will discuss further.

(i) **Chlorpyrifos**

Chlorpyrifos (CPF) is agriculture's most widely used organophosphorus pesticide to control pests and boost production [66]. Its relatively brief to moderate persistence can be attributed to various dissipation mechanisms, such as volatilization, photolysis, and microbial degradation [67]. In specific ways, aptamers outperform antibodies as potential recognition probes. Their distinctive benefits, such as their extraordinary affinity and specificity, easy modification, and durable stability, have put them on the frontier of recognizable components [68]. Of particular note, aptamer-based biosensors have been extensively used in detecting organic compounds, Pesticides, insecticides, and other proteins, using their outstanding sensitivity, quick reaction times, simple operation, and low cost [69]. Carbon black (CB) and graphene oxide@Fe_3O_4 were prepared to detect chlorpyrifos. Yancui Jiao *et al* [70] aimed to enhance the current signal of an aptasensor through the utilization of chitosan (CS) functionalized CB, which enables the capture of more graphene oxide@Fe_3O_4. The CS functionalized CBs possess high specific surface area, excellent dispersibility, and good electrical conductivity, which makes them an ideal candidate for the proposed application. The resulting graphene oxide@Fe_3O_4 nanocomposite exhibited a robust synergistic effect, producing a single sensing film. The uniform deposition of Fe_3O_4 onto the graphene oxide substrate, facilitated by the significant surface area provided by the latter, enabled effective electron transfer, making it possible to detect chlorpyrifos with exceptional selectivity and a low detection limit. This study demonstrated the potential of the proposed approach in developing a highly sensitive and selective aptasensor for detecting chlorpyrifos. Due to the special synergistic effects of graphene oxide@Fe_3O_4, the immobilization of the probe Apt on the electrode was considerably enhanced. To create a unique biosensing device, graphene oxide@Fe_3O_4 nanocomposite was combined with the biomolecule chlorpyrifos aptamer. The optimized aptasensor offered a dynamic range of 0.1–105.0 ng ml^{-1} with a detection limit of 0.033 ng ml^{-1} under the optimum circumstances. The selectivity, repeatability, and stability of the aptasensor were good. The proposed aptasensor can also be used to monitor. Although the constructed aptasensor showed excellent selectivity against CPF, it is essential to show that the suggested aptasensor can be used in real-world scenarios. Due to their high risk of pesticide residue, some green vegetables, such as cabbage, lettuce, leek, and pakchoi, are highly regulated goods in food analysis. Therefore, it is crucial to find CPF in these vegetables. They were first homogenized in a blender to a puree that flowed freely. The homogenate was centrifuged for 20 min at 1000 rpm to remove the particulates. 0.22 mm membrane was used to filter the supernatant. The recoveries for the sample extraction solutions were assessed using the conventional addition procedure. Three different concentrations of the CPF standard solution were mixed with these sample solutions. Based on triplicate studies at each concentration, the recovery rates ranged from 96% to 106%, while the relative standard deviation (RSD) ranged from 1.21% to 3.70%. These findings suggested that the aptasensor had many possible practical uses.

(ii) **Parathion**

Parathion is a highly effective insecticide with a wide range of applications for controlling various insect species and protecting crops. It is used as a preharvest soil fumigant and as a foliage treatment for many plants grown in open fields. Its broad-spectrum activity makes it a popular choice among experts in the field [71]. The fact that parathion demonstrates significant toxicity through a variety of exposure routes, including ingestion, skin contact, and inhalation, all of which have tragically resulted in fatal outcomes, must be noted as a serious hazard to human health. Like other pesticides made of organophosphorus, parathion permanently inhibits the enzyme AChE. An enzyme biosensor that uses amperometry was developed to test for parathion directly. The biosensor is built with a parathion hydrolase derived from Pseudomonas species isolated from polluted soil. This enzyme is mounted on a carbon electrode surface and catalyzes the hydrolysis of parathion. As a result of this enzymatic activity, p-nitrophenol is formed, which is then detected using anodic oxidation [72].

T.H Vignesh *et al* [73] developed a biosensor to detect methyl parathion (MP). This biosensor uses glutaraldehyde (Glu) cross-linked with AChE to achieve selective detection. Semiconducting-SWCNTs wrapped with bovine serum albumin are used to immobilize the AChE. The biosensor, BSA/AChE-Glu-s-SWCNTs/GCE, was tested using FTIR, CV, EIS, and SWV. The proposed biosensor showed excellent sensitivity and selectivity for detecting MP compared to other biosensors such as BSA/AChE-s-SWCNTs/GCE, s-SWCNTs/GCE, and bare GCE. The s-SWCNTs in this biosensor play a significant role in facilitating electron transfer and provide an increased surface area for the successful assembly of Glu/AChE/BSA. The composite of AChE-Glu-s-SWCNTs had a bovine serum albumin (BSA) layer that functioned as an exceptional protection barrier. This layer sheltered the AChE enzyme from byproducts generated during hydrolysis, especially acetic acid. In the presence of MP, the interaction between AChE and MP is effective. This interaction leads to a complex of MP-AChE on the surface of GCE. The formation of this complex results in the degradation of the electron transport properties of the electrode, which causes a decrease in overall performance and conductivity. To detect varied concentrations of MP, SWV utilized a composite modified electrode consisting of BSA, AChE, and Glu-s-SWCNTs, leveraging this interaction. The proposed biosensor exhibited a wide linear range for the MP target in 100 mM phosphate buffered saline solution (PBS) (pH 7.4) from 1.0×10^{-10} M to 5.0×10^{-6} M with LOD of 3.75×10^{-11} M. Furthermore, the BSA/AChE-Glu-s-SWCNTs-modified GCE, biosensor demonstrated high repeatability and reproducibility when detecting MP. In addition, the suggested biosensor showed improved electrode stability when stored at 4 °C.

In another study, Kaur *et al* [74] developed an electrochemical sensing device that uses a unique bioelectrode containing the redox-active protein hemoglobin (Hb) for the exact detection of MP. This bioelectrode is carefully manufactured by immobilizing Hb on biocompatible coatings of electrochemically reduced graphene oxide-chitosan (ERGO-CS/Hb/FTO). The concentration of redox moiety on the surface of the electrochemical biosensor is higher (2.92×10^{-9} mol cm^{-2}) and there is a favorable heterogeneous electron transfer rate constant (0.0032 s^{-1}), indicating better surface coverage and charge transfer properties. This sophisticated sensor has a low detection limit of 79.77 nM and a high sensitivity of 45.77 A cm^{-2} μM^{-1}, with good repeatability.

(iii) **Malathion**

Malathion is used in residential, public health, and agricultural settings as an organophosphate pesticide. [75]. Overuse of insecticides contaminates agricultural land, water, and air. This chemical dissolves readily in most organic solvents but is less soluble in water, mineral oils, and petroleum ether. The distribution of these pesticides in the environment, including the air, water, soil, and animals, is influenced by physical, chemical, and biological processes [76]. He *et al* [77] established an electrochemical biosensor by anchoring AChE onto core–shell nanostructured HCS@PANI nanocomposite. This nanocomposite shows qualities such as its hollow nanostructure, electrochemical solid activity, and amino functionality. It gives a strong bio-affinity for AChE and, in turn, enables the development of a stable electrochemical biosensor that can quickly and quantitatively detect malathion. The electrochemical results showed that the electrochemical AChE biosensor that was produced had good malathion sensitivity, with LODs of 0.71 ng · ml^{-1} (2.15 pM) and 0.16 ng · ml^{-1} (0.48 pM) for CV and SWV, respectively, the concentration range of malathion from 1.0 ng · ml^{-1} to 10 μg · ml^{-1}. In addition, the produced biosensor portrayed good reproducibility, acceptable stability, and selectivity

In a study by Wang *et al* [78], a unique composite structure made of covalent organic framework (COF) was utilized to create an electrochemical biosensor for detecting malathion. COF combined with MWCNTs, known as COF@MWCNTs, were synthesized by forming

COF-DhaTab (Dha-2,5-dihydroxyterephthalaldehyde) (1,3,5-tris(4-aminophenyl)benzene on the surface of MWCNTs via in situ using solvothermal technique. This composite material has a dual purpose, acting as an excellent matrix for immobilizing AChE and increasing electrochemical signals. The biosensor made of AChE/COF@MWCNTs/GCE could quantitatively measure malathion with a low detection limit of 0.5 nM. This biosensor also showed a broad linear measurement range from 10^{-9} to 10^{-5} M.

4.6.3 Electrochemical sensing of carbamates

Carbamate insecticides are widely adopted in agriculture due to their robust insecticidal properties [79]. However, these substances block the activity of AChE, an indispensable enzyme that regulates acetylcholine, a neurotransmitter essential for proper nervous system functioning. Even sublethal levels of carbamate pesticides in the environment can seriously threaten ecosystems and human health. Therefore, developing techniques to detect carbamate insecticide residues is of paramount importance. Enzyme-based electrochemical biosensors have emerged as the most promising alternative to conventional detection techniques for carbamate residues in recent years. These biosensors offer several advantages, including high sensitivity, rapid response, and ease of use. Thanks to their specificity, selectivity, and accuracy, they have gained considerable attention from researchers and regulators alike. Overall, developing sensitive and reliable methods for detecting carbamate residues is essential for ensuring the safety of the environment and human health.

(i) **Carbaryl**

Qian Liu and colleagues covalently immobilized AChE on MWCNTs/graphene oxide nanoribbons (MWCNTs/GONRs) nanostructures. The film has better catalytic activity due to the covalent binding method and is superior to MWCNTs. The biosensor has a strong affinity for acetylthiocholine with a Michaelis–Menten constant value of 0.25 mM. After a 30-day storage period, the sensor maintained 86% of its initial current response, indicating high stability. They proposed a successful method for monitoring carbaryl based on the inhibition of carbaryl on the immobilized AChE activity. They obtained a broad linear relationship between inhibition and log[carbaryl] from 5.0 nM up to 5000.0 nM, with a low detection limit of 1.7 nM (S/N = 3). Using this approach, they demonstrated the feasibility of directly analyzing pertinent samples to meet the challenges in toxicity analysis, environmental monitoring, food quality control, and military investigation [80].

Li *et al* have developed a highly sensitive electrochemical biosensor using AChE immobilized on an electrochemically induced porous graphene oxide network (e-pGON). The e-pGON was constructed by scanning the GO-modified electrode with a successive CV method, which makes the substrate more accessible to AChE's active centers and increases the electron transfer rate. The biosensor has a remarkable affinity for acetylthiocholine and a low

Michaelis–Menten constant of 0.45 mmol l^{-1}. It precisely correlates the amount of carbaryl inhibited with its concentration between 0.3 and 6.1 ng ml^{-1}. The biosensor also has a reasonable detection limit (LOD) of 0.15 ng ml^{-1} and acceptable stability and repeatability [81].

4.6.4 Detection of multiple pesticides

Guler *et al* [82] fabricated a sensitive and selective AChE electrochemical biosensor using a GCE modified with Nafion as a protective membrane, an Ag@rGO-NH_2 nanocomposite, and GA as a cross-linking agent. This study shows that adding Ag@rGO-NH_2 significantly increased the electron transfer rate, which produced the ideal conditions for AChE immobilization. An apparent Michaelis–Menten constant (K_m) of 20.5 mM suggested that the resultant NA/Ag@rGO-NH_2/AChE/GCE biosensor had a high affinity for acetylthiocholine and showed acceptable repeatability, sensitivity, and reproducibility. The biosensor confirmed the ability to precisely measure the quantities of methidathion, malathion, and chlorpyrifos ethyl within linear ranges of 12.0–105.0 ng ml^{-1} for methidathion, 21.0–122.0 ng ml^{-1} for chlorpyrifos ethyl, and 6.3–77.0 ng ml^{-1} for malathion. On the other hand, Vishwanathan *et al* [83] fabricated an electrochemical biosensor to detect MP and chlorpyrifos, members of the organophosphorus insecticide class. The biosensor used a nanoscale polyaniline matrix to immobilize AChE. This matrix was created by covering a gold substrate with self-assembled monolayers of SWCNTs wrapped in thiol-terminated single-strand oligonucleotide (ssDNA) terminals. When detecting MP and chlorpyrifos, the biosensor showed a dynamic range from 1.0×10^{-11} to 1.0×10^{-6} M, with good stability and repeatability ($0.6 < SD < 3.5$). The biosensor demonstrated good sensitivity; it shows a LOD of 1.0×10^{-12} M for both pesticides.

Yang *et al* [84] constructed an amperometric biosensor by modifying GCE with NiO nanoparticles (NiO NPs), carboxylic graphene (CGR), and Nafion (NiO NPs-CGR-NF) for the detection of MP, chlorpyrifos, and carbofuran. This nanocomposite has a highly hydrophilic surface that enhances AChE adhesion and good properties such as enhanced conductivity, catalytic activity, and biocompatibility. The biosensor depicted affinity for ATCl and successfully catalyzes its hydrolysis, with an apparent Michaelis–Menten constant of 135.0 μM. The improved biosensor identified MP and chlorpyrifos within linear ranges of 1.0×10^{-13} to 1.0×10^{-10} M and 1.0×10^{-10} to 1.0×10^{-8} M, respectively, with detection limits as low as 5.0×10^{-14} M. While the linear ranges for carbofuran were 1.0×10^{-12} to 1.0×10^{-10} M and 1.0×10^{-10} to 1.0×10^{-8} M, with a LOD of 5.0×10^{-13} M (table 4.1).

4.7 Conclusion

In this chapter, we discussed the functions of a traditional biosensor's components using various electrochemical techniques. This chapter has introduced the basics of biosensors and types of bioreceptors. After thoroughly discussing immobilization techniques, selecting a specific application for immobilizing bioreceptor molecules is

Table 4.1. Summary of carbon-based biosensors developed for pesticides.

Analyte	Bioreceptor	Sensing material	Biosensor type	Linear range	Limit of detection	Real samples validation	References
Chlorpyrifos	Chlorpyrifos Aptamer	GO@Fe_3O_4	Aptasensor	0.1–10^5 ng ml^{-1}	00.033 ng ml^{-1}	Vegetable sample	[85]
MP	AChE	BSA/AChE-Glu-s-SWCNT/GCE	Electrochemical biosensor	1.0 $\times 10^{-10}$ M–5.0 $\times 10^{-6}$ M	.75 $\times$ 10^{-11} M	Strawberry and apple Juice	[73]
MP	Hemoglobin	ERGO-CS/Hb/FTO	Electrochemical biosensor	—	779.77 nM	Vegetable sample	[74]
Carbaryl	AChE	AChE-MWCNTs/GONRs	Amperometric	5.0 nM–5000.0 nM	11.7 nM	Cabbage	[80]
Carbaryl	AChE	AChE-e-pGON-GCE	Amperometric	0.3–6.1 ng ml^{-1}	0.15 ng ml^{-1}	Spinach and cabbage sample	[81]
Malathion	AChE	AChE/HCS@PANI	Electrochemical biosensor	1.0 ng.ml^{-1}–10.0 μg.ml^{-1}	0.16 ng · ml^{-1}	Fruits and vegetables	[77]

crucial in developing biosensors that can significantly improve sensitivity, selectivity, quick response, and low cost by incorporating nanomaterials.

The development of biosensors has been aided by the utilization of nanostructured materials in the immobilization of receptors. Nanomaterials present inherent properties that are conducive to the creation of biosensors. These materials can facilitate surface chemistry, which results in the formation of an effective bio-nano interface. This interface can detect even the minutest concentration of target molecules of interest. By linking the bioreceptor, such as an enzyme, antibody, ssDNA, or cell, with nanostructured materials, the biosensors can function optimally in agriculture to detect metal ions, fungicides, and pesticides (as discussed). Carbon nanomaterials are becoming increasingly significant in creating biosensors for detecting pesticides. Their exceptional physical, mechanical, electrical, and multifunctional properties make them essential for enhancing the sensitivity, specificity, and overall performance of biosensors. Carbon-based nanomaterials have thus led to significant advancements in biosensor technology, enabling the creation of more sensitive probes and expanding their applications across various fields. These nanomaterials influence the entire sensor design process, from immobilizing recognition elements to processing signals, and they work well with any detecting mechanism or platform. It is essential to acknowledge that there are still significant challenges that must be addressed in the field of biosensing. The complex interactions between biological molecules and nanomaterials present a formidable hurdle. The arrangement and amount of biomolecules on nanomaterial surfaces play a crucial role in determining the analytical performance of biosensors based on nanomaterials. Furthermore, the practical application of nanomaterial-based biosensors is hindered by the difficulty of creating stable and reproducible devices. Despite these obstacles, the future of biosensing with nanomaterials looks promising. However, addressing these challenges and advancing the field will require focused interdisciplinary efforts.

References

[1] Kaur H, Bhosale A and Shrivastav S 2018 Biosensors: classification fundamental characterization and new trends: a review *Int. J. Health Sci. Res.* **8** 315–33

[2] Cho I H, Kim D H and Park S 2020 Electrochemical biosensors: perspective on functional nanomaterials for on-site analysis *Biomater. Res.* **24** 6

[3] Clark L C and Lyons C 1962 Electrode systems for continuous monitoring in cardiovascular surgery *Ann. N Y Acad. Sci.* **102** 29–45

[4] Mehrota P 2016 Biosensors and their applications—a review *J. Oral Biol. Craniofac. Res.* **6** 153–9

[5] Mehrota P 2016 *Biosensor and its Applications* (Springer)

[6] Arora N 2013 Recent advances in biosensors technology: a review *Octa J. Biosci.* **1** 147–50

[7] Grieshaber D, MacKenzie R, Vörös J and Reimhult E 2008 Electrochemical biosensors-sensor principles and architectures *Sensors (Basel)* **8** 1400–58

[8] Justino C I L, Duarte A C and Rocha-Santos A P 2017 Recent progress in biosensors for environmental monitoring: a review *Sensors (Basel)* **17** 2918

[9] Zhou Y, Fang Y and Ramasamy R P 2019 Non-covalent functionalization of carbon nanotubes for electrochemical biosensor development *Sensors (Basel)* **19** 392
[10] Zhang W, Asiri A M, Liu D, Du D and Lin Y 2014 Nanomaterial-based biosensors for environmental and biological monitoring of organophosphorus pesticides and nerve agents *TrAC Trends Anal. Chem.* **54** 1–10
[11] O'Hara T and Singh B 2021 Electrochemical biosensors for detection of pesticides and heavy metal toxicants in water: recent trends and progress *ACS EST Water* **1** 462–78
[12] Ronkainen N J, Halsall H B and Heineman W R 2010 Electrochemical biosensors *Chem. Soc. Rev.* **39** 1747–63
[13] Halsall H B and Heineman W R 1990 Electrochemical immunoassay: an ultrasensitive method *J. Int. Fed. Clin. Chem.* **2** 179–87
[14] Tajik S *et al* 2021 Recent developments in voltammetric and amperometric sensors for cysteine detection *RSC Adv.* **11** 5411–25
[15] Pohanka M and Skládal P 2008 Electrochemical biosensors—principles and applications *J. Appl. Biomed.* **6** 57–64
[16] Yoshinobu T *et al* 2005 The light-addressable potentiometric sensor for multi-ion sensing and imaging *Methods* **37** 94–102
[17] Karunakaran C, Rajkumar R and Bhargava K 2015 Introduction to biosensors *Biosensors and Bioelectronics.* ed C Karunakaran, K Bhargava and R Benjamin (Amsterdam: Elsevier) ch 1 pp 1–68
[18] Hernandez-Vargas G, Sosa-Hernández J E, Saldarriaga-Hernandez S, Villalba-Rodríguez A M, Parra-Saldivar R and Iqbal H M N 2018 Electrochemical biosensors: a solution to pollution detection with reference to environmental contaminants *Biosensors* **8** 29
[19] Umezawa Y, Umezawa K and Sato H 1995 Selectivity coefficients for ion-selective electrodes: recommended methods for reporting $K_{A,B}^{pot}$ values (technical report) *Pure Appl. Chem.* **67** 507–18
[20] Lindner E, Tóth K and Pungor E 1986 Definition and determination of response time of ion selective electrodes *Pure Appl. Chem.* **58** 469–79
[21] Thevenot D R, Tóth K, Durst R A and Wilson G S 1999 Electrochemical biosensors: recommended definitions and classification *Pure Appl. Chem.* **71** 2333–48
[22] Scholz F 2013 *Electroanalytical Methods: Guide to Experiments and Applications* (Berlin: Springer)
[23] Barker G C 1958 Square wave polarography and some related techniques *Anal. Chim. Acta* **18** 118–31
[24] Osteryoung J G and Osteryoung R A 2002 *Square Wave Voltammetry* (Washington, DC: ACS Publications)
[25] Crew A, Lonsdale D, Byrd N, Pittson R and Hart J P 2011 A screen-printed, amperometric biosensor array incorporated into a novel automated system for the simultaneous determination of organophosphate pesticides *Biosens. Bioelectron.* **26** 2847–51
[26] Labuda J, Brett A M O, Evtugyn G, Fojta M, Mascini M, Ozsoz M, Palchetti I, Paleček E and Wang J 2010 Electrochemical nucleic acid-based biosensors: concepts, terms, and methodology (IUPAC technical report) *Pure Appl. Chem.* **82** 1161–87
[27] Justino C I L, Freitas A C, Pereira R, Duarte A C and Rocha Santos T A P 2015 Recent developments in recognition elements for chemical sensors and biosensors *TrAC, Trends Anal. Chem.* **68** 2–17
[28] BelBruno J J 2019 Molecularly imprinted polymers *Chem. Rev.* **119** 94–119

[29] Daprà J, Lauridsen L H, Nielsen A T and Rozlosnik N 2013 Comparative study on aptamers as recognition elements for antibiotics in a label-free all-polymer biosensor *Biosens. Bioelectron.* **43** 315–20
[30] Zhou Y and Ramasamy R P 2015 Phage-based electrochemical biosensors for detection of pathogenic bacteria *ECS Trans.* **69** 1
[31] Putzbach W and Ronkainen N J 2013 Immobilization techniques in the fabrication of nanomaterial-based electrochemical biosensors: a review *Sensors* **13** 4811–40
[32] Homaei A A, Sariri R, Vianello F and Stevanato R 2013 Enzyme immobilization: an update *J. Chem. Biol.* **6** 185–205
[33] Niknejad H and Mahmoudzadeh R 2015 Comparison of different crosslinking methods for preparation of docetaxel-loaded albumin nanoparticles *Iran. J. Pharm. Res. IJPR* **14** 385–94
[34] Zucca P and Sanjust E 2014 Inorganic materials as supports for covalent enzyme immobilization: methods and mechanisms *Molecules* **19** 14139–94
[35] Sandhyarani N 2019 Surface modification methods for electrochemical biosensors *Electrochemical Biosensors* ed A A Ensafi (Amsterdam: Elsevier) ch 3 pp 45–75
[36] Bhakta S A, Evans E, Benavidez T E and Garcia C D 2015 Protein adsorption onto nanomaterials for the development of biosensors and analytical devices: a review *Anal. Chim. Acta* **872** 7–25
[37] Imam H T, Marr P C and Marr A C 2021 Enzyme entrapment, biocatalyst immobilization without covalent attachment *Green Chem.* **23** 4980–5005
[38] Park B-W, Yoon D-Y and Kim D-S 2010 Recent progress in bio-sensing techniques with encapsulated enzymes *Biosens. Bioelectron.* **26** 1–10
[39] Vasconcelos H, Coelho L C C, Matias A, Saraiva C, Jorge P A S and de Almeida J M M M 2021 Biosensors for biogenic amines: a review *Biosensors* **11** 82
[40] Malhotra B D and Ali M A 2018 Nanomaterials in biosensors: fundamentals and applications *Nanomaterials for Biosensors* (Elsevier) pp 1–74
[41] Xiang L, Zhao C and Wang J 2011 Nanomaterials-based electrochemical sensors and biosensors for pesticide detection *Sens. Lett.* **9** 1184–9
[42] Hu Y, Huang Y, Tan C, Zhang X, Lu Q, Sindoro M, Huang X, Huang W, Wang L and Zhang H 2017 Two-dimensional transition metal dichalcogenide nanomaterials for biosensing applications *Mater. Chem. Front.* **1** 24–36
[43] Panwar N, Soehartono A M, Chan K K, Zeng S, Xu G, Qu J, Coquet P, Yong K-T and Chen X 2019 Nanocarbons for biology and medicine: sensing, imaging, and drug delivery *Chem. Rev.* **119** 9559–656
[44] Khalaj Z, Monajjemi M and Diudea M V 2017 Main allotropes of carbon: a brief review *Sustainable Nanosystems Development, Properties, and Applications* (Hershey, PA: IGI Global) pp 185–213
[45] Yang W, Ratinac K R, Ringer S P, Thordarson P, Gooding J J and Braet F 2010 Carbon nanomaterials in biosensors: should you use nanotubes or graphene? *Angew. Chem. Int. Ed.* **49** 2114–38
[46] Fang Y and Wang E 2013 Electrochemical biosensors on platforms of graphene *Chem. Commun.* **49** 9526–39
[47] Hwang H, Jeong J, Kim Y and Chang M 2020 Carbon nanomaterials as versatile platforms for biosensing applications *Micromachines* **11** 814
[48] Ajayan P M 1999 Nanotubes from carbon *Chem. Rev.* **99** 1787–800

[49] Lin Z, Wu G, Zhao L and Lai K W C 2019 Carbon nanomaterial-based biosensors: a review of design and applications *IEEE Nanotechnol. Mag.* **13** 4–14

[50] Heller I, Kong J, Heering H A, Williams K A, Lemay S G and Dekker C 2005 Individual single-walled carbon nanotubes as nanoelectrodes for electrochemistry *Nano Lett.* **5** 137–42

[51] Jacobs C B, Peairs M J and Venton B J 2010 Review: carbon nanotube based electrochemical sensors for biomolecules *Anal. Chim. Acta* **662** 105–27

[52] Swamy B E K and Venton B J 2007 Carbon nanotube-modified microelectrodes for simultaneous detection of dopamine and serotonin *in vivo Analyst* **132** 876–84

[53] Bardhan N M, Ghosh D and Belcher A M 2014 Carbon nanotubes as *in vivo* bacterial probes *Nat. Commun.* **5** 4918

[54] Wang Z and Dai Z 2015 Carbon nanomaterial-based electrochemical biosensors: an overview *Nanoscale* **7** 6420–31

[55] Geim A K and Novoselov K S 2007 The rise of graphene *Nat. Mater.* **6** 183–91

[56] Peigney A, Laurent C, Flahaut E, Bacsa R R and Rousset A 2001 Specific surface area of carbon nanotubes and bundles of carbon nanotubes *Carbon* **39** 507–14

[57] Yang Y, Yang X, Yang Y and Yuan Q 2018 Aptamer-functionalized carbon nanomaterials electrochemical sensors for detecting cancer relevant biomolecules *Carbon* **129** 380–95

[58] Zhao F, Wu J, Ying Y, She Y, Wang J and Ping J 2018 Carbon nanomaterial-enabled pesticide biosensors: design strategy, biosensing mechanism, and practical application *TrAC, Trends Anal. Chem.* **106** 62–83

[59] Raja I S, Song S-J, Kang M S, Lee Y B, Kim B, Hong S W, Jeong S J, Lee J-C and Han D-W 2019 Toxicity of zero- and one-dimensional carbon nanomaterials *Nanomaterials* **9** 1214

[60] Zhang Q, Huang J-Q, Qian W-Z, Zhang Y-Y and Wei F 2013 The road for nanomaterials industry: a review of carbon nanotube production, post-treatment, and bulk applications for composites and energy storage *Small* **9** 1237–65

[61] Terrones M *et al* 2010 Graphene and graphite nanoribbons: morphology, properties, synthesis, defects and applications *Nano Today* **5** 351–72

[62] Abbasi E, Aval S F, Akbarzadeh A, Milani M, Nasrabadi H T, Joo S W, Hanifehpour Y, Nejati-Koshki K and Pashaei-Asl R 2014 Dendrimers: synthesis, applications, and properties *Nanoscale Res. Lett.* **9** 247

[63] Karadurmus L, Cetinkaya A, Kaya S I and Ozkan S A 2022 Recent trends on electrochemical carbon-based nanosensors for sensitive assay of pesticides *Trends Environ. Anal. Chem.* **34** e00158

[64] Mulchandani A, Chen W, Mulchandani P, Wang J and Rogers K R 2001 Biosensors for direct determination of organophosphate pesticides *Biosens. Bioelectron.* **16** 225–30

[65] Kumaran A, Vashishth R, Singh S, Surendran U, James A and Velayudhaperumal Chellam P 2022 Biosensors for detection of organophosphate pesticides: current technologies and future directives *Microchem. J.* **178** 107420

[66] Guardino X, Obiols J, Russell M G, Farran A and Serra C 1998 Determination of chlorpyrifos in air, leaves and soil from a greenhouse by gas-chromatography with nitrogen–phosphorus detection, high-performance liquid chromatography and capillary electrophoresis *J. Chromatog.* A **823** 91–6

[67] Ge J, Lu M, Wang D, Zhang Z, Liu X and Yu W 2016 Dissipation and distribution of chlorpyrifos in selected vegetables through foliage and root uptake *Chemosphere* **144** 201–6

[68] Zhou L, Wang J, Li D and Li Y 2014 An electrochemical aptasensor based on gold nanoparticles dotted graphene modified glassy carbon electrode for label-free detection of bisphenol a in milk samples *Food Chem.* **162** 34–40
[69] Zhu Y, Chandra P, Song K-M, Ban C and Shim Y-B 2012 Label-free detection of kanamycin based on the aptamer-functionalized conducting polymer/gold nanocomposite *Biosens. Bioelectron.* **36** 29–34
[70] Jiao Y, Hou W, Fu J, Guo Y, Sun X, Wang X and Zhao J 2017 A nanostructured electrochemical aptasensor for highly sensitive detection of chlorpyrifos *Sens. Actuators* B **243** 1164–70
[71] Kim T-S, Kim J-K, Choi K, Stenstrom M K and Zoh K-D 2006 Degradation mechanism and the toxicity assessment in TiO_2 photocatalysis and photolysis of parathion *Chemosphere* **62** 926–33
[72] Pedrosa V A, Caetano J, Machado S A S and Bertotti M 2008 Determination of parathion and carbaryl pesticides in water and food samples using a self assembled monolayer/acetylcholinesterase electrochemical biosensor *Sensors* **8** 4600–10
[73] Kumar T H V and Sundramoorthy A K 2019 Electrochemical biosensor for methyl parathion based on single-walled carbon nanotube/glutaraldehyde crosslinked acetylcholinesterase-wrapped bovine serum albumin nanocomposites *Anal. Chim. Acta* **1074** 131–41
[74] Kaur R, Rana S, Lalit K, Singh P and Kaur K 2020 Electrochemical detection of methyl parathion via a novel biosensor tailored on highly biocompatible electrochemically reduced graphene oxide-chitosan-hemoglobin coatings *Biosens. Bioelectron.* **167** 112486
[75] Azizan M A I, TAufik S, Norizan M N and Abdul Rashid J I 2023 A review on surface modification in the development of electrochemical biosensor for malathion *Biosens. Bioelectron.* X **13** 100291
[76] Raghu P, Madhusudana Reddy T, Reddaiah K, Kumara Swamy B E and Sreedhar M 2014 Acetylcholinesterase based biosensor for monitoring of Malathion and Acephate in food samples: a voltammetric study *Food Chem.* **142** 188–96
[77] He L, Cui B, Liu J, Song Y, Wang M, Peng D and Zhang Z 2018 Novel electrochemical biosensor based on core–shell nanostructured composite of hollow carbon spheres and polyaniline for sensitively detecting malathion *Sensors Actuators* B **258** 813–21
[78] Wang X, Yang S, Shan J and Bai X 2022 Novel electrochemical acetylcholinesterase biosensor based on core–shell covalent organic framework@multi-walled carbon nanotubes (COF@MWCNTs) composite for detection of Malathion *Int. J. Electrochem. Sci.* **17** 220543
[79] Song Y, Zhang M, Wang L, Wan L, Xiao X, Ye S and Wang J 2011 A novel biosensor based on acetylecholinesterase/prussian blue–chitosan modified electrode for detection of carbaryl pesticides *Electrochim. Acta* **56** 7267–71
[80] Liu Q, Fei A, Huan J, Mao H and Wang K 2015 Effective amperometric biosensor for carbaryl detection based on covalent immobilization acetylcholinesterase on multiwall carbon nanotubes/graphene oxide nanoribbons nanostructure *J. Electroanal. Chem.* **740** 8–13
[81] Li Y, Shi L, Han G, Xiao Y and Zhou W 2017 Electrochemical biosensing of carbaryl based on acetylcholinesterase immobilized onto electrochemically inducing porous graphene oxide network *Sensors Actuators* B **238** 945–53
[82] Guler M, Turkoglu V and Basi Z 2017 Determination of malation, methidathion, and chlorpyrifos ethyl pesticides using acetylcholinesterase biosensor based on Nafion/Ag@rGO-NH_2 nanocomposites *Electrochim. Acta* **240** 129–35

[83] Viswanathan S, Radecka H and Radecki J 2009 Electrochemical biosensor for pesticides based on acetylcholinesterase immobilized on polyaniline deposited on vertically assembled carbon nanotubes wrapped with ssDNA *Biosens. Bioelectron.* **24** 2772–7

[84] Yang L, Wang G, Liu Y and Wang M 2013 Development of a biosensor based on immobilization of acetylcholinesterase on NiO nanoparticles–carboxylic graphene–nafion modified electrode for detection of pesticides *Talanta* **113** 135–41

[85] Jiao Y, Hou W, Fu J, Guo Y, Sun X, Wang X and Zhao J 2017 A nanostructured electrochemical aptasensor for highly sensitive detection of chlorpyrifos *Sensors Actuators* B **243** 1164–70

IOP Publishing

Electrochemical Interfaces for the Detection of Agricultural Pollutants

Chandra Sekhar Rout

Chapter 5

Emerging agricultural and environmental pollutants: their impact on public health

G Manasa, B R Karishma and Chandra Sekhar Rout

This chapter provides a comprehensive overview of emerging agricultural pollutants, delving into their sources and potential environmental and public health impacts. Key pollutants include pesticides, fertilizers, heavy metals, and volatile organic compounds (VOCs). Predominantly sourced from advanced agricultural practices, such as improper waste management and inadvertent runoff events, these contaminants are currently being detected at increasing concentrations in soil, air, and aquatic systems. Consequent ecotoxicological effects include disruptions to soil and aquatic microbiota, bioaccumulation, and loss of aquatic biodiversity. In addition, pollutants such as heavy metals in potable water sources present potential human health implications, including endocrine disruption and long-term chronic illnesses. At the same time, volatilization of specific ions like ammonia from fertilizers leads to particulate matter (PM) pollution, posing severe respiratory concerns. This chapter emphasizes the urgent need for a deeper understanding of these agrochemicals and their associated ecophysiological effects to develop enhanced monitoring techniques and mitigation strategies.

5.1 Introduction

Since the start of human civilization, the discovery of agriculture has shaped our history. Agriculture has undoubtedly been the foundation of humanity's sustenance, epitomizing the remarkable marriage between man and nature. However, as the world embraced modern farming practices to increase productivity, agricultural pollution emerged as an unintended consequence. The delicate balance between people and nature seemed in jeopardy as ecosystems suffered the effects of chemical-intensive agriculture.

doi:10.1088/978-0-7503-5879-8ch5

The development of the agricultural sector is inevitably intertwined with world history itself. The First World War, the depression of the 1930s, and the Second World War all contributed to a sequence of events that redirected agriculture, leading to changes in production, labor dynamics, technology adaption, and government policies [1]. Paramount importance was given to increasing crop and livestock production to support the post-war effort, as a result of which the Food and Agricultural Organization (FAO) was created in 1945 as a specialized body of the United Nations to improve the global standard of living [2]. Eventually, the demand to maximize yields and surpluses peaked during the 1960s, and farmers gradually adopted synthetic fertilizers, pesticides, and intensive farming practices, leading to environmental degradation and soil erosion [3]. Over the last 50 years, there has been an aggressive upsurge in agricultural production, up to three times more than earlier, due to the ever-expanding population coupled with increased land availability and complimenting technological contributions [4]. According to the latest reports, agriculture contributes to massive production, averaging 23.7 food tons per day worldwide [4]. However, this situation has also brought about a significant increase in environmental degradation, biodiversity loss, and climate change. Agriculture has also been found to be responsible for 21% of greenhouse gas emissions in recent years according to the FAO [5].

Throughout the latter half of the twentieth century, several scientific studies contributed to our understanding and identification of agricultural pollution. Studies have long indicated the effects of agricultural practices on water quality, ecosystems, and soil integrity. However, only in the modern era, with advanced scientific understanding, have the precise impacts and solutions to agricultural pollution been broadly acknowledged. Therefore, in a similar attempt to understand the roots of agricultural pollution and reduce its detrimental outcomes, this chapter aims to discuss the numerous sources, effects, types, and transmission of these agricultural pollutants into our ecosystem.

5.2 Agricultural pollution

Agricultural waste refers to the byproducts, residues, and discarded materials generated from farming practices and various agricultural activities such as harvesting, pruning, threshing, milling, slaughtering, and packaging. It includes biodegradable matter, such as crop residues, animal manure, and leftover food and feed, as well as non-biodegradable wastes like packaging materials, plastics, and agrochemical containers. Based on this, agricultural wastes are broadly classified into four types, as described in table 5.1.

The difference between agricultural waste and agricultural pollutants lies in their nature and the potential impact they have on the environment. Agricultural wastes are an inevitable outcome of crop production systems and can be managed and utilized in an environmentally responsible manner. While these wastes can pose challenges regarding disposal and management, not all agricultural waste is inherently polluting. Proper management and disposal can minimize their potential to become pollutants and even allow for their beneficial use in areas such as

Table 5.1. Types of agricultural wastes, their sources, and examples [6, 7].

Type of agricultural wastes	Sources	Examples
Crop production wastes	Solid wastes generated from agricultural activities.	Bagasse, husks, roots, molasses, shells, skins, stems, pruning, and trimming residues, etc.
Animal production wastes	Wastes that are generated from animal husbandry and livestock breeding.	Animal excreta, bedding/litter, animal carcasses, damaged feeders, water trough, etc.
Processing wastes	Residues produced during agricultural commodities' processing, handling, and transformation into value-added products.	Packaging materials, Vegetable peels, seeds, cores, grain processing byproducts like bran, husks, or spent grains from brewing, etc.
Chemical wastes	Wastes originate from pesticides, insecticides, herbicides, veterinary medicines, animal health products, etc.	Unused or expired pesticides, empty agrochemical containers, disinfectants, sanitizers, etc.

composting and energy generation [4]. On the other hand, agricultural pollutants are substances released into the environment due to agricultural activities and can potentially cause environmental degradation. These pollutants can include nutrients, pesticides, herbicides, fungicides, antibiotics, hormones, and other chemicals used in agricultural practices, as shown in table 5.1. When agricultural pollutants are not properly managed, they can contaminate soil, water, and air, adversely affecting ecosystems, wildlife, and human health.

5.3 Emerging agricultural pollutants

Chemistry provides a powerful lens through which we can examine and understand the complex issue of agricultural pollution. As elucidated in table 5.1, many of the listed pollutants in chemical wastes pose severe threats to our ecosystem and human health. Pesticide and herbicide runoffs can contaminate water bodies, leading to environmental disruptions and harm to aquatic organisms. The accumulation of these chemicals can have long-term effects on the health of their immediate surroundings and the biodiversity they support. Additionally, excessive use of agrochemicals can degrade soil quality, leading to nutrient imbalances and reduced soil fertility, affecting plant growth and the natural food chain [8].

These hazards also extend to human health, particularly for farmers, farmworkers, and pesticide applicators who handle these chemicals directly. Occupational exposure to agrochemicals can lead to various health issues, such as skin irritation, respiratory problems, and an increased risk of certain types of cancers. Moreover, there are concerns about toxic residues in food products, which can impact consumers' health. Regulatory agencies set maximum residue limits (MRLs) to ensure food safety, but proper monitoring and adherence to these limits are essential to minimize risks [9]. Another concern is the development of pesticide resistance. Pests and weeds can develop resistance to agrochemicals, necessitating increased pesticide use to achieve the same level of control. This can lead to a vicious cycle where pests become even more resistant, posing challenges to crop protection and increasing the risk of environmental contamination [10].

Moreover, a predominantly agrarian economy, India has substantially increased pesticide use since the Green Revolution. A total of 293 pesticides are registered for use in India, out of which 130 are banned in other parts of the world, and 39 of them are categorized as highly hazardous pesticides by Pesticides Action Network (PAN) International and the World Health Organization (WHO) [11]. Organochlorine pesticides like DDT, aldrin, hexachlorocyclohexane, and dieldrin are low-cost and have a wide range of effects on various pests, so they are popularly used in India. Over the years, the Indian government has banned or restricted several pesticides deemed hazardous. Recently, in 2018, the Ministry of Agriculture issued a draft order proposing a ban on 27 unsafe pesticides, consisting of acephate, atrazine, benfuracarb, butachlor, captan, carbendazim, carbofuran, chlorpyriphos, deltamethrin, dicofol, dimethoate, dinocap, diuron, malathion, mancozeb, methomyl, monocrotophos, oxyfluorfen, pendimethalin, quinalphos, sulfosulfuron, thiodicarb, thiophanate methyl, thiram, zineb, and ziram [12]. The Indian Government has also taken significant measures in terms of integrated pest management since 1985 to build an eco-friendly strategy for pest containment. It has also modified and passed a Fertilizer Control Order under the Essential Commodities Act [12].

Therefore, understanding the chemical nature of these pollutants and analyzing their potential effects becomes crucial to pacify and develop strategies for effectively reducing agricultural pollution. Hence, the following section describes the chemical classification of agricultural pollutants as illustrated in figure 5.1. It also discusses some of the relevant research studies on these emerging pollutants.

5.3.1 Inorganic agricultural pollutants

Inorganic agricultural pollutants include a range of non-biodegradable substances released through farming activities. Notable examples include nitrates and phosphates from synthetic fertilizers, heavy metals from contaminated irrigation water or soil amendments, and residues from certain pesticides. These compounds, stemming from various agricultural sources, present substantial environmental health and sustainability challenges, as discussed in this section.

5.3.1.1 Heavy metals

Heavy metals are naturally occurring elements found in the Earth's crust, known for their ability to possess extraordinarily high density. While some heavy metals, such as copper and zinc, are essential micronutrients for plant growth, excessive concentrations of heavy metals in agricultural soils can lead to environmental pollution. Tchounwou *et al* divided the sources of heavy metal pollution into two

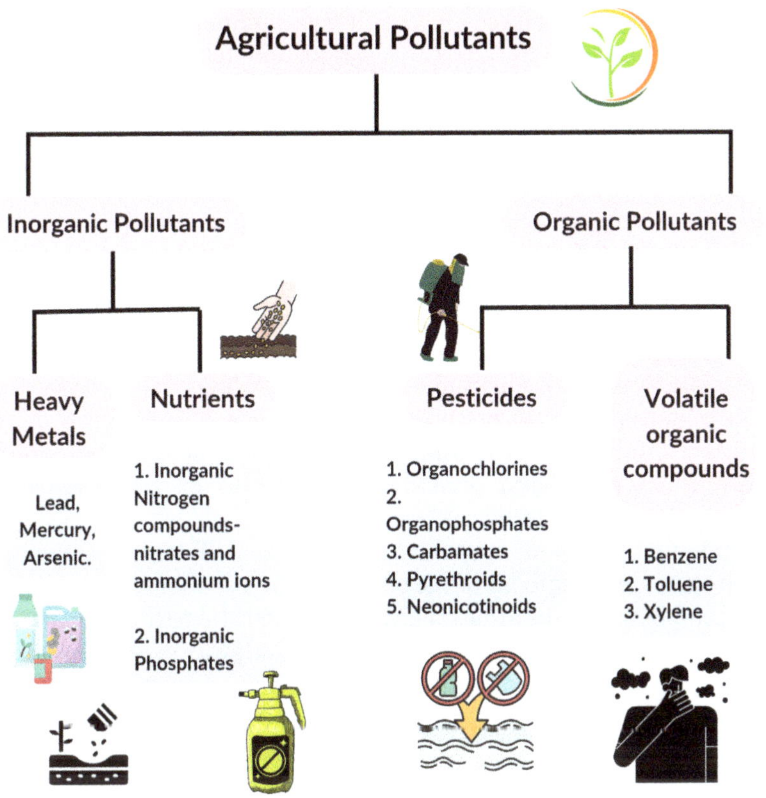

Figure 5.1. Classification of agricultural pollutants.

categories, which are natural and anthropogenic [11]. While the former arises due to volcanic eruptions, rock weathering, sedimentary rocks, and soil formations, the latter results from mining activities, industrial emissions, and the use of agro-chemicals [11].

Agricultural ecosystems serve as a host for various toxic trace elements as some of these metals, such as copper (Cu), iron (Fe), selenium (Se), magnesium (Mg), zinc (Zn), manganese (Mn), molybdenum (Mo), have been reported as essential nutrients for plant growth, deficiency of which could lead to various disorders and syndromes [12]. Therefore, these metals are supplied as constituents of fertilizers. They also play vital roles in critical metabolic processes, including the regular functioning of enzymes, cytochromes, and cofactors of various redox reactions. However, excessive use of fertilizers has become the principal reason for heavy metal accumulation and their detrimental effects.

Inorganic phosphate fertilizers and liming materials release these toxic metals, which cause irreparable damage to the soil fertility because these heavy metals reduce the bioavailability of other essential macronutrients, not just obstructing plant growth but also entering the food chain and posing significant threats to human health [13]. Arsenic (As), mercury (Hg), cadmium (Cd), lead (Pb), and chromium (Cr) have been listed as established carcinogens by the United States Environmental Protection Agency (U.S. EPA) and the International Agency for Research on Cancer (IARC) [11]. Addressing heavy metal pollution in agriculture requires a multifaceted approach encompassing research, technological advancements, and policy development, which will be further discussed in the following sections.

5.3.1.2 Inorganic nitrogen compounds

Though nitrogen is abundantly available in our atmosphere, it is least accessible in the soil, mediated mainly by soil bacteria to the plants. Nevertheless, nitrogen is a quintessential macronutrient for plant nourishment, which is why synthetic nitrogen fertilizers are employed in farming. Since the onset of the Haber–Bosch process in the early-twentieth century, ammonium nitrate (NH_4NO_3) has been used as a chief constituent of nitrogen fertilizers because it provides 34% nitrogen directly compared to other equivalents [10]. Like heavy metal pollution, inorganic nitrogen compounds are also released predominantly due to excessive application and inefficient management of fertilizers.

Both ammonium ions and nitrates are classified as pollutants because they release reactive nitrogen species into all of the environment's spatial scales, which can react with other compounds in the atmosphere to form delicate particulate matter ($PM_{2.5}$) and ground-level ozone (O_3) [14]. According to a Galloway *et al* study, between 1860 and 2000, the reactive nitrogen production rate increased from approximately 15 Tg to about 165 Tg yr^{-1}, with about five times more nitrogen coming from agricultural production than from energy production [15]. Excessive deposition of these reactive species causes serious hazards to aquatic ecosystems through eutrophication and nitrate leaching.

Moreover, elevated nitrate levels in drinking water sources can pose health risks, especially for infants and vulnerable populations, because excessive nitrate consumption can lead to methemoglobinemia or blue baby syndrome [16]. Likewise, ammonium ions have been reported to cause soil acidification. They are subject to ammonia volatilization, a process in which ammonium is converted to gaseous ammonia and released into the atmosphere, potentially impacting air quality and human health [17].

5.3.1.3 Inorganic phosphates

Phosphorous, one of the most indispensable macronutrients, ensures healthy root development, flowering, and fruiting. Hence, maintaining an adequate level of inorganic phosphates in the soil is regulated through various natural processes, such as mineral dissolution, rock weathering, and mycorrhizal symbiosis, as well as human-induced processes, such as the application of fertilizers and manures, all of which constitute the Earth's complex phosphorous cycle. However, the phosphorous cycle, which occurs naturally, like the nitrogen cycle, has been altered and misbalanced due to various anthropogenic activities, the foremost of which is agricultural practices [18].

Inorganic phosphates, such as monoammonium phosphate and diammonium phosphate, are acidic. Their application can lower soil pH, making it more acidic. This can be beneficial in alkaline soils because it helps to neutralize excessive soil alkalinity. Still, excessive use of phosphates can further acidify the soil, leading to soil pH imbalances and nutrient availability issues [19]. Additionally, excessive buildup of phosphate ions in soil elevates their potential runoffs to aquatic bodies, which in turn gets heavily impaired mainly due to processes such as eutrophication [19].

Soil compaction is another alarming effect of the application of inorganic phosphates. Since these fertilizers are employed through heavy machinery or improper soil management practices, they most often lead to compacted soils having reduced pore space, limiting water infiltration and root penetration [20]. As discussed earlier, they threaten public sanitation, like heavy metals and inorganic nitrates.

5.3.2 Organic pesticides

The term 'pesticide' encompasses various products and chemicals designed to control and eliminate pests, including insects, weeds, fungi, bacteria, rodents, and other organisms that can harm crops. Based on their target pests and chemical composition, pesticides are classified into three categories [21]:

(i) *Insecticides:* These pesticides are formulated to kill or control insects. They can be further categorized based on the specific group of insects they target, such as organophosphates, pyrethroids, neonicotinoids, and carbamates.

(ii) *Herbicides:* Herbicides eliminate weeds and unwanted plants. They can be selective, targeting specific types of plants, or nonselective, which kills all vegetation they come into contact with. Common herbicide includes glyphosate and atrazine.

(iii) *Fungicides:* Fungicides prevent and control fungal diseases that affect crops. They work by inhibiting or killing the fungi responsible for the condition. Examples of fungicides include copper-based compounds, triazoles, and strobilurins.

In the late-nineteenth century, the development of synthetic organic compounds like DDT revolutionized pesticide chemistry, providing broad-spectrum insecticide activity [22]. However, the discovery of its detrimental environmental impacts marked a turning point in the understanding and regulation of pesticide use. It was first brought to public attention by Rachel Carson in her influential book 'Silent Spring' published in 1962. Carson highlighted the bioaccumulation of DDT in ecosystems and its impacts on wildlife, particularly birds [23]. DDT belongs to the class of pesticides called organochlorines, which is highly persistent in the environment, and its chemical properties enable it to bioaccumulate in organisms over time. This leads to biomagnification, resulting in elevated DDT levels in top predators, such as birds of prey and fish, leading to eggshell thinning and reproductive defects [24].

Similarly, organophosphate-based insecticides such as malathion and glyphosate are well-established soil degraders and water contaminators, like organochlorines [25]. In addition, they also harm nontarget organisms such as bees and butterflies, which are pollinators. Exposure to these pesticides can result in reduced foraging efficiency, impaired navigation, and negative impacts on colony health and productivity [26]. Tetrachlorvinphos, an insecticide used to control fleas, lice, ticks, insect larvae, and various flies, is banned in the European Union because of the risks associated with chronic health effects, including neurological disorders, developmental abnormalities, and cancers, even upon low levels of exposure [27].

Carbamates are another class of pesticides that are well-known for inhibiting the enzyme acetylcholinesterase and blocking the intermitting signaling of neurological messages. Widely used as insecticides, carbamates have been reported to exert high risks to human health, especially to agricultural workers, pesticide applicators, and individuals living near treated areas. Direct exposure through inhalation, dermal contact, or ingestion can result in acute poisoning symptoms, such as nausea, headaches, and respiratory distress [28]. Common carbamates such as fenobucarb, carbofuran, and carbendazim have also been shown to have low volatility, leading to air pollution, including photodegradation, reaction with atmospheric oxidants, and surface deposition [29].

As mentioned earlier, pyrethroids are an exciting class of pesticides extracted from chrysanthemum flowers and have been used as an insecticide for centuries. Synthetic analogs of pyrethrum, with improved stability and effectiveness, were developed throughout the twentieth century. Synthetic pyrethroids, such as DDT, were initially believed to be less persistent in the environment than organochlorines. However, recent studies have shown that some pyrethroids can persist in soil and water due to their resistance to degradation due to the high degree of halogenation and the presence of ester groups [30]. Additionally, pyrethroids have a peculiar transportation mode through air and water as drift, leading to unintentional contamination of nontarget areas. Rise occurs during aerial spraying and depends on factors like air currents, spray droplet size, application techniques, and operator skills. This can be reduced by using drift-reducing nozzles and proper spraying equipment calibration and maintenance [30].

The last class of synthetic organic pesticides is neonicotinoids, which are chemically similar to nicotine and are mainly used to impair the nervous systems of insects to control their effects on crop growth. They bind to nicotinic acetylcholine receptors in the nervous system of insects, causing paralysis and ultimately leading to their death, making them effective against a wide range of pests. Though they have low soil persistence, they enter water bodies through runoff from treated fields, increasing the risk of leaching into groundwater and surface water. Improper use or over-application of common nenonicotinoids such as acetamiprid can result in residues exceeding the allowable limits, leading to various chronic health diseases. Therefore, countries such as the United States and Canada strictly regulated MRLs of acetamiprids to as low values as 0.2–3 ppm due to their potential neurotoxic effects in mammals, including impacts on learning and memory, as well as endocrine disruption [31].

5.3.3 Volatile organic compounds

VOCs are a group of carbon-based compounds that quickly evaporate at room temperature and pressure, such as benzene, xylene, formaldehyde, methanol, hexane, etc. VOCs play a significant role in the formation of ground-level ozone and smog. When VOCs react with nitrogen oxides in the presence of sunlight, they contribute to the formation of ozone, a harmful pollutant. Ground-level ozone can cause respiratory problems, eye irritation, and damage to vegetation [32]. The Intergovernmental Panel on Climate Change estimates that agriculture contributes to approximately 14% of global anthropogenic VOC emissions [33]. A study conducted by McDonald *et al* in 2011 supports that these emissions include VOCs released from applying pesticides and fertilizers, livestock operations, biomass burning, equipment and machinery, etc [34]. Precision agriculture technologies, such as remote sensing, GPS, and variable rate application systems, enable farmers to apply pesticides and fertilizers more accurately and efficiently [35]. In addition, adopting conservation tillage practices, such as no-till or reduced tillage, helps to retain crop residues on the soil surface, preventing the breakdown of organic matter and the release of VOCs [36]. Such a targeted approach mitigates unnecessary chemical applications, minimizing VOC emissions.

5.4 Transportation of agricultural pollutants

Another essential tool to help us better understand these pollutants is the modes of transportation through which they progress into numerous natural domains, which are discussed in this section. Realizing the transportation patterns of these agricultural pollutants becomes crucial in developing analysis methods, mitigation strategies, and control measures to achieve sustainable agriculture. Considering this, sources of pollution are broadly categorized into 'point and non-point pollution' based on their specific characteristics.

Point pollution in agriculture refers to discharging pollutants from specific and identifiable sources. These sources are usually associated with a single-entry point into the environment, making them easier to locate and monitor. Examples of point pollution in agriculture include [37, 38]:

(i) *Agricultural processing facilities:* Wastewater and effluents discharged from food processing plants, slaughterhouses, and other agricultural processing facilities can contain high levels of nutrients, pesticides, and fertilizers, posing risks to water bodies.
(ii) *Storage and handling of agricultural chemicals:* Inadequate storage or improper disposal of pesticides, herbicides, fertilizers, and other agricultural chemicals can result in point source pollution, especially when these toxins enter water bodies directly.
(iii) *Animal waste management:* Poorly managed animal feeding operations, such as concentrated animal feeding operations, can generate large quantities of manure that, if not correctly stored, treated, and utilized, contaminate nearby water sources.

Alternatively, non-point pollution in agriculture refers to the diffuse and scattered release of pollutants from multiple sources, making it challenging to identify and pinpoint a specific origin. Unlike point pollution, non-point pollution does not have a single-entry point into the environment, making it more difficult to control and manage. Examples of non-point pollution in agriculture include [37, 38]:

(i) *Runoff from agricultural fields:* Excessive use of fertilizers, pesticides, and herbicides on agricultural fields can result in the runoff of these substances during rainfall events. This runoff carries pollutants into nearby water bodies, contributing to water pollution.
(ii) *Soil erosion:* Improper land management practices, such as over-tilling, deforestation, and improper irrigation techniques, can lead to soil erosion. Eroded soil can contain pollutants such as sediment, nutrients, and pesticides, which can be transported by runoff and wind, affecting water quality and ecosystems downstream.
(iii) *Agricultural drainage systems:* Artificial drainage systems, such as ditches and tile drains, can facilitate the transport of nutrients, pesticides, and sediments from fields into streams, rivers, and groundwater, contributing to non-point pollution.

It is imperative to recognize the nature and properties of these agricultural pollutants to gain more profound insights into their negative impacts on the various environmental compartments. The following subsections discuss further evidence, research studies, and the influences of these listed agrochemical pollutants on air, water, and soil ecosystems in detail.

5.5 Agricultural pollutants and ecosystem

5.5.1 Contamination of soil

Soil, the foundation of agriculture, provides vital ecosystem services and supports plant growth. Unfortunately, the extensive use of agrochemicals, improper waste management, and unsustainable farming practices have resulted in soil contamination, posing significant threats to human health and ecological balance. As discussed in the previous subsections, toxic metals and pesticides are widely reported and studied regarding soil contamination due to their potential toxicity and physicochemical properties, allowing them to have high mobility and persistence in the environment. This chapter discusses the direct impact of pollutant residues in the soil and highlights various research studies related to the same.

Among the many pollutants that were discussed previously, a recent 2023 study by Yao *et al* revealed that organophosphates and pyrethroids constituted maximum levels of residues in soil and were found to have LOD–991 ng g^{-1} and 8.76–2810 ng g^{-1}, respectively [39]. Among the organophosphates, dimethoates were observed to be the predominant contaminants, while fenpropathrins were major pollutants among pyrethroids [40].

Dimethoate is known to have adverse effects on soil microbial communities. Since microorganisms play a crucial role in maintaining soil fertility, nutrient cycling, and overall soil health, their destruction can disrupt the balance of microbial populations, reduce diversity in the soil, and inhibit their metabolic activities. Chemically known as O,O-dimethyl S-methyl carbamoyl methyl phosphorodithioate, dimethoate is used as an effective insecticide but can also act as an acetylcholinesterase (AChE) inhibitor. According to a study conducted by Martikainen *et al* in 2019, changes in microbial cell structures, enzymatic activities, and functional gene expression were confirmed in response to dimethoate contamination [40]. Similarly, Miglani *et al* in their 2019 study, analyzed the adverse effects it had on earthworm survival, reproduction, and behavior, which are essential soil organisms involved in soil structure formation and nutrient cycling [41]. Another such experiment carried out by Huang *et al* correlated the mechanism of dimethoate to its structure because it has a phosphorus atom bonded to two oxygen atoms (forming the phosphate group), two sulfur atoms (forming the dithioate group), and a carbamate group. This structure allows them to have non-covalent and steric interactions with AChE enzymes in both target pests and nontarget organisms. With AChE inhibited, acetylcholine builds up in the synaptic clefts of nerve cells of nontarget organisms. It interferes with the regulation of ion channels, disrupts membrane potential, and impairs neurotransmitter-mediated signal transduction pathways, causing severe damage to soil microbiota, with certain sensitive microbial groups being disproportionately affected [42].

Likewise, fenpropathrins are reported to interact with GABA receptors in both pests and nontarget organisms, blocking their effective nerve impulse transmission and eventually leading to paralysis and death. Fenpropathrins, like other pyrethroids, also work by binding to and modifying sodium channels, leading to their prolonged opening and delayed closure. This results in the continuous influx of sodium ions, which leads to repetitive nerve firing and overstimulation of the nervous system [30, 43]. In addition to disrupting the biodiversity of soil ecosystems, repeated applications of fenpropathrins can result in the buildup of soil residues. Though it is not very soluble in water to be carried as runoffs, fenpropathrins can adhere to soil particles and organic matter, leading to its bioaccumulation over time owing to its high persistence in sediments [30].

The organochlorine compounds are another infamous class of pesticides that are highly insoluble in water, like fenpropathrins. Organochlorines' most extensive application as insecticides peaked from the late-1940s to the early-1960s. Paul Muller, who discovered DDT's insecticidal properties, was even awarded a Nobel Prize for its immense impact in eliminating mosquitoes, allowing approximately one billion individuals to live without the constant threat of malaria [44]. With a half-life of 2–15 years, DDT has high persistence abilities in the soil [45]. Even though DDT was banned in many countries decades ago, it is still illegally used in most developing countries. Other organochlorines, such as diazion, aldrin, dicofol, endosulfan, lindane, methoxychlor, polychlorinated biphenyls, chlordane, etc, share similar properties of high persistence, low polarity, low aqueous solubility, and increased lipid solubility. These properties cause them to disrupt microbial activity, interfere with nutrient cycling, damage soil fertility, and ultimately pose risks to plant and animal health. Organochlorine pesticides like endosulfan and methylchlorophenoxyacetic acid (MCPA) intermediates such as 4-chloro-o-cresol, 4-chlorophenoxyacetic acid, and 4-chloro-2-methylphenol that are still used in developed countries such as the United States are reported to have more extended periods of persistence and bioaccumulation, because of which the 2004 Stockholm convention labeled most of these organochlorines as persistent organic pollutants

(POPs) [46]. By utilizing the ultra-sonication technique combined with GC–MS analysis, Goncalves *et al* detected a relatively high presence of endosulfan and endosulfan sulfate, ranging from 0.002 to 0.039 $\mu g\ g^{-1}$ in soil samples obtained from a horticulture area in Portugal [47]. The study highlights an interesting take on the possibility of biodegradation of endosulfan by soil bacteria, leading to the synthesis of sulfated endosulfan, which is highly pernicious and resistant compared to the former [48].

Organochlorines, organophosphates, and pyrethroids discussed above impede a healthy soil environment by affecting the crucial functions of soil microorganisms and invertebrates. On the other hand, heavy metal contamination in soil directly affects its physical attributes, leading to soil compaction, reduced soil porosity, and impaired water infiltration [11, 12]. According to the 2019 Ministry of Ecology and Environment of China survey, the prevalence of soil pollution exceeding regulatory standards is 16.1%. Specifically, the rates of heavy metal contamination exceeding standards are significant, with cadmium (Cd), arsenic (As), mercury (Hg), lead (Pb), and chromium (Cr) exhibiting rates as high as 7.00%, 2.70%, 1.60%, 1.50%, and 1.10%, respectively [49].

A study by Salam *et al* investigated mercury contamination in soil using a next-generation shotgun metagenomic approach from soil samples from Mandate estate, Ilorin, Nigeria. The study showed that after mercury contamination, the physico-chemical properties of the soil underwent notable changes. The soil pH, measured initially at a neutral level of 6.99 ± 0.001, shifted towards acidity, measuring approximately 5.96 ± 0.25. Additionally, the moisture content of the soil declined significantly, reaching levels below 4% [50]. Furthermore, accumulated mercury drastically boosted the growth of phylum *Planctomycetes* in the soil, which is not reported to be involved in mercury detoxification and is also responsible for inhibiting other soil organisms [50].

Unlike other metal contaminants, As exhibits distinct behavior that deviates from the typical patterns. At the same time, most other heavy metals tend to be soluble around acidic conditions, exhibiting high solubility in basic to neutral pH (6.6–7.8) and moderately soluble at acidic pH, making their properties complicated to understand [51]. Inorganic forms of As with two oxidation states, As (III) and As (V), are prevalent, and As (III) is reported to be 60 times more toxic than As (V) because the former is highly mobile and pollutes groundwater [52]. Uptake of As is a severe concern for plant health because it leads to various phytotoxic effects, including inhibited growth, degradation of chlorophyll, depletion of nutrients, and oxidative stress [53]. A recent study by Chauhan *et al* also confirmed that heavy metal stress and fertility indicators, such as the activity of soil enzymes, and growth-limiting factors, such as soil nitrogen and phosphorus, are negatively correlated [54].

Generally, exposure of plants to heavy metals results in oxidative stress, leading to cellular damage. Additionally, plants' accumulation of metal ions disturbs the ions' balance within the cells [55]. When plants absorb toxic metals like Pb, Cd, etc, through capillary action, it negatively affects seed germination by slowing it down and inhibiting the growth of seedlings. It also reduces various parameters, including germination percentage, index, root/shoot length, tolerance level, and the dry mass of both roots and shoots [56, 57]. Because of the risks posed by these heavy metals, phytoremediation technology is now utilized in plants to extract, stabilize, or degrade heavy metals from soil. Certain plant species, known as hyperaccumulators, can accumulate high levels of heavy metals without significant adverse effects, in which case phytoremediation offers a sustainable and cost-effective method for soil cleanup [55].

5.5.2 Contamination of air

Air pollution is a pressing environmental issue that affects individuals' health and well-being worldwide. While industrial emissions and vehicular exhaust are commonly recognized sources of air pollution, the role of agriculture in contributing to this problem should not be overlooked. While the application of pesticides and fertilizers can lead to the emission of VOCs and nitrogen oxides (NO_x), the practice of burning crop residues, such as rice straw, after harvest contributes to the release of harmful pollutants, such as PM and carbon monoxide (CO).

Among various such gases entering the atmosphere, ammonia has been widely regarded as a significant threat to air quality. Once released, ammonia reacts with other pollutants in the air, contributing to the formation of delicate PM ($PM_{2.5}$) and ground-level ozone (smog). These pollutants have severe implications for human health and the environment. According to a study by Lamarque *et al* in 2010, the global emissions of ammonia doubled from 23 to 60 Tg yr^{-1} in the past 70 years, with agricultural fertilizers contributing to a total of 33% [58]. Gaseous ammonia is the notorious cause of the formation of several inorganic aerosols, such as ammonium sulfate, ammonium bisulfate, ammonium nitrate, etc. These are the main precursors for the construction of the deadly $PM_{2.5}$. Excess inhalation makes the exposed population vulnerable to chronic obstructive pulmonary disease (COPD), such as asthma, and weakens the immune system [59]. It is also reported to enter the bloodstream and cause inflammation, which may lead to the formation of plaques in the arteries, increasing the risk of heart attacks, strokes, and other cardiovascular problems [59].

Most nitrogen fertilizers or manures in agricultural lands lead to ammonium ion (NH_4^+) formation. Livestock excreta containing urea and uric acid are also easily decomposed to ammonia through the action of soil bacteria, which further evolves ammonium ions as follows [60].

$$C_5H_4O_3N_4 + 1.5\,O_2 + 4H_2O \rightarrow 5CO_2 + 4NH_3$$

$$CO(NH_2)_2 + H_2O \rightarrow CO_2 + 2NH_3$$

The volatilization of these ammonium ions mainly depends on the pH of the soil and the compound; under higher pH or alkaline conditions, the NH_4^+ undergoes a reaction with water (H_2O), leading to the formation of ammonia and a hydroxide ion (OH^-). Once ammonia is formed, it can escape into the air as a gas due to its high vapor pressure and low molecular weight. While the pH of the soil plays a crucial role in releasing ammonia into the air, factors such as temperature, soil moisture, and soil texture play minor roles in the ammonia escape [61]. Warmer temperatures and dry conditions favor the volatilization rate, while adequate soil moisture and soils with higher clay content can help retain ammonium ions, reducing volatilization [61].

This ammonia emitted acts as a base, facilitating the neutralization of acidic compounds, such as sulfuric acid and nitric acid, in the atmosphere, forming ammonium sulfate and nitrate aerosols. Neutralization leads to the formation of ammonium ions from these aerosols, which serve as nuclei for particle growth. Nucleated particles further collide and aggregate through coagulation, forming larger clusters. Condensation of volatile compounds onto the particles' surfaces leads to further development, eventually creating the harmful $PM_{2.5}$. Studies have shown that $PM_{2.5}$ particles exhibit acidity due to partially neutralizing acidic sulfates and nitrates [62–64]. Several research studies from the late 1990s to the early 2000s indicate that aerosol acidity can potentially impact pH-sensitive heterogeneous atmospheric processes, such as the oxidation of sulfur dioxide to sulfate and the creation of nitrate and secondary organic aerosol [65, 66].

Altered nutrient cycles due to $PM_{2.5}$ can cause reduced photosynthesis in plants, which has cascading effects on wildlife and biodiversity. Moreover, high concentrations of $PM_{2.5}$ and its deposition contribute to reduced visibility, causing smog and haze, and impacting transportation and outdoor activities [67]. $PM_{2.5}$ can scatter and absorb sunlight in the atmosphere, reducing the amount of solar radiation reaching the Earth's surface. This leads to a cooling effect known as solar dimming. However, the extent of this effect can vary depending on the composition and concentration of $PM_{2.5}$ particles. Based on an irradiation data analysis conducted by Song *et al* it was observed that when $PM_{2.5}$ concentrations exceeded $33.5\ \mu g\ m^{-3}$, global horizontal irradiance decreased by over 5% in most months [68]. Additionally, it was also found that $PM_{2.5}$ had a significant attenuation on photovoltaic solar energy production. Song *et al* reported that throughout the experiment, the energy output of crystalline silicon and thin-film photovoltaic systems experienced average losses of up to 7.00% and 9.73%, respectively, due to $PM_{2.5}$-related factors [68].

Such an effect of aerosol pollution directly reduces the electricity generated from solar panels. This can lead to energy shortages and may require increased reliance on alternative energy sources, such as fossil fuels or grid electricity, to meet energy demands. Decreased solar power generation can have economic consequences, particularly for solar energy producers and businesses that depend on consistent and predictable energy sources. It can also lead to price fluctuations in energy markets, potentially causing energy prices to rise during reduced solar power availability [69].

Another potential threat posed by $PM_{2.5}$ particles is their ability to act as cloud condensation nuclei or ice nuclei, which influences cloud formation and properties. A 2017 study by Zhao *et al* on aerosol-cloud interactions in China revealed that $PM_{2.5}$ particle pollution changes in cloud cover, cloud optical properties, and precipitation patterns. In some cases, increased $PM_{2.5}$ concentrations can also lead to the formation of more numerous but smaller cloud droplets, which can affect cloud lifetime, cloud albedo (reflectivity), and radiative properties [32].

Apart from ammonia, another class of compounds called nitrogen oxides (NO_x) is a group of highly reactive gases that include nitric oxide (NO) and nitrogen dioxide (NO_2), contributing to several effects on air quality. Nitrogen oxides enter the atmosphere through agricultural processes such as fertilizer application, manure management, biomass burning, and animal waste. NO_x emissions contribute to the formation of ground-level ozone, also called tropospheric ozone, a secondary air pollutant constituted mainly of NO_x and VOCs. Ground-level ozone is a potent greenhouse gas that contributes to climate change. While it has a relatively short atmospheric lifetime compared to carbon dioxide, its warming effect on a per-molecule basis is significantly higher. This makes it a concern regarding global temperature rise and climate-related impacts [70].

Taking into account the alterations in atmospheric stability and temperature driven by climate changes, Bell *et al* in their 2007 study, predicted that by 2050, the increase in temperature alone might lead to a 68% rise in the number of days exceeding ozone standards in the eastern United States [71]. Another research study has forecasted that the combination of regional climate shifts and the global increase in ozone levels will result in elevated ground-level ozone concentrations across most of the United States. Specifically, the study anticipates that the 95th percentile for daily 8 h maximum ozone levels will elevate from 79 parts per billion (ppb) in 2012 to 87 ppb by 2050 [72]. Exposure to ground-level ozone can lead to various adverse health effects, including respiratory irritation, decreased lung function, and worsening respiratory conditions like asthma. Prolonged or repeated exposure to elevated ozone levels can have particularly detrimental effects, leading to chronic respiratory problems and reduced quality of life. Vulnerable populations, such as children, older people, and individuals with pre-existing respiratory conditions, are at a heightened risk. Moreover, ground-level ozone can harm vegetation, damage crops, and disrupt ecosystems, impacting agriculture and biodiversity [70].

In conclusion, air pollution resulting from agricultural contaminants is a multifaceted environmental challenge with far-reaching consequences. The release of ammonia, nitrous oxide, VOCs, and PM from farming practices significantly impacts air quality, leading to respiratory issues, smog formation, and ecosystem damage. As we seek sustainable and environmentally responsible agricultural practices, we must employ advanced technologies, improved manure management techniques, and better land-use planning to mitigate the harmful effects of these contaminants.

5.5.3 Contamination of water

The issue of water contamination stemming from agricultural practices is a complex and urgent concern within environmental chemistry. Agricultural activities introduce various contaminants exhibiting a potential for long-term presence in water bodies, significantly impacting water quality and posing substantial risks to aquatic ecosystems and human health. Nitrates from agricultural activities are the prevalent chemical pollutants found in groundwater aquifers worldwide [16]. Nitrates from fertilizers and livestock manure can percolate through the soil and enter groundwater, contaminating drinking water sources. Especially in the case of infants, they can lead to methemoglobinemia or 'blue baby syndrome,' which reduces the blood's ability to carry oxygen [73]. Apart from nitrates, many other pesticides, such as DDT, carbamates, benzene hexachloride (BHC), and endosulfan, are also known to contaminate groundwater, and cause surface water pollution and eutrophication. The following section discusses various potential contaminants and their effects on aquatic environments.

Abascal *et al* recently reviewed the global analysis of nitrates present in ground waters among 292 regions around the world and found that 109 of them were reported to have a higher concentration of nitrates, up to 100–160 ppm. In contrast, the standard established by WHO is just 50 ppm. Among the continents, Africa stands first, followed by Asia, Europe, and America, which have high agricultural density in these regions [74]. From a worldwide perspective, crop production is the most significant factor affecting the nitrogen cycle. According to Liu *et al* nearly half of the total annual nitrogen influx into croplands, which amounts to 136.6 Tg N, is attributed to nitrogen-based fertilizers [75, 76]. They further project that out of the total nitrogen outflows of 148 Tg N per year, approximately 23 Tg N per year is lost through leaching, while 24 Tg N per year results from soil erosion. When soil conditions are aerobic, nitrogen readily transforms into nitrate, and a substantial portion of unutilized nitrate dissolves in precipitation and irrigation water [75]. Eventually, this nitrate infiltrates the soil, reaching underlying aquifers or surface waters or evaporating into harmful gases such as ammonia. This leads to many problems, as outlined in the scheme below (figure 5.2) [77].

Elevated nitrate levels in surface waters can stimulate algae growth, leading to algal blooms. When these blooms die and decompose, they deplete oxygen levels in the water, causing 'dead zones' where aquatic life cannot survive. A research study by Camargo and Alonso found that high nitrate concentrations adversely affected fish by impairing their respiratory functions, reducing growth rates, and increasing

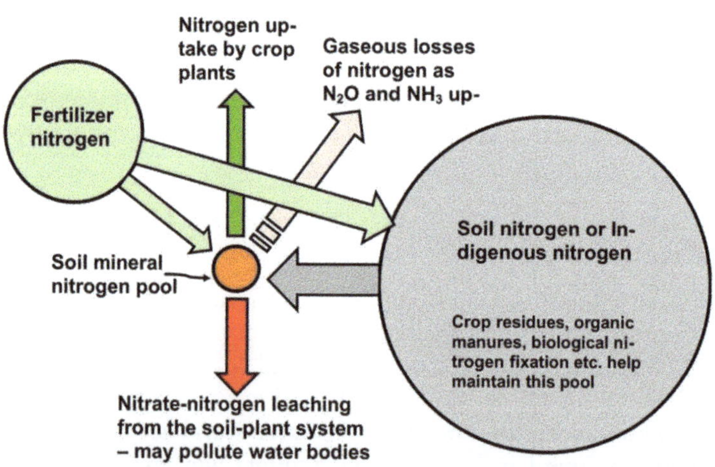

Figure 5.2. Fate of nitrate fertilizers in the environment. Reproduced from [77]. CC BY 4.0.

mortality rates [76]. Martyniuk and Denslow employed the use of omics technologies to investigate how nitrates disrupted androgen signaling in teleost fishes and discovered that fishes in systems near feedlots and farmlands were found to have cellular responses to inhibition of androgenic activation, including apoptosis, lipid transport, and oxidation, hormone synthesis, and transport, immune response, protein metabolism, and cell proliferation, reflecting the effect of nitrate toxicity on their reproductive health [77].

A similar study conducted by Fulton *et al* on grass shrimps revealed that exposure to organochlorine pesticides, such as DDT, endosulfan, toxaphene, etc, and phenylpyrazoles such fipronil can disrupt hormone systems in fish, leading to reproductive abnormalities. Adult shrimp mortality occurred within 24 hours of exposure, whereas larval mortality occurred around 96 hours, indicating the high reproductive risks associated with insecticide contamination in water bodies [78]. Another interesting study conducted by Ankley *et al* evaluated the influence of organochlorines on the androgenic and estrogenic effects of fathead minnows, and it was demonstrated that they exert significant reproductive toxicity, eventually leading to shifts in community composition and ecosystem dynamics [79]. Tongo *et al* investigated pesticide contamination in the Ikpoba river ecosystem in Southern Nigeria. They assessed pesticide concentrations, bioaccumulation, and biomagnification in various food web components, including lower trophic-level organisms. They discovered that Aldrin was the predominant pesticide, with sediment having the highest concentrations. *Commelina erecta*, a macrophyte, exhibited the highest pesticide levels, indicating its role as a significant pesticide reservoir, potentially contributing to the transfer of pesticides up the food web [80]. Through bioaccumulation, these chemicals gradually accumulate in the tissues of aquatic organisms, concentrating as they move up the food chain. In addition to bioaccumulation, biomagnification exacerbates this issue by causing a substantial increase in pesticide concentrations in predators at higher trophic levels. Humans can also be exposed to these contaminants by consuming contaminated fish and seafood, raising concerns about potential health risks [81, 82].

Apart from fishes and other invertebrates, a recent study by Michelle *et al* on the effects of neonicotinoids in pollinators and aquatic insects shed light on the nontarget disruption of these insecticides in beneficial organisms such as honeybees, which also results in an explicit impact on human food supply and economy [83]. As discussed in the above sections, it can be concluded that pollutants arising from agricultural practices have adverse impacts, rippling through ecosystems and endangering various aspects of the environment and human health. The following subsections further discuss the consequences of agricultural pollutants on public health and epidemiology.

5.5.4 Effects of agricultural pollutants on public health

Public health stands at the intersection of human well-being and environmental sustainability. It is one of the most challenging issues we are dealing with in the pervasive impact of agricultural pollutants. As discussed earlier, the consequences of agricultural practices are widely interconnected through ecosystems, infiltrating air, water, and soil, and ultimately affecting the health of populations on a global scale. Recent research illuminates the profound implications of these pollutants, from the neurotoxic effects of pesticides to the antibiotic resistance bred in livestock farming. In this section, we will explore the numerous impacts of agricultural contaminants on public health by shedding light on recent research studies (figure 5.3).

Rusiecki *et al* studied the impact of organic pollutants on global DNA methylation in samples extracted from 70 Greenlandic Inuit [84]. DNA hypomethylation refers to reducing the methylation of cytosine residues within DNA molecules. Hypomethylation, or reduced methylation, can affect gene expression, genome stability, and cellular functions. The researchers performed in-vitro and animal studies. They reported that DNA methylation patterns were adversely affected by several agricultural pollutants, with the highest hypomethylation observed in plasmas exposed to organochlorine pesticides such as DDT and β-hexachlorocyclohexane (HCH), followed by polychlorinated biphenyls (PCB), oxychlordane, and mirex [90]. This impact can lead to various severe conditions such as autoimmune disorders, cancer progression, and even activation of some retroviruses in the system. Hypomethylation can also disrupt gene imprinting, leading to biallelic expression causing developmental disorders [85–87]. A study conducted by Freire *et al* and Richardson *et al* also reported an increased risk of Parkinson's disease with pesticide exposure, especially among the classes of chloropyrifos, organochlorines, and pyrethroids, respectively [88, 89]. Organochlorines have drawn much attention

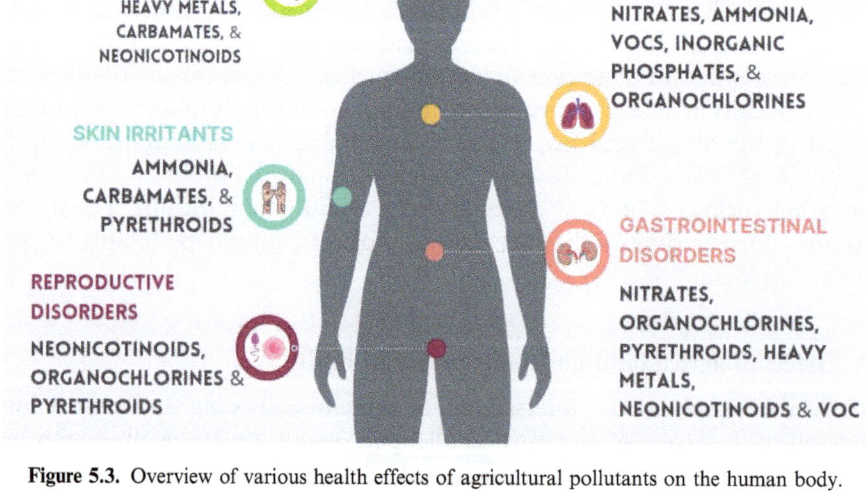

Figure 5.3. Overview of various health effects of agricultural pollutants on the human body.

concerning human hazards because they disrupt the endocrine system by mimicking or blocking hormones, leading to genetic, neurotoxicity, and reproductive disorders [44, 90]. Another recent study published by Ehrenstein *et al* reported that prenatal exposure to DDT was associated with an increased risk of autism in children, too [91].

Neurotoxicity is a widespread consequence of carbamate exposure due to its ability to inhibit acetylcholinesterase, leading to an accumulation of acetylcholine at nerve synapses, resulting in overstimulation of cholinergic receptors. Li *et al* investigated the impact of different carbamate pesticides, ziram, and thiram, on human natural killer cells. They found that ziram and thiram induced apoptosis and necrosis in these cells in a time- and dose-dependent manner, with thiram exhibiting the most substantial effect [92]. They proposed the mechanism of apoptosis involving the activation of caspase-cascade and mitochondrial cytochrome-c pathways. These findings highlight that carbamate pesticides can trigger programmed cell death in natural killer cells, resulting in tissue atrophy, organ dysfunction, immune suppression, and autoimmune disorders [93, 95, 96]. Fenitrothion, belonging to the class of organophosphates, is also widely reported to be involved in blocking nerve impulse transmission, entering the human system through contaminated drinking water [97]. Ghany *et al* studied the effect of oral administration of fenitrothion in rats for some time. They observed an elevation in bilirubin and a reduction of hepatic glycogen and albumin, indicating severe deterioration of the lungs [97].

Phenyl urea compounds are another class of herbicide compounds that are sustained in water runoffs and polluting groundwater systems, causing public health concerns. Diuron, Fenuron, and Fenfuram are widely known for their effects on organs such as the kidney and liver, and they hold a high potential to be carcinogenic upon excessive human contact [98]. Their lipophilicity and high stability result in easy environmental transport [98].

As discussed in the previous sections, runoffs from water bodies containing heavy metals, inorganic fertilizers, and organic pesticides tend to enter the groundwater systems and contaminate the public drinking water. Chen *et al* studied the association between chronic exposure to arsenic-contaminated drinking water and adverse health outcomes, including cardiovascular diseases and diabetes. They revealed higher stroke and myocardial infarction risks were observed upon arsenic exposure [94, 99]. Similarly, many research studies have emphasized the vulnerability of fertilizer dust, ammonia, PM and VOCs constituting several chronic respiratory diseases, such as lung cancer, pulmonary hypertension, and bronchiectasis [100–102].

Highly toxic quaternary ammonium herbicides, such as Paraquat, are also reported to cause oxidative stress in terrestrial and aquatic microorganisms, leading to pulmonary fibrosis and other organ failures. Dong *et al* studied the effect of Paraquat poisoning in rats and observed that the poisoned organism shows reduced appetite and pancreatic injury. At the same time, Blanco *et al* also reported evidence of reproductive diseases in rural women exposed to Paraquat due to the high amount of free radicals as a result of their oxidative stress [103, 104]. Other heterocyclic derivatives in herbicides, such as amitrole and bentazone, and fungicides, such as fenfuram and thiabendazole, are also widely studied for acting as carcinogens owing to their ability to bind to active sites on DNA with their triazole and benzimidazole [105].

As reviewed over the past few sections, improper application and introduction of these toxic agricultural chemicals reach humans through various environmental means. Table 5.2. highlights some of the most common agricultural pollutants and their effect on human health.

Table 5.2. Classes of agricultural pollutants, their sources, and impact on public health with examples.

Class of agricultural pollutants	Examples	Means of exposure	Impact on human health and public
Heavy metals	Lead, cadmium, arsenic, mercury.	Contaminated water sources from fertilizer runoffs pollute drinking water and groundwater systems.	A neurological disorder, cancer, bone and joint disorder, liver damage, and renal dysfunction.
Inorganic nitrogen fertilizers	Nitrates (ammonium nitrate, calcium ammonium nitrate, potassium nitrate, etc).	Inorganic nitrate fertilizers enter soil and water bodies.	Methemoglobinemia (Blue Baby Syndrome), thyroid malfunctions, explosive.
	Ammonia.	Volatilizes into the air, causing the formation of PM.	Cardiovascular disorders, allergies, eye and skin irritation, regional climate shifts.
Inorganic phosphates fertilizers	Single super phosphate, triple super phosphates.	Water contamination, direct inhalation.	Direct inhalation can cause acute poisoning, results in algal blooms, and lowers other nutrient uptake in plants.
Organochlorine pesticides	DDT, methoxychlor, dieldrin, chlordane, toxaphene, etc.	Direct inhalation, dietary exposure, contaminated soil, agricultural runoff in water.	Neurotoxicity, endocrine disruption, cancer, kidney and liver damage, respiratory and developmental disorders.
Carbamates	Carbyl, oxamyl, carbofuran, thiodicarb, methomyl.	Through the skin, consumption of contaminated water and food, and inhalation.	Skin irritation, cholinergic effects, and neurological effects—tremors and seizures increase susceptibility to infections.

Pyrethroids	Allethrin, resmethrin, permethrin, cyfluthrin, esfenvalerate.	Residues in food, transportation, and drift, agricultural runoff.	Persistence and bioaccumulation, resistant development, toxicity to nontarget insects, aquatic toxicity.
Neonicotinoids	Acetamiprid, clothianidin, dinotefuran, imidacloprid, nitenpyram.	Agricultural runoffs, off-target food items, persist in soil.	Muscle tremors, lower testosterone levels, altered insulin regulation, changes to fat metabolism, birth defects.
VOCs	Benzene, toluene, xylene, formaldehyde.	Volatilizes into air, runoffs and leaching, soil emission, through fumigations.	COPD, headaches, dizziness, asthma, liver and kidney damage, and cardiovascular problems.

5.6 Conclusion

Over the years, the intensification of agricultural practices with the widespread use of fertilizers, pesticides, and insecticides has led to significant environmental and public health challenges, as discussed throughout this chapter. Research studies on these toxic agrochemicals and their effects on various ecosystems have been a focus point for the last few decades. They are crucial in understanding and developing newer, more advanced mitigation strategies, policies, and sustainable farming practices. Therefore, broadening our analysis methods and employing knowledge from various areas to determine the qualitative and quantitative effects of these agricultural pollutants on different natural systems is extremely important. However, adopting an affordable and accurate method of analyte determination is challenging. Developing sensors to determine these pollutants can be a promising solution to monitor the impacts of these chemicals. These sensors offer real-time monitoring and data-driven insights, enabling farmers to optimize resource use, minimize the over-application of pesticides and fertilizers, and promptly detect pollution events (figure 5.4).

In this realm, electrochemical sensors have emerged as effective candidates. Unlike conventional methods of analysis, such as chromatography and spectroscopy, which are time-consuming and sophisticated, electrochemical sensors provide rapid and on-site analysis. This real-time detection is crucial for immediate decision-making in agricultural practices and contamination control. Moreover, electrochemical sensors are susceptible and selective, capable of detecting even minute concentrations of contaminants, enabling specific analysis of residues from soil and water samples. Their low operational costs and compact design make them a cost-effective solution for regular monitoring, especially in resource-limited settings. By enhancing precision agriculture and promoting sustainable practices, such as

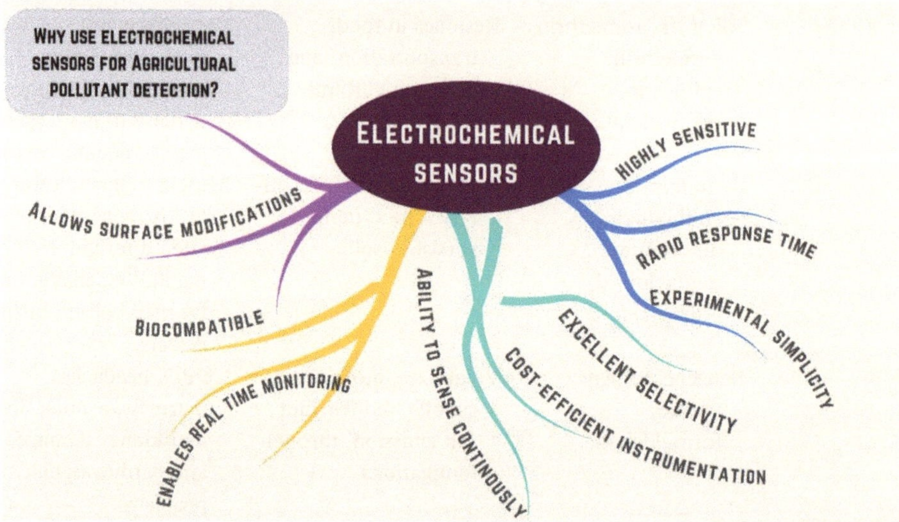

Figure 5.4. Electrochemical sensors as a practical solution for agricultural contaminants determination.

reduced chemical inputs and improved soil management, these sensors can play a pivotal role in protecting ecosystems, conserving vital resources, ensuring food safety, and contributing to a more sustainable and resilient agricultural sector that can meet the needs of a growing global population while minimizing its environmental footprint. Consequently, the next few chapters are dedicated to reviewing electrochemical sensors for detecting various fertilizers and pesticides, and their potential efficacy in accomplishing precise information to enable sustainable and safe farming practices.

References

[1] Bradley P, Segers Y and Van Molle L 2012 *War, Agriculture, and Food* (Milton Park: Routledge)

[2] Bozzoli C and Brück T 2009 Agriculture, poverty, and postwar reconstruction: micro-level evidence from Northern Mozambique *J. Peace Res.* **46** 377–97

[3] Evenson R E and Gollin D 2003 Assessing the impact of the green revolution, 1960 to 2000 *Science* **300** 758–62

[4] Duque-Acevedo M, Belmonte-Ureña L J, Cortés-García F J and Camacho-Ferre F 2020 Agricultural waste: review of the evolution, approaches, and perspectives on alternative uses *Glob. Ecol. Conserv.* **22** e00902

[5] Myers S, Fanzo J, Wiebe K, Huybers P and Smith M 2022 Current guidance underestimates risk of global environmental change to food security *Brit. Med. J.* **378** e071533

[6] Oluseun Adejumo I and Adebukola Adebiyi O 2021 Agricultural solid wastes: causes, effects, and effective management *Strategies of Sustainable Solid Waste Management* ed H M Saleh (London: IntechOpen)

[7] Nagendran R 2011 Agricultural waste and pollution *Waste* (Amsterdam: Elsevier) pp 341–55

[8] Eissa F, Al-Sisi M and Ghanem K 2022 Occurrence and ecotoxicological risk assessment of pesticides in sediments of the Rosetta branch, Nile river, Egypt *J. Environ. Sci.* **118** 21–31

[9] Pretty J 2008 Agricultural sustainability: concepts, principles and evidence *Philos. Trans. R. Soc. B Biol. Sci.* **363** 447–65

[10] Tripathi S, Srivastava P, Devi R S and Bhadouria R 2020 Influence of synthetic fertilizers and pesticides on soil health and soil microbiology *Agrochemicals Detection, Treatment and Remediation* (Amsterdam: Elsevier) pp 25–54

[11] Pandey J K 2023 Use of Hazardous chemical pesticides in India: a review *Proc. Natl Acad. Sci. India* B **93** 523–37

[12] Abhilash P C and Singh N 2009 Pesticide use and application: an Indian scenario *J. Hazard. Mater.* **165** 1–12

[13] Tchounwou P B, Yedjou C G, Patlolla A K and Sutton D J 2012 Heavy metal toxicity and the environment *Molecular, Clinical and Environmental Toxicology* Experientia Supplementum Vol. 101 ed A Luch (Basel: Springer) pp 133–64

[14] Alloway B J 2013 *Heavy Metals in Soils: Trace Metals and Metalloids in Soils and their Bioavailability* **vol 22** (Dordrecht: Springer)

[15] Kabata-Pendias A and Mukherjee A B 2007 *Trace Elements from Soil to Human* (Berlin: Springer)

[16] Galloway J N, Aber J D, Erisman J W, Seitzinger S P, Howarth R W, Cowling E B and Cosby B J 2003 The nitrogen cascade *BioScience* **53** 341

[17] Rotiroti M, Sacchi E, Caschetto M, Zanotti C, Fumagalli L, Biasibetti M, Bonomi T and Leoni B 2023 Groundwater and surface water nitrate pollution in an intensively irrigated system: sources, dynamics and adaptation to climate change *J. Hydrol.* **623** 129868

[18] Knobeloch L, Salna B, Hogan A, Postle J and Anderson H 2000 Blue babies and nitrate-contaminated well water *Environ. Health Perspect.* **108** 675–8

[19] Withers P J A and Jarvie H P 2008 Delivery and cycling of phosphorus in rivers: a review *Sci. Total Environ.* **400** 379–95

[20] Stutter M I, Shand C A, George T S, Blackwell M S A, Bol R, MacKay R L, Richardson A E, Condron L M, Turner B L and Haygarth P M 2012 Recovering phosphorus from soil: a root solution? *Environ. Sci. Technol.* **46** 1977–8

[21] Bouray M, Moir J L, Lehto N J, Condron L M, Touhami D and Hummel C 2021 Soil pH effects on phosphorus mobilization in the rhizosphere of *Lupinus angustifolius Plant Soil* **469** 387–407

[22] Sharma S, Kumar S, Kumar V and Sharma R 2023 Pesticides and vegetables: ecological and metabolic fate with their field and food significance *Int. J. Environ. Sci. Technol.* **20** 2267–92

[23] Hassaan M A and El Nemr A 2020 Pesticides pollution: classifications, human health impact, extraction and treatment techniques *Egypt. J. Aquat. Res.* **46** 207–20

[24] Carson R 1962 *Silent Spring-Rachel Carson-1962* (Houghton Mifflin)

[25] Smith D 1999 Worldwide trends in DDT levels in human breast milk *Int. J. Epidemiol.* **28** 179–88

[26] Whitacre D M (ed) 2010 *Reviews of Environmental Contamination and Toxicology 205* (New York: Springer)

[27] Lamb R W, McAlexander H, Woodley C M and Shukla M K 2021 Towards a comprehensive understanding of malathion degradation: theoretical investigation of degradation pathways and related kinetics under alkaline conditions *Environ. Sci. Process. Impacts* **23** 1231–41

[28] IARC Working Group on the Evaluation of Carcinogenic Risks to Humans 2017 *Some Organophosphate Insecticides and Herbicides* (Lyon: International Agency for Research on Cancer)
[29] Kumar S, Baggi T R and Zughaibi T 2022 Forensic toxicological and analytical aspects of carbamate poisoning—a review *J. Forensic Leg. Med.* **92** 102450
[30] Rüdel H 1997 Volatilisation of pesticides from soil and plant surfaces *Chemosphere* **35** 143–52
[31] Weston D P and Lydy M J 2010 Urban and agricultural sources of pyrethroid insecticides to the Sacramento-San Joaquin Delta of California *Environ. Sci. Technol.* **44** 1833–40
[32] Pfeil R 2014 Pesticide residues: pyrethroids *Encyclopedia of Food Safety* (Amsterdam: Elsevier) pp 31–4
[33] Zeinali M, McConnell L L, Hapeman C J, Nguyen A, Schmidt W F and Howard C J 2011 Volatile organic compounds in pesticide formulations: methods to estimate ozone formation potential *Atmosph. Environ.* **45** 2404–12
[34] Zhang J J, Wei Y and Fang Z 2019 Ozone pollution: a major health hazard worldwide *Front. Immunol.* **10** 2518
[35] Intergovernmental Panel on Climate Change 2007 *Mitigation of Climate Change* (Cambridge: Cambridge University Press)
[36] Wang H, Zhao Z, Winiwarter W, Bai Z, Wang X, Fan X, Zhu Z, Hu C and Ma L 2021 Strategies to reduce ammonia emissions from livestock and their cost-benefit analysis: a case study of Sheyang county *Environ. Pollut.* **290** 118045
[37] Xiang C, Wang Y and Liu H 2017 A scientometrics review on nonpoint source pollution research *Ecol. Eng.* **99** 400–8
[38] Chang D, Lai Z, Li S, Li D and Zhou J 2021 Critical source areas' identification for nonpoint source pollution related to nitrogen and phosphorus in an agricultural watershed based on SWAT model *Environ. Sci. Pollut. Res.* **28** 47162–81
[39] Wang J, Zhao J, Lei X and Wang H 2019 An effective method for point pollution source identification in rivers with performance-improved ensemble Kalman filter *J. Hydrol.* **577** 123991
[40] Shen Z, Liao Q, Hong Q and Gong Y 2012 An overview of research on agricultural nonpoint source pollution modelling in China *Sep. Purif. Technol.* **84** 104–11
[41] Yao R, Yao S, Ai T, Huang J, Liu Y and Sun J 2023 Organophosphate pesticides and pyrethroids in farmland of the Pearl river Delta, China: regional residue, distributions and risks *Int. J. Environ. Res. Public. Health* **20** 1017
[42] Martikainen E, Haimi J and Ahtiainen J 1998 Effects of dimethoate and benomyl on soil organisms and soil processes—a microcosm study *Appl. Soil Ecol.* **9** 381–7
[43] Miglani R and Bisht S S 2019 World of earthworms with pesticides and insecticides *Interdiscip. Toxicol.* **12** 71–82
[44] Martikainen E, Haimi J and Ahtiainen J 1998 Effects of dimethoate and benomyl on soil organisms and soil processes – a microcosm study *Appl. Soil Ecol.* **9** 381–7
[45] Soderlund D M 2010 Toxicology and mode of action of pyrethroid insecticides *Hayes' Handbook of Pesticide Toxicology* (Amsterdam: Elsevier) pp 1665–86
[46] Jayaraj R, Megha P and Sreedev P 2016 Organochlorine pesticides, their toxic effects on living organisms and their fate in the environment *Interdiscip. Toxicol.* **9** 90–100
[47] Jarman W M and Ballschmiter K 2012 From coal to DDT: the history of the development of the pesticide DDT from synthetic dyes till silent spring *Endeavour* **36** 131–42

[48] Jayaraj R, Megha P and Sreedev P 2016 Review article. organochlorine pesticides, their toxic effects on living organisms and their fate in the environment *Interdiscip. Toxicol.* **9** 90–100

[49] Goncalves C and Alpendurada M 2005 Assessment of pesticide contamination in soil samples from an intensive horticulture area, using ultrasonic extraction and gas chromatography–mass spectrometry *Talanta* **65** 1179–89

[50] Kumar M, Lakshmi C V and Khanna S 2008 Biodegradation and bioremediation of endosulfan contaminated soil *Bioresour. Technol.* **99** 3116–22

[51] Salam L B, Shomope H, Ummi Z and Bukar F 2019 Mercury contamination imposes structural shift on the microbial community of an agricultural soil *Bull. Natl. Res. Cent.* **43** 163

[52] Guo M *et al* 2012 Genome sequences of three species in the family Planctomycetaceae *J. Bacteriol.* **194** 3740–1

[53] Shrivastava A, Ghosh D, Dash A and Bose S 2015 Arsenic contamination in soil and sediment in India: sources, effects, and remediation *Curr. Pollut. Rep.* **1** 35–46

[54] Al-Makishah N H, Taleb M A and Barakat M A 2020 Arsenic bioaccumulation in arsenic-contaminated soil: a review *Chem. Pap.* **74** 2743–57

[55] Moreno-Jiménez E, Esteban E and Peñalosa J M 2012 The fate of arsenic in soil-plant systems *Reviews of Environmental Contamination and Toxicology* vol 215 ed D M Whitacre (New York: Springer) pp 1–37

[56] Chauhan P S, Mishra S K, Misra S, Dixit V K, Pandey S, Khare P, Khan M H, Dwivedi S and Lehri A 2018 Evaluation of fertility indicators associated with arsenic-contaminated paddy fields soil *Int. J. Environ. Sci. Technol.* **15** 2447–58

[57] Collin S *et al* 2022 Bioaccumulation of lead (Pb) and its effects in plants: a review *J. Hazard. Mater. Lett.* **3** 100064

[58] Gidlow D A 2015 Lead toxicity *Occup. Med.* **65** 348–56

[59] Lamarque J-F *et al* 2010 Historical (1850–2000) gridded anthropogenic and biomass burning emissions of reactive gases and aerosols: methodology and application *Atmos. Chem. Phys.* **10** 7017–39

[60] Henze D K, Seinfeld J H and Shindell D T 2009 Inverse modeling and mapping US air quality influences of inorganic $PM_{2.5}$ precursor emissions using the adjoint of GEOS-Chem *Atmos. Chem. Phys.* **9** 5877–903

[61] Sharma S, Chandra M and Kota S H 2020 Health effects associated with $PM_{2.5}$: a systematic review *Curr. Pollut. Rep.* **6** 345–67

[62] Wyer K E, Kelleghan D B, Blanes-Vidal V, Schauberger G and Curran T P 2022 Ammonia emissions from agriculture and their contribution to fine particulate matter: a review of implications for human health *J. Environ. Manage.* **323** 116285

[63] Pan B, Lam S K, Mosier A, Luo Y and Chen D 2016 Ammonia volatilization from synthetic fertilizers and its mitigation strategies: a global synthesis *Agric. Ecosyst. Environ.* **232** 283–9

[64] Jang M, Czoschke N M, Lee S and Kamens R M 2002 Heterogeneous atmospheric aerosol production by acid-catalyzed particle-phase reactions *Science* **298** 814–7

[65] Keeler G J, Spengler J D and Castillo R A 1991 Acid aerosol measurements at a suburban Connecticut site *Atmos. Environ. Part Gen. Top.* **25** 681–90

[66] Kim H-S, Huh J-B, Hopke P K, Holsen T M and Yi S-M 2007 Characteristics of the major chemical constituents of $PM_{2.5}$ and smog events in Seoul, Korea in 2003 and 2004 *Atmos. Environ.* **41** 6762–70

[67] Seinfeld J H, Pandis S N and Noone K 1998 Atmospheric chemistry and physics: from air pollution to climate change *Phys. Today* **51** 88–90
[68] Selokar A, Ramachandran B, Elangovan K N and Dattatreya Varma B 2020 $PM_{2.5}$ particulate matter and its effects in Delhi/NCR *Mater. Today Proc.* **33** 4566–72
[69] Song Z, Wang M and Yang H 2022 Quantification of the impact of fine particulate matter on solar energy resources and energy performance of different photovoltaic technologies *ACS Environ. Au* **2** 275–86
[70] Del Hoyo M, Rondanelli R and Escobar R 2020 Significant decrease of photovoltaic power production by aerosols. The case of Santiago de Chile *Renew. Energy* **148** 1137–49
[71] Zhao B *et al* 2017 Enhanced $PM_{2.5}$ pollution in China due to aerosol-cloud interactions *Sci. Rep.* **7** 4453
[72] Bell M L, Goldberg R, Hogrefe C, Kinney P L, Knowlton K, Lynn B, Rosenthal J, Rosenzweig C and Patz J A 2007 Climate change, ambient ozone, and health in 50 US cities *Clim. Change* **82** 61–76
[73] Pfister G G, Walters S, Lamarque J-F, Fast J, Barth M C, Wong J, Done J, Holland G and Bruyère C L 2014 Projections of future summertime ozone over the U.S.: projections of future U.S. surface ozone *J. Geophys. Res. Atmos.* **119** 5559–82
[74] Li P, Karunanidhi D, Subramani T and Srinivasamoorthy K 2021 Sources and consequences of groundwater contamination *Arch. Environ. Contam. Toxicol.* **80** 1–10
[75] Abascal E, Gómez-Coma L, Ortiz I and Ortiz A 2022 Global diagnosis of nitrate pollution in groundwater and review of removal technologies *Sci. Total Environ.* **810** 152233
[76] Liu J, You L, Amini M, Obersteiner M, Herrero M, Zehnder A J B and Yang H 2010 A high-resolution assessment on global nitrogen flows in cropland *Proc. Natl Acad. Sci.* **107** 8035–40
[77] Bijay-Singh and Craswell E 2021 Fertilizers and nitrate pollution of surface and ground water: an increasingly pervasive global problem *SN Appl. Sci.* **3** 518
[78] Camargo J A and Alonso Á 2006 Ecological and toxicological effects of inorganic nitrogen pollution in aquatic ecosystems: a global assessment *Environ. Int.* **32** 831–49
[79] Martyniuk C J and Denslow N D 2012 Exploring Androgen-regulated pathways in teleost fish using transcriptomics and proteomics *Integr. Comp. Biol.* **52** 695–704
[80] Jensen C S, Garsdal L and Baatrup E 1997 Acetylcholinesterase inhibition and altered locomotor behavior in the carabid beetle *Pterostichus cupreus.* A linkage between biomarkers at two levels of biological complexity *Environ. Toxicol. Chem.* **16** 1727–32
[81] Ankley G T, Jensen K M, Kahl M D, Korte J J and Makynen E A 2001 Description and evaluation of a short-term reproduction test with the fathead minnow (*Pimephales promelas*) *Environ. Toxicol. Chem.* **20** 1276–90
[82] Tongo I, Onokpasa A, Emerure F, Balogun P T, Enuneku A A, Erhunmwunse N, Asemota O, Ogbomida E, Ogbeide O and Ezemonye L 2022 Levels, bioaccumulation and biomagnification of pesticide residues in a tropical freshwater food web *Int. J. Environ. Sci. Technol.* **19** 1467–82
[83] Tanabe S 2002 Contamination and toxic effects of persistent endocrine disrupters in marine mammals and birds *Mar. Pollut. Bull.* **45** 69–77
[84] Hladik M L, Main A R and Goulson D 2018 Environmental risks and challenges associated with neonicotinoid insecticides *Environ. Sci. Technol.* **52** 3329–35

[85] Rusiecki J A, Baccarelli A, Bollati V, Tarantini L, Moore L E and Bonefeld-Jorgensen E C 2008 Global DNA hypomethylation is associated with high serum-persistent organic pollutants in greenlandic inuit *Environ. Health Perspect.* **116** 1547–52
[86] Esteller M 2008 Epigenetics in cancer *N. Engl. J. Med.* **358** 1148–59
[87] Baylin S B and Jones P A 2011 A decade of exploring the cancer epigenome—biological and translational implications *Nat. Rev. Cancer* **11** 726–34
[88] Reik W, Dean W and Walter J 2001 Epigenetic reprogramming in mammalian development *Science* **293** 1089–93
[89] Freire C and Koifman S 2012 Pesticide exposure and Parkinson's disease: epidemiological evidence of association *NeuroToxicology* **33** 947–71
[90] Wagner-Schuman M, Richardson J R, Auinger P, Braun J M, Lanphear B P, Epstein J N, Yolton K and Froehlich T E 2015 Association of pyrethroid pesticide exposure with attention-deficit/hyperactivity disorder in a nationally representative sample of U.S. children *Environ. Health* **14** 44
[91] McGovern V 2006 PCBs are endocrine disruptors: mixture affects reproductive development in female mice *Environ. Health Perspect.* **114** A368–9
[92] Taiwo A M 2019 A review of environmental and health effects of organochlorine pesticide residues in Africa *Chemosphere* **220** 1126–40
[93] Von Ehrenstein O S, Ling C, Cui X, Cockburn M, Park A S, Yu F, Wu J and Ritz B 2019 Prenatal and infant exposure to ambient pesticides and autism spectrum disorder in children: population based case-control study *Brit. Med. J.* **364** 1962
[94] Li Q, Kobayashi M and Kawada T 2014 Carbamate pesticide-induced apoptosis and necrosis in human natural killer cells *J. Biol. Regul. Homeost. Agents* **28** 23–32
[95] Li Q, Kobayashi M and Kawada T 2015 Carbamate pesticide-Induced apoptosis in human T lymphocytes *Int. J. Environ. Res. Public. Health* **12** 3633–45
[96] Ramirez-Priego P, Estévez M-C, Díaz-Luisravelo H J, Manclús J J, Montoya Á and Lechuga L M 2021 Real-time monitoring of fenitrothion in water samples using a silicon nanophotonic biosensor *Anal. Chim. Acta* **1152** 338276
[97] Abdel-Ghany R, Mohammed E, Anis S and Barakat W 2016 Impact of exposure to fenitrothion on vital organs in rats *J. Toxicol.* **2016** 5609734
[98] Mahmood I, Imadi S R, Shazadi K, Gul A and Hakeem K R 2016 Effects of pesticides on environment *Plant, Soil and Microbes* ed K R Hakeem, M S Akhtar and S N A Abdullah (Cham: Springer International Publishing) pp 253–69
[99] Chen Y, Santella R M, Kibriya M G, Wang Q, Kappil M, Verret W J, Graziano J H and Ahsan H 2007 Association between arsenic exposure from drinking water and plasma levels of soluble cell adhesion molecules *Environ. Health Perspect.* **115** 1415–20
[100] Mamane A, Baldi I, Tessier J-F, Raherison C and Bouvier G 2015 Occupational exposure to pesticides and respiratory health *Eur. Respir. Rev.* **24** 306–19
[101] Nordgren T M and Bailey K L 2016 Pulmonary health effects of agriculture *Curr. Opin. Pulm. Med.* **22** 144–9
[102] Sigsgaard T *et al* 2020 Respiratory diseases and allergy in farmers working with livestock: a EAACI position paper *Clin. Transl. Allergy* **10** 29
[103] Dong X-S, Xu X-Y, Sun Y-Q, Wei-Liu , Jiang Z-H and Liu Z 2013 Toll-like receptor 4 is involved in myocardial damage following paraquat poisoning in mice *Toxicology* **312** 115–22

[104] Blanco-Ayala T, Andérica-Romero A C and Pedraza-Chaverri J 2014 New insights into antioxidant strategies against paraquat toxicity *Free Radic. Res.* **48** 623–40
[105] Lee Y T, Tan Y J and Oon C E 2023 Benzimidazole and its derivatives as cancer therapeutics: the potential role from traditional to precision medicine *Acta Pharm. Sin.* B **13** 478–97

Chapter 6

Carbon-based electrochemical sensor assisted environmental analysis for fertilizer contamination

G Manasa and Chandra Sekhar Rout

Agricultural fertilizers are indispensable for enhancing crop yields and ensuring food security. NPK nutrients are crucial for plant growth and are often used through fertilizers. Soil nutrients vary spatially, leading to inefficient plant growth. Excess nutrients cause harm to humans and biodiversity, and have a substantial economic impact. The urgent need to identify and lower the adverse effects of agricultural fertilizers on pollution to the environment and public health is highlighted. An affordable system is needed to monitor soil conditions and real-time nutrient movement. This chapter underscores the critical need to develop effective detection methods to identify and mitigate the impact of agricultural fertilizers on environmental pollution and human well-being. Therefore, we have prioritized the electrochemical methods for detecting agro-fertilizers drawn from the existing literature. In particular, we examine the current state of knowledge regarding fertilizer pollution and the requirement for advanced detection strategies. Nitrate, nitrite, urea, phosphate, and potassium carbon-based sensors are investigated for their sensing performances. The utilization of carbon nanotubes (CNTs) is gaining significance in advancing cutting-edge sensing technologies, particularly in electrochemical sensors. CNTs possess unique structural and electrical characteristics that make them highly advantageous for various sensing applications, such as identifying pollutants, biomolecules, and pesticides. This chapter highlights several fundamental attributes of carbon-based sensors that are especially pertinent for monitoring fertilizers.

doi:10.1088/978-0-7503-5879-8ch6

6.1 Introduction

Agriculture is the primary provider of food for the world's population and is crucial to ensuring global food security [1, 2]. However, the growing population and the changing climate have made it challenging to produce enough food, which poses a threat to food security. Modern agricultural practices have resulted in an increase in the use of agrochemicals due to rapid urbanization and industrialization, which, in turn, has caused the accumulation of new contaminants in the agricultural system [3]. Due to the high demand for food, there is pressure to overproduce by applying chemicals to high-yielding crops [4]. Agricultural pollution stems from various factors, including excessive fertilization, agrochemical use (i.e., pesticides, fungicides, and herbicides), inadequate animal waste management, post-harvest handling, and conventional irrigation methods. Salts, organic matter, pathogens, sediments, pesticides, heavy metals, nutrients, and other emerging contaminants are released due to certain practices. These contaminants are released through processes such as erosion, runoff, leaching, and atmospheric deposition. Ultimately, these contaminants end up in water bodies, which results in a compromise of their quality [5]. Globally, agriculture alone consumes 70% of all surface water supplies, making it the single largest user of freshwater resources. One of the primary contributors to water pollution is agriculture. Although recycled water is reintroduced to surface water and groundwater, except for water lost through evapotranspiration [6], farming practices can lead to salination and waterlogging of irrigated land, soil erosion due to inadequate farming techniques, and the release of pollutants and sediment into surface and groundwater [7]. In many countries, the agro-food-processing industry also significantly contributes to organic pollution [8]. The health of waterways is threatened by nutrient runoff from agriculture, which can result in intricate and long-lasting consequences for both the environment and human populations. Therefore, it is comprehensible that agriculture exists with a symbiosis of water and land, which is in recent years a problem of concern that is attributed to the following hazards [7, 8]:

(i) Environmental impact:
- Water and soil pollution due to persistent organic pollutants cause global contamination. Contamination of marine ecosystems and/or groundwater resources from land-based activities can result in ecosystem dysfunction and loss of biodiversity. This, in turn, can cause further harm to the environment [9].
- Pollution of air through the release of ammonia and nitrous oxide from fertilizers. Respiratory issues have been associated with ammonia emissions, while atmospheric ozone and climate change are negatively impacted by nitrous oxide, which is a potent greenhouse gas.

(ii) Human impact:
- Agricultural pollution has both direct and indirect human impacts. A substantial number of people die annually from water-borne diseases stemming from fertilizer application [10]. Excessive spraying has resulted in detecting pesticide residues in food that can potentially affect health.

- The literature also supports the contention that inhalation of ammonia from fertilizers can lead to respiratory issues and exacerbate pre-existing conditions. Additionally, fertilizer pollutants have been linked to cardiovascular diseases, emphasizing the significance of minimizing human exposure [10].

6.2 Need for the detection of fertilizers and nutrients

Recently, certain substances that were previously unregulated are now being recognized as potential environmental pollutants, which are referred to as emerging contaminants. These contaminants can come from various sources, including agricultural practices, pharmaceutical discharges, industries, and urban runoffs. Agricultural pollutants, in particular, can arise from agrochemicals, fertilizers, exhaust fumes, methane, and sedimentation. Long-term fertilizer use can lead to soil nitrification, acidification, and water eutrophication due to fertilizer runoff. One of the primary concerns when addressing agricultural pollution control is the impact on soil fertility and the physical and chemical properties of the land.

Fertilizers are a crucial ingredient in modern agriculture because they provide essential nutrients to plants, enhancing crop yield. Chapter 5 explored the primary purpose and the adverse effects of their use. In brief, fertilizers are substances applied to soil or plants to supply essential nutrients for plant growth and development. Non-organic fertilizers primarily include nitrogen (N), phosphorous (P), and potassium (K), and are commonly denoted as NPK. Fertilizers may also contain secondary nutrients and micronutrients required in smaller quantities for optimal plant growth. However, the indiscriminate use of agricultural fertilizers comprising NPK compounds has become a primary environmental concern [11]. Additionally, the use of fertilizers is believed to be a source of heavy metal (Cd, Hg, Pb, As, Ni, Cu) and natural radionuclides (^{210}Po, ^{232}Th, ^{230}U) contaminants buildup that is ultimately absorbed and may enter the food chain, leading to soil, water, and air pollution [12]. Governing bodies all over the world are currently investigating the matter of nutrient runoff and mitigation strategies to identify various ways to prevent environmental damage caused by excessive agricultural fertilization. Therefore, the lack of detection and monitoring implementation is due to the skepticism of the landowners who are hesitant to adopt it without substantial incentives, resulting in a fundamental lack of cost or benefit analysis. This research gap and issues that have been identified can be remedied or prevented by globally adopting the mitigation strategies that have been reviewed by the governing bodies. Therefore, the governing bodies look forward to researching cost-effective and efficient strategies for different site situations. In this scenario, electrochemical sensors are promising because of their miniaturized, portable, reliable, and economically efficient methodology.

According to the WHO, the 'intensification of farming practice' is to blame for the rise in nitrogen levels in groundwater in many regions of the world [13]. In several nations, nitrate in drinking water has increased to over the recommended 10 mg l^{-1}. The WHO established the drinking water guidelines to prevent methemoglobinemia, to which newborns are particularly susceptible [14]. Table 6.1 represents the various agricultural activities that lead to pollution and their impact on the biosphere. In this chapter, we have prioritized the degradation of the water, soil, and air quality from agricultural practices, such as applying fertilizers, that cause nutrient loss from the soil and its introduction to surface and groundwater. This overabundance of nutrients (especially N and P) in water sources causes eutrophication, which is linked to the rapid growth of aquatic plants and algae. The decomposition of these organisms is a consequence of decreased dissolved oxygen, from which other aquatic life-forms are dependent. Conversely, high nitrate concentrations cause toxicity in water for livestock and human consumption [15].

Table 6.1. The impact of different agricultural activities on the biosphere and the pollution caused by them.

Agricultural activity	Impact	Pollution
Herbicides/pesticides/ insecticides: These chemicals can effectively killed weeds, pests, and other unwanted fauna and flora.	They can become too effective and can harm other species that feed upon the affected plants and animals. (i) *Per se*, the bee population has been declining globally in recent years due to the widespread application of neonicotinoids [16]. This has adversely affected their crucial role as pollinators, making their loss particularly problematic. (ii) Runoff leads to contamination of water bodies and biota, dysfunction of the ecological system, loss of top predators due to reproductive failure, and growth inhibition.	Water and soil
Fertilizers: These chemicals bolster the yield of crops.	Unfortunately, these chemicals have not been applied sparingly. The vast majority of the product is sprayed on fields and is not all absorbed by the intended crop. The excess amounts gradually contaminate the soil or are washed away into nearby water bodies, thereby exerting pressure on that biota (by disturbing the delicate balance of nutrients in them). Manure spreading: A fertilizer activity leading to soil and water contamination that receives metals, pathogens, nitrogen, and phosphorous [17].	Soil and water—eutrophication

Sedimentation: This is one of the less well-known forms of farming-related pollution.	Overfilling the farmland is a common practice in industrial farming methods, which degrades soil quality, promotes runoffs, and causes soil erosion. This soil eventually finds its way into the nearby streams, lakes, rivers, and coastal seas, where its muddiness and turbidity can adversely affect wildlife and flora by depriving them of sunlight and disrupting their regular cycles of life [18].	
Gases [19]:	Agriculture emissions are dominated by methane (CH_4), nitrous oxide (N_2O), and carbon dioxide (CO_2).	Air—attributed to green Greenhouse effect
CH_4: In a country like India, not all farmers are privileged to use machinery for agriculture. Hence, cattle are their best friend when plowing the fields.	On average, each cow releases up to 100 kg of methane into the atmosphere annually, even before considering other ruminant animals. Given that dairy and livestock are among the primary sources of methane emissions, it should come as no surprise that agriculture has a poor reputation.	
N_2O: A major agricultural pollutant —Agrochemical fertilizers that contain nitrogen and animal waste decomposition both release this gas.	Manure, a fertilizer commonly used on organic farms, is rich in nitrogen due to its animal origins. However, excess nitrogen in manure can result in the release of NO_2 into the atmosphere when microbes break down the animal waste. Additionally, as atmospheric nitrogen is transformed into forms of nitrogen that plants can use, N_2O is a naturally occurring by-product of the nitrogen cycle. Microbes start to degrade nitrogen when agrochemical fertilizers are applied to a field, frequently in excess. As a result, far more N_2O is released into the atmosphere than would typically be conceivable in natural ecosystems.	

(*Continued*)

Table 6.1. (*Continued*)

Agricultural activity	Impact	Pollution
Exhaust fumes: The quantity of human intervention in agriculture has decreased because of farmyard machinery and equipment, making farmers' lives considerably easier.	Many machines are powered by diesel or petrol engines, releasing harmful gases through exhaust fumes. This affects the environment. It is the most well-known contaminant, but many others harm human health.	Exhaust fumes The quantity of human intervention in agriculture has decreased because of farmyard machinery and equipment, making farmers' lives considerably easier.

The current literature emphasizes the need for sophisticated detection methods to monitor and mitigate fertilizer pollution. Although several ion-selective membranes exist for NPK, they can only measure one target at a time, with significant interference during the detection process and a lack of portable detection methods and equipment [20]. In this scenario, electrochemical sensors are promising because they can detect multianalytes simultaneously, or many sensors can be integrated into a chip to provide simultaneous detection. It is crucial to check nitrate levels to avoid the adverse effects of excessive nitrate in the environment. Frequent measurements at a high spatial resolution over a large area are needed to understand the nitrate problem better and adjust nitrogen fertilizer inputs in agriculture. This can be achieved by setting up a network of sensors distributed across the area, as shown in figures 6.1(a) and (b). The ecosystem would benefit from real-time concentration data, which could be provided by nitrate sensors located at points where nitrate enters and accumulates. Each of these sensors can be represented by a white circle. Electrochemical sensors also facilitate inexpensive, real-time, field-deployable, and miniaturized sensors for monitoring NPK salts in various actual samples. This technique will benefit the agriculture industry (by using optimum pesticides, fertilizers, etc) and environmental regulators by furnishing reliable and accessible sensing capabilities for monitoring nutrients, bringing out better evaluation and control of these pollutants [21].

6.2.1 Benefits of employing electrochemical sensors for fertilizer detection

By maximizing food production and enabling higher yields with fewer fertilizers, applying sensors in agriculture boosts farmer earnings, addresses food insecurity, and enhances agriculture sustainability. There are significant environmental advantages to using sensors in agriculture. Approximately 30% of the nitrate fertilizer used

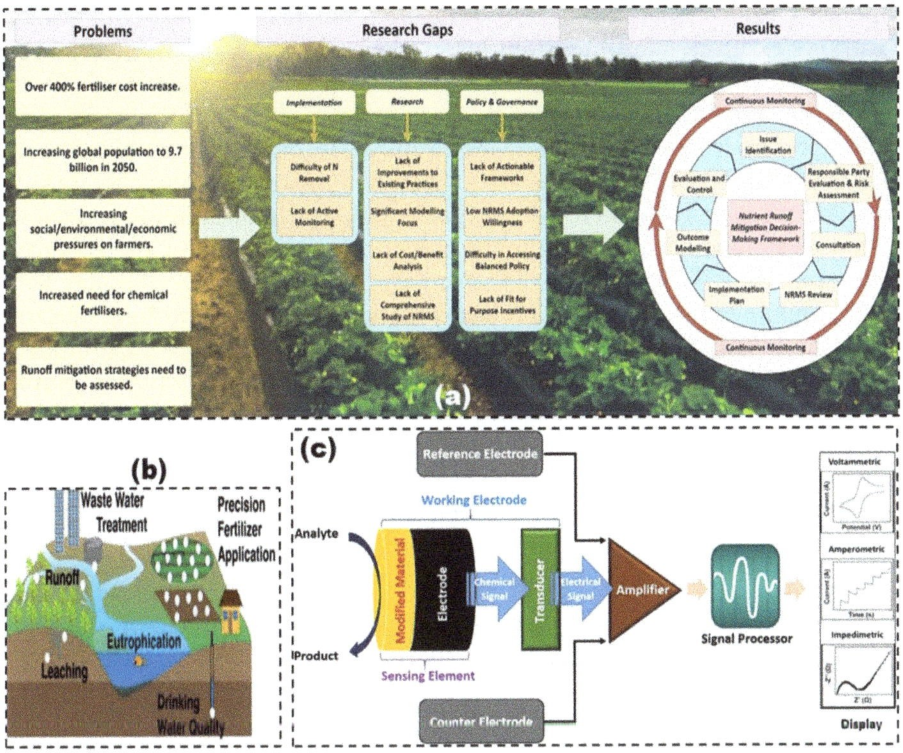

Figure 6.1. (a) Electrochemical sensor data could enable a site-specific nutrient runoff management framework with tailored recommendations for policymakers. Reprinted from [21], Copyright (2023), with permission from Elsevier. (b) One potential solution for mapping nitrate flow from fertilizer application to runoff is to use large-scale electrochemical sensors. These sensors can accurately measure and monitor nutrient levels, providing valuable data for researchers, policymakers, and farmers alike. Reproduced from [30]. CC BY 4.0. (c) A schematic diagram of a conventional electrochemical sensor provides a comprehensive representation of the sensor's internal structure and the critical components that enable it to detect the presence of a target analyte. Reprinted from [23], Copyright (2021), with permission from Elsevier.

on crops is thought to be washed away and contaminates lakes, streams, and seas. Thus, sensors can determine the exact quantity of fertilizer required, reducing the excess runoff and subsequent environmental contamination. The irrigation procedures can be optimized by using the data from sensors to determine when and how much water crops need at any time.

Agro-pollutants have been detected and monitored using voltage-calibrated techniques. These techniques utilize glassy carbon electrodes (GCEs), which enable continuous detection without requiring extra agents. Over time, various substrates have been studied to enhance electrode performance and facilitate voltammetric detection. These substrates include copper, nickel, boron-doped diamond (BDD), platinum, carbon, cadmium, alloys, gold, lead, and indium tin oxide [22]. The operation of electrochemical sensors is based on converting chemical information into electrical signals. These sensor systems typically comprise several key components, each crucial in detection. It includes the modifying material (catalyst), the working electrode substrate (transducer), the amplifier, and the signal processor (figure 6.1(c)) [23]. Despite these advances, a drawback was discovered: the bare electrode has a low electron transfer rate, and species generated during the electrochemical process tend to contaminate the electrode, leading to electrode passivation. Hence, modifying the surface is the most promising approach to improve sensitivity and selectivity significantly. Different organic and inorganic catalysts and enzymes can be used as modifiers to promote the reduction or oxidation of agro-pollutants, thereby enhancing the sensitivity and selectivity of electrodes. An emerging field in sensor technology is using carbon-based nanomaterials in working electrodes [24–29]. These nanomaterials include zero-dimensional (0D) carbon quantum dots (CQDs), one-dimensional (1D) CNTs, two-dimensional (2D) graphene, graphene oxide (GO), reduced graphene oxide (rGO), and three-dimensional (3D) carbon nanofibers. This chapter provides a brief overview of voltammetry as a practical sensing technique. It then describes how incorporating carbon-based nanomaterials in the fabrication process enhances sensitivity and limits detection in electrochemical sensors.

6.3 Necessity for detecting agricultural fertilizers/nutrient contamination from environmental samples

Inorganic fertilizers and organic fertilizers are the two main classifications of fertilizers. NPK is an example of an inorganic fertilizer, while compost, green manure, and bone meal are examples of organic fertilizers. NPK blends are the most commonly used mineral fertilizers in agriculture. They vary depending on the type of soil and crop [31–33]. They are often enriched with magnesium, calcium, and micronutrients such as manganese, iron, zinc, molybdenum, copper, and boron. These elements work together to improve plant metabolism, leading to increased crop growth and production [34]. Nutrient pollution is a phenomenon in which excessive amounts of nutrients, mainly nitrogen and phosphorus, are introduced into bodies of water. This nutrient overload acts as a fertilizer and causes an overgrowth of algae, known as eutrophication. As a result, the aquatic life in the affected water bodies is adversely affected [18]. Nutrients can runoff of land from (i) agricultural lands during the watering process or rain and (ii) urban areas where lawn and garden fertilizers are applied. Inorganic fertilizers often provide the three crucial macronutrients that crops require, i.e., NPK.

(i) **Phosphate fertilizers:** The growth of the plant's roots is aided by phosphorous fertilizers. Many soils in their natural state are low in readily available phosphorous and thus require fertilization to obtain the maximum possible yield. Phosphates are classified as organic phosphates, orthophosphates, and condensed phosphates (e.g., pyrometaphosphate and other polyphosphates). The two condensed phosphates are irrelevant to water quality regulation studies because they rapidly hydrolyze, converting to orthophosphates in natural waters [35]. Plants take up phosphorous in a water-soluble form of orthophosphates represented by the radicals PO_4^{3-}, HPO_4^{2-}, and $H_2PO_4^-$. Consequently, to meet the demand, fertilizer industries use around 95% of the approximately 150 million tons of phosphate rock worldwide yearly [36]. Phosphate rocks are naturally occurring mineral formations that contain calcium and phosphorus related to the apatite family. These ores contain traces of metal contamination, and the amount of metals in rock phosphate varies according to where they come from [37]. While sedimentary rocks have higher concentrations, igneous rocks have lower concentrations [38]. Thus, phosphorus fertilizers may contain heavy metals because heavy metals can exist as impurities in natural materials and minerals [39]. This heavy metal contamination from agricultural activities and its detection will be discussed in chapter 8. Reports indicate that mineral fertilizers have a major impact on contaminating agricultural soils. The accumulation of Cd in farming soils and watersheds is mainly caused by the application of mineral phosphate fertilizers. Likewise, many other heavy metal ions are introduced into the farmlands through mineral fertilizers, and recently the natural radioactivity and radiation hazards associated with mineral phosphate fertilizer production were also highlighted [40]. However, in the last few decades, we have seen a marked increase in research addressing the issues surrounding diffuse losses from agricultural land through leaching and surface runoffs possessing detrimental effects on environmental and water quality. Although agronomically the amount of phosphate lost per annum in runoff is generally inconsequential, from the water quality perspective even a minimal phosphorous concentration can cause water eutrophication.

(ii) **Potassium fertilizers:** K is a crucial fertilizer that aids in strengthening plants' disease resistance and protects the plant from harm during dry spells by bolstering its root system and preventing wilting. It is also an essential nutrient for photosynthesis. Despite soil containing over 20 000 ppm of potassium, plants can only use exchangeable potassium ions (K^+) found in soil (surface of soil particles) and water. The majority of field crops require 60–120 ppm of available K^+. It is interesting to note that insufficient potassium levels may lead to limited plant growth, decreased blooming, meager harvests, and substandard produce. Conversely, excessive water-soluble K^+ ions can impede seed sprouting and prevent the absorption of other vital nutrients. In numerous agrosystems, potassium is applied in the form of potassium chloride (KCl, muriate of potash) and potassium sulfate (K_2SO_4) [41], although potassium nitrate is rare. KCl is the widely applied potassium on farms, which is mined from rock deposits left by evaporites. Heavy crop production can rapidly deplete soil potassium, necessitating fertilizers to maintain crop yield quality. It is essential to monitor the soil's K^+ content to optimize fertilizer usage because different crops require a narrow range of usable soluble K^+. When leached from the farmlands, K^+ is known to cause salinization of the water process, affecting local fauna composition [42]. Attributed to its effect on salinity, K^+ acts indirectly in the toxicity even though it is present in minute concentration [43].

(iii) **Nitrogen fertilizers:** Unlike phosphorous and potassium, which are mineral forms, nitrogen is usually found in organic substances. Fertilizers, both inorganic and organic, contain sources of nitrogen. Nitrogen fertilizers are essential for plant growth, particularly in the middle of a plant's life when it requires support to keep growing big and produce new leaves [44]. When present in a water-based solution, nitrogen undergoes a three-stage transformation into ammonia, nitrite, and nitrate. The three ions are toxic to aquatic life-forms when these nutrients are deposited in excess [45]. Hence, detecting fertilizers is crucial for safeguarding the environment, human health, and food safety and promoting sustainable agriculture. The developed electrochemical sensors in the literature for these species are discussed below.

6.4 Carbon-based electrochemical sensors for nitrate, nitrite, urea, phosphate, and potassium

6.4.1 Nitrate sensing

Nitrate is a key fertilizer component in agriculture, often in nitrate (NO_3-N). Depending on the crop and field conditions, growers may apply several hundred pounds of nitrogen per acre, which can be expensive, with prices increasing rapidly. Despite studies showing that nitrate concentration in soil can vary significantly, fertilizer is typically applied uniformly across a field. Precision agriculture practitioners are designing site-specific management zones for more efficient nitrogen application, but measurement tools are limited. Nitrate ions are vital to the nitrogen cycle and necessary for plant growth and development. They are most frequently present in soil as roots absorb nitrogen and transfer it to leaves for photosynthesis. The natural nitrogen fixation process transforms nitrogen into a form that plants can utilize. Because they guarantee that crops can access the minerals they need, nitrate ions are also essential for soil fertility and agricultural output. The increased nitrate deposition in the used soil and water evaporation were caused by irrigated agricultural land in several arid and semiarid locations. The amount of nitrate that accumulated or leached varied depending on the circumstances. It has been detected in the soil depths because microorganisms nitrify fertilizers, converting them to nitrate. In addition, because nitrate is negatively charged, it can contaminate groundwater. Even during ideal conditions, plants utilize 50% of the nitrogenous fertilizers that are added to the soil, 2%–20% is lost via evaporation, 15%–25% reacts with organic compounds in the clay soil, and the remaining 2%–10% interferes with surface and groundwater [45]. Because nitrates dissolve in water, they move through the soil like soil water does. Hence, rain will wash nitrates down from the soil profile and may end up in other water bodies, such as rivers, lakes, ponds, estuaries, etc. This contamination comprises carcinogenic chemicals such as nitrosamines, particularly with hazardous buildup of nitrate (NO_3), nitrite (NO_2), and ammonia (NH_3) [44]. However, controlling nitrate ions can be difficult, necessitating close attention to crop management and soil testing. While it is possible to estimate the amount of nitrogen in growing plant material using optical remote sensing, assessing the NO_3-N content in soil involves collecting a soil sample and conducting a laboratory analysis using time-consuming chromatography or spectrographic methods. Due to its high mobility, nitrate concentrations vary over time, which makes it very difficult to obtain accurate measurements. There are models available that can estimate nitrate fluxes based on measurements taken at the beginning and end of a season; however, these models rely on many estimations and assumptions. Hence, portable and user-friendly electrochemical sensors are reviewed in this section to detect nitrate. Here, let us discuss the carbon-based nitrate electrochemical sensors reported in the literature.

Hussein *et al* [46] have fabricated an electrochemical sensor for nitrate using commercially available screen-printed electrodes (SPEs) coated with carbon, either carbon nanofibers (CNF) or single-walled carbon nanotubes (SWCNT). Both these carbon SPEs were modified by employing spontaneous Pd deposition followed by the next step, the galvanostatic electrodeposition of copper. The two electrodes were designated as Pd–Cu modified SWCNT SPE and Pd–Cu modified CNF SPE, respectively. The Pd–Cu modified SWCNT-SPE was fabricated, and the electrode regions initially formed a compact covering of aggregated Pd nanoparticles (NPs). This reduced the accessible carbon surface for copper nucleation and growth and resulted in a significantly higher Pd/Cu volume ratio in the SWCNT instance. As a consequence, in addition to the large micrometer-sized copper crystals that first appeared in the macro defects of the carbon structure, a finer copper deposit grew on the surface of Pd-modified SWCNT. Due to this, and the possibility of close contact between Cu and Pd in the Pd NP-populated areas, a stable and sensitive electro-analytical signal for nitrate reduction was developed. Comparatively, while fabricating Pd–Cu modified CNF, the large-sized, well-separated Cu particles nucleated and grew on the CNF-based bi-metal modified electrode. However, they remained unstable upon exposure to nitrate ions. The scanning electron microscope (SEM) images show two types of bi-metal modified electrodes, CNF and SWCNT, showing a significant difference in the distribution of the two metallic phases (figures 6.2(a) and (b)). In the case of SWCNT, the amount of Pd is three times as much as that in CNF. A possible reason for this difference is the under-potential deposition of Cu, which is known to occur on Pd and not on carbon electrodes. As in the case of SWCNT-SPE, upon the significant coverage of Pd, the under-potential deposition process will presumably dominate initially and consume the available Cu ions, thus impeding the nucleation and growth on the Pd-free carbon surface. Therefore, the designed and constructed bi-metal modified SWCNT-SPE represented a more significant opportunity for the electroanalytical determination of nitrate in acidic solutions with a wide linear range and limit of detection (LOD) of 52.0 μmol dm^{-3} (figure 6.2(c)). The Langmuir equation was used to model the nitrate reduction currents' non-linear concentration dependency, which was then applied to recovery calculations. The sensitivity, reproducible signal, and stability of the metallic phases over extended nitrate reduction determination series were higher in Pd–Cu modified SWCNT-SPE.

Ali *et al* [47] have developed a bio-impedimetric nitrate sensor based on poly(3,4-ethylenedioxythiophene) (PEDOT) nanofibers (NFs) and GO composite. The PEDOT NFs surface strongly interacted with the GO sheets due to pi–pi and

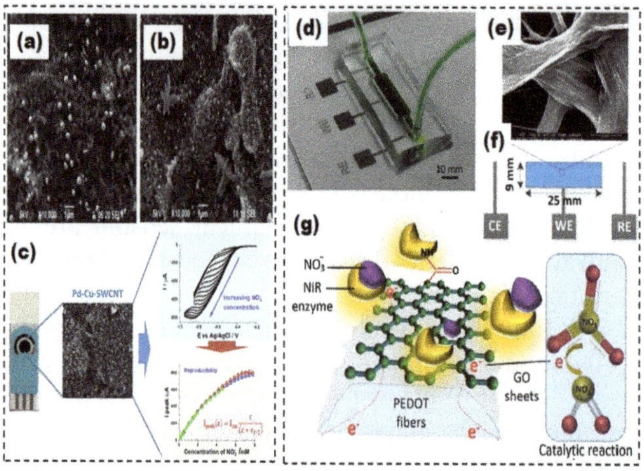

Figure 6.2. SEM images of (a) Pd–Cu modified CNF and (b) Pd–Cu modified SWCNT. (c) Graphical representation of Pd–Cu modified SWCNT-SPE for nitrate detection. Reprinted from [46], Copyright (2023), with permission from Elsevier. (d) Photograph of the constructed sensor using PEDOT NFs-GO. (e) SEM image of PEDOT NFs-GO composite. (f) Layout and the geometry of the working electrode. (g) Illustration of the surface-immobilized PEDOT NFs-GO with NiR enzyme sensor. Reprinted from [47], Copyright (2017), with permission from Elsevier.

electrostatic interactions on which nitrate reductase (NiR) was immobilized. The constructed sensor was labeled NiR/PEDOT NFs-GO films (figure 6.2(d–g)). The NiR enzyme molecules immobilized onto the PEDOT NFs-GO surface favored specific detection of nitrate ions, even when other interfering species from agriculture soils were present. The strong covalent coupling of the NiR enzyme molecules with the several functional groups on GO produced an elevated R_{ct} value. The PEDOT NFs-GO composite's wide electrochemical surface area enhanced the working electrode's NiR enzyme loading capacity, extending the sensor's range of dynamic detection concentrations. The sensitivity was improved over the test range of 0.044–442.0 mg l^{-1} (7.09–7128.0 μM) nitrate ions because of the GO incorporation. The sensor displayed excellent selectivity, stability, and repeatability. The prospect of this work is to construct an array of electrodes with specific recognition molecules, and attempts are being made to employ microfluidic technology to detect multiple ions.

6.4.2 Nitrite sensing

Nitrite contamination in water, food, and environmental samples is a severe risk to human health because it can transform into cancer-causing substances. Given its profound ecological and physiological effects, accurate and sensitive nitrite surveillance is crucial to address the detrimental impact on terrestrial and aquatic ecosystems. Therefore, we reviewed the literature to find the following reports on nitrite sensing using electrochemical sensors. Many 0D, 1D, 2D, and 3D nanomaterials with excellent chemical and physical traits have modified the GCE to promote catalytic and electron transport properties.

6.4.2.1 0D nanocatalysts

CQDs 0D carbon nanomaterials with size <10 nm boast exceptional characteristics that make them highly desirable for various applications. These include their low toxicity, chemical stability, favorable biocompatibility, affordability of raw materials for synthesis, and ability to serve as electron donors and acceptors. As a result, they have been widely and effectively utilized in electrochemical sensors.

Multiple studies have confirmed that composites made by combining highly conductive conducting polymers with carbon materials can significantly improve the conductivity of carbon materials [48, 49]. These composites also enhance the selectivity and sensitivity of sensors that use them. Building on these findings, Li *et al* [48], via a one-pot technique, synthesized a composite comprised of polyethyleneimine (PEI), a conducting polymer, and CQDs (PEI-CQDs). During the production of CQDs, a water-soluble cationic polyelectrolyte called PEI, which contained the required N atom and amino group (-NH_2), was used as a precursor. The amino functionalization and N-doping of the CQDs were carried out simultaneously. This composite served as the foundation for a susceptible electrochemical sensor for nitrite. As a result of N-doping, the electrocatalytic activity of the CQDs was enhanced, while their electrical conductivity and dispersibility were improved due to amino functionalization. Additionally, the numerous amino-functional groups on the surface of the prepared PEI-CQDs are beneficial for the selective detection of nitrite due to the interaction between the nitrite and amino groups. The results demonstrate the excellent nitrite detection performance of the proposed electrochemical sensor based on PEI-CQDs. The sensor's sensitivity and selectivity were improved in slightly acidic conditions through electrostatic contact and hydrogen bonding between the protonated amino groups of PEI-CQDs and nitrite. The sensor operated with a linear range of 0.0–1000.0 and 20.0–380.0 μM, with a low detection limit of 2.87 and 1.16 μM. It has strong selectivity for nitrite detection and remarkable repeatability, and it can be stored for long periods without losing stability. This sensor successfully measured nitrite levels in milk samples, bottled drinking water, and tap water, indicating its potential for detecting nitrite in food, the environment, and other applications.

Feng *et al* [50] constructed a sensitive electrochemical sensor for nitrite detection using an Au@CQDs-MXene nanocomposite. Xylan-derived CQDs were utilized as environmentally-friendly in situ reducing agents to synthesize AuNPs and produce a nanocomposite. Afterward, the Au@CQDs were affixed to the surface of MXene, resulting in the formation of the Au@CQDs-MXene nanocomposite. Notably, no chemical-reducing agents were employed throughout the green one-pot synthesis of this nanocomposite. Researchers used CQDs to avoid harmful chemicals and produce gold nanoparticles (AuNPs). CQDs possess hydroxyl groups, allowing them to reduce chemicals sustainably and effectively. This makes them a good choice for lowering agents in green chemistry. CQDs can also be used as a site to grow AuNPs in a controlled manner. Despite its nanophase properties, Au@CQDs tend to agglomerate easily, requiring attachment sites to prevent this from occurring. However, MXene is a novel 2D inorganic compound with a unique layered structure [51]. This arrangement offers a vast specific surface area with numerous functional groups on its surface. These groups can function as a fixed foundation to distribute Au@CQDs. Furthermore, the high electronic conductivity property of MXene can aid in constructing a modified electrode of Au@CQDs-MXene nanomaterial, which is highly sensitive. Meanwhile, Au@CQDs can prevent the aggregation of MXene. Furthermore, creditable to its excellent conductivity, Au@CQDs overcome the adverse effects of excess oxygen-containing functional groups on MXene. The Au@CQDs-MXene nanocomposite aided in the oxidation reaction of nitrite. Its synthesis involved a one-pot method with as-prepared CQDs and MXene, making it easy and convenient to operate. The sensor shows a good linear correlation between nitrite concentration and differential pulse voltammetric peak current, and is divided into two linear ranges based on nitrite concentration. The first detection range is between 1.0 and 500.0 μM, while the second range is between 500.0 and 3200.0 μM. The estimated detection limit for nitrite concentration was 0.078 μM. Notably, the sensor was found to be effective in the detection of nitrite in tap water and salted vegetables. Thus, the Au@CQDs-MXene/GCE sensor holds promise for the accurate and rapid detection of nitrite in various environmental and food samples.

6.4.2.2 1D nanocatalysts

Mounesh *et al* [52] have prepared a nickel tetra-substituted 6-bromobenzothiazole carboxamide nickel (II) phthalocyanine (NiTBBTCAPc)-MWCNTs catalyst for investigating the nitrite oxidation reaction. The sensor was fabricated by drop coating the NiTBBTCAPc-MWCNTs onto the priorly polished GCE to obtain a film-modified electrode. A reasonable charge transfer behavior was observed for NiTBBTCAPc-MWCNTS, which is creditable to the enhanced surface area (possessing more excellent edge basal/plane ratio) and high electrical conductivity of MWCNTs. An improved catalytic response was attributed to the sensor's good stability, high proton conductivity, and possible multi-charge transfer. The CV and DPV results demonstrated that the modified electrode portrays good electroanalytical performance with a lower detection limit (CA: 6.0 nM) and greater sensitivity with a linear range from 50.0 to 500.0 nM. The sensor demonstrated selectivity for nitrite in the presence of excess organic molecules and inorganic ions. It was successfully validated in drinking water and food samples for real-time applications. The same group (Mounesh *et al*) [53] subsequently developed a tetra-4-(2-methoxyphenoxy) carboxamide cobalt(II) amide bridged phthalocyanine (CoTMePhCAPc) with composite MWCNTs for the simultaneous detection of nitrite and hydrogen peroxide (H_2O_2). The sensor was constructed by scattering the CoTMePh CAPc/MWCNTs suspension onto the GCE surface and allowed to dry. The developed sensor was an effective promoter of kinetics, i.e., the electrochemical oxidation of nitrite with good stability and potential for multi-charge transfer trait. MWCNTs contributed to the enhanced sensitive and selective electrocatalytic sensing of nitrite ions (figure 6.3(a)). On the other hand, Lu *et al* [54] have also employed cobalt(II) phthalocyanine (CoPc) as the catalyst for nitrite sensing; however, their LOD value (2.11 μM using the DPV technique) was not significant compared to the CoTMePh CAPc/MWCNTs/GCE.

Salhi *et al* [55] constructed a sensor by electropolymerized 1,8-diamino naphthalene (1,8-DAN) onto the functionalized MWCNT/carbon paste electrode

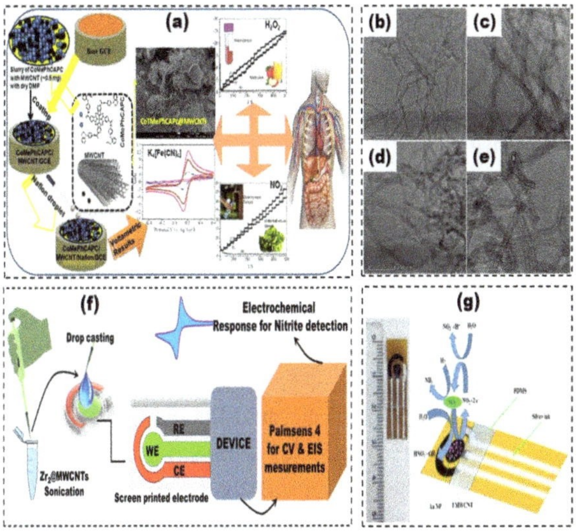

Figure 6.3. (a) Schematic illustrations of CoTMePh CAPc/MWCNTs/GCE fabrication and its application for nitrite sensing. Reprinted with permission from [53]. Copyright (2023) American Chemical Society. TEM images: (b) and (c) before 1,8-DAN polymerization, (d) and (e) after 1,8-DAN polymerization. Reproduced from [55]. CC BY 4.0. (f) Schematics of SPE modification with ZrO_2@MWCNTs catalyst and the electrochemical setup. (g) A photograph of the fabricated modified LIG sensor and the possible mechanism of nitrite oxidation at LIG/f-MWNCT-AuNPs. Reprinted from [57], Copyright (2021), with permission from Elsevier.

(1,8-DAN/f-MWCNT/CPE). Figure 6.3 depicts the TEM images before (figures 6.3(b) and (c)) and after (figures 6.3(d) and (e)) 1,8-DAN polymerization onto the f-MWCNTs. Electrocatalytic effects of 1,8-DAN/f-MWCNT/CPE towards nitrite were noted. Likewise, reports from Zhen *et al*, Rajalakshmi *et al*, Huang *et al*, and Arulraj *et al* [58–61] elucidate the synergistic effect of MWCNTs combined with conducting polymers that promote nitrite sensing.

Rajab *et al* [56] developed an electrochemical assay employing a disposable nanosensor chip with a catalyst ZrO_2@MWCNTs that portrayed good conductivity, electrocatalytic activity, sensitivity, and selectivity (figure 6.3(f)). The voltammetric (lower overpotential), impedimetric patterns (least charge transfer), and chronoamperograms (dynamic linear range: 5.0–100.0 μM and LOD: 0.94 μM) supported the excellent performance of the sensor. The sensor's reproducibility and stability were satisfactory, and the natural water and food sample analyses were reliable for their accuracy. The MWCNT composite sensor shows potential for developing portable analysis systems that can be used for direct on-site determination of nitrite levels, based on the available data. Additionally, no previous experience is necessary to operate the system. This disposable SPE had the extra advantage of preventing contamination by sample impurities, and a lower sample volume was sufficient for analysis. Nasraoui *et al* [57] reported a laser-induced graphene (LIG) electrode patterned onto a flexible poly(imide) substrate. Subsequently, they modified by carboxylic functionalized MWCNT (f-MWCNT) and Au nanoparticles (AuNPs) film. The study developed 3D porous carbonaceous co-planar electrodes using a laser source and motorized stage. LIG-patterned electrodes were designed on a Kapton into black, and a 3D carbonaceous material was generated with a thickness greater than 10.0 μM. The prepared LIG was then modified by drop coating f-MWCNT and subsequently with AuNP suspension and designated as LIG/f-MWNCT-AuNPs (figure 6.3(g)). Excellent synergies between MWCNT and AuNPs favored catalytic oxidation of nitrite and were insensitive to the presence of common interfering species. The LIG/f-MWNCT-AuNPs portrayed a dynamic range from 10.0 to 140.0 μM with an LOD of 0.9 μM. Thus, modified LIG can be used for nitrite on-site monitoring while circumventing more traditional and costly analytical techniques like chromatography and spectrophotometry. More interestingly, they are prepared more cost-efficiently using a flexible platform.

MWCNTs have been proposed as metal catalyst support for electrocatalytic and sensing of nitrite ascribed to their high chemical stability and surface-to-volume ratio, with unique electrical properties. Metal particles decorated MWCNTs such as silver-electrode coated CNTs-epoxy composite (Ag-CNT electrode) [62] and carboxymethyl cellulose (CMC) stabilized Cu nanoparticles decorated MWCNTs (carboxylic functionalized) (Cu/MWCNTs/GC) are the metal supported MWCNTs composite sensors developed for nitrite quantification [63].

Thus, MWCNTs decorated with phthalocyanines, conducting polymers, and metal nanoparticles were prepared to introduce additional functionality to MWCNTs and enhance the available surface for catalysis.

6.4.2.3 2D nanocatalysts

2D graphene-based composites exhibit good physiochemical features, including ease of modification or functionalization, variable form, and size. We will next examine the sensing capabilities of graphene and further explore its unique traits for its potential nitrite sensing applications. Hence, initially, we investigate GO-polymer composite followed by rGO-polymer composite, and subsequently nanoparticles and enzyme.

Valsalakumar *et al* [64] synthesized an electroactive polyaniline-graphene oxide composite, which includes hexagonal zirconium phosphate disks (PGZrP), that served as the basis for a sophisticated electrochemical sensor that can accurately detect nitrite in a variety of biological and aqueous environments. PGZrP-modified GCE displayed a sharp and precise anodic peak with good electroconductive and electrocatalytic proficiency in determining nitrite ions. The response signals demonstrate that the PG composite facilitated excellent anchoring sites for nanoparticles (ZrP) and provided more electroactive sites for the anodic nitrite reaction (figure 6.4(a)). The synergy between the PG and ZrP resulted in an enhanced electrochemical sensing capability with a linear operational range from 0.124 μM to 4000.0 μM and an LOD of 80.0 nM. Furthermore, the proposed sensor was validated to precisely quantify nitrite concentrations from aquatic and biological real samples. These results indicated an enhanced electrochemical performance of PGZrP/GCE characterized by commendable operational stability, robust repeatability, and reproducibility. Furthermore, Li *et al* [65] have constructed non-enzymatic electrochemical sensors for nitrite based on methyl red and GO

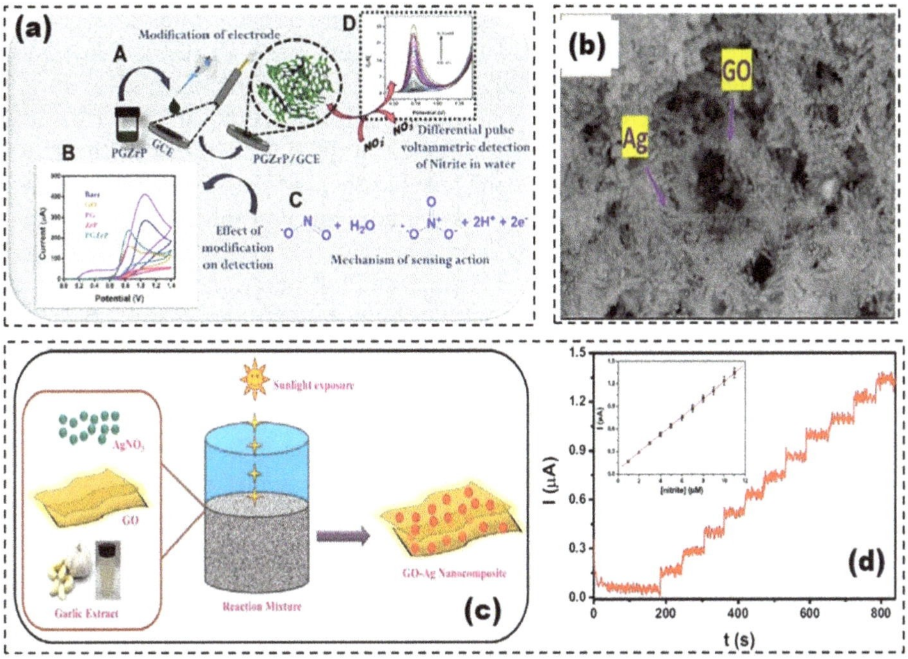

Figure 6.4. (a) Construction of PGZrP-modified GCE: A. GCE modified with PGZrP, B. Cyclic voltammetric response of nitrite at various electrodes used in the study, C. Possible mechanism of nitrite oxidation at the proposed electrode, D. Quantification of nitrite employing DOV technique. Reprinted with permission from [64]. Copyright (2023) American Chemical Society. (b) SEM image of GC/GO/Ag NPs: a catalyst for nitrite sensing. [66]. CC BY 4.0. (c) Preparation of GO-Ag composite. (d) Amperometric *i–t* curve obtained at GC/GO-Ag modified electrode for subsequent addition of 1.0 μM nitrite in 0.1 M PBS at a regular interval of 60 s. Inset: Calibration curve: I_{pa} versus concentration of nitrite. Reprinted from [67], Copyright (2015), with permission from Elsevier.

nanocomposite-modified carbon paste electrodes (MR/GO/CPE). The MR/GO composite was prepared via ultrasonic dispersion, composed of 5 mg of GO and 2 mg of MR in 4 ml DMF. Subsequently, the resultant suspension was drop-coated and dried under infrared irradiation. Next, to construct MR/rGO/CPE, the modified electrode was introduced into an aqueous colloidal solution in the presence of NaCl, wherein the GO sheets were electrochemically reduced with a reduction peak potential of −1.2 V. The electrochemical reduction of GO led to an enhancement in the performance of MR/GO/CPE. The reliable reaction between GO sheets and MR is indicated by the more significant catalytic response current. This suggests that the oxygen-containing functional groups on GO play a crucial role in the reaction. The functional groups on the surface of rGO were decreased following the electrochemical reduction of GO. This lowers the interaction between the amino group of MR and the carboxyl and oxygen functional groups on rGO, reducing MR's loading and stability on rGO nanosheets. Because of this, MR/rGO/CPE is less stable and has a lower electrocatalytic current than MR/GO/CPE. Amperometric quantification yielded a wide linear range from 5.0 to 7000.0 μM with an LOD of

0.011 μM. Attributed to hydrophilic oxygenated functional groups (–OH, –C–O–C–, –COOH) present on GO favor its monolayer sheets dispersion in aqueous solutions, making it amphiphilic with hydrophobic basal planes and hydrophilic edges. Consequently, MR/GO/CPE was more stable when crosslinked with the MR cationic dye and synergistically enabled electrocatalytic activity for nitrite ions. In addition, the FESEM micrographs depicted that the surface of MR/GC with high-density holes and crevasses was created as a consequence of the assembly of MR on the GO sheets. This enables greater surface area available at MR/GO/CPE for nitrite determination. Furthermore, MR/GO/CPE displayed a good anti-interference trait against a few organic molecules and several inorganic species. The proposed sensor was evaluated for good recoveries from real samples, validating its proficient practical application.

On the contrary, Guo *et al* [68] constructed a composite electrode consisting of a paste electrode made of reduced graphene oxide (rGO-PE) and poly-neutral red (pNR), which could be used as an accurate and sensitive electrochemical sensor to measure the amount of nitrate. The electropolymerization method was employed to produce pNR/rGO-PE. SEM and x-ray diffraction (XRD) analyses confirmed that the electropolymerization of neutral red on rGO-PE was successful. Electrochemical experiments using CV and amperometry demonstrated that adding rGO nanosheets to the conducting NR polymer resulted in an improved electrochemical response of the modified electrode with exceptional selectivity and sensitivity of 0.015 11 μA μM^{-1}. Moreover, the modified electrode exhibited a stable and wide linear range from 0.0 to 14 000.0 μM. The sensor detected low nitrite levels, with a detection limit of 17.0 nM, attributed to the electrode's electrochemical responsiveness enhanced by adding rGO nanosheets to conducting NR polymers with synergistic effects. For the amperometric real sample analysis, the obtained relative standard deviation (RSD) values (3.56%–4.78%) and recovery values (90.00%–96.66%) were satisfactory, indicating validity and practical usability.

To determine nitrite in real water samples, a sensitive and straightforward electrochemical sensor was proposed by Ezzat *et al* [66] to prepare silver nanoparticles through a green synthesis approach and coat them onto GO support. Upon SEM confirmation, the sensor was designated as GC/GO/Ag NPs (figure 6.4(b)). This is attributable to the synergism of GO sheets and Ag NPs and their unique traits as modifying agents that magnified the nitrite electrochemical response current. GO in silver composite amplified the surface area and charge transfer process. Using a chronoamperometric (CA) approach, this sensor reported satisfactory LOD values for nitrite detection in acidic, neutral, and alkaline mediums. GC/GO/Ag NPs also demonstrated anti-fouling characteristics in the presence of various organic and inorganic substances. Additionally, the sensor was validated for its effective performance in detecting nitrites from tape and wastewater samples.

Ikhsan *et al* [67] reported a simple method for the synthesis of Ag NPs on GO sheets through the use of an aqueous garlic extract and exposure to bright sunlight. The garlic extract functioned as both a reducing and stabilizing agent for Ag NPs during the sunlight-induced process, while the GO sheets provided effective stabilization for the growth of Ag NPs (figure 6.4(c)). The GO-Ag composite modified GCE (GC/GO-Ag) was constructed by drop coating GO-Ag dispersion. GO-Ag composite modified electrode facilitated fast charge transfer kinetics, the synergistic catalytic effect of Ag NPs, and GO towards nitrite anodic reaction. The sensor represented good selectivity for nitrite ions in the presence of other common interferents, such as inorganic ions. Amperometric *i–t* curve quantification presented a LOD value of 37.0 nM, which is well below the World Health Organization (WHO) guidance level of 65.0 μM for the short term and a provisional guidelines concentration of 4.3 μM over the long term for nitrite ions (figure 6.4(d)). Finally, GC/GO-Ag was verified for practical applicability with a good recovery percentage from real lake water samples.

The above studies expressed graphene-based composites using conducting polymers and nanoparticles (metal oxide). Xu *et al* [69] designed and developed a wireless, portable, cost-efficient smartphone-based electrochemical sensor employing CV and CA techniques. The sensor was fabricated via in situ electrochemical modification of a screen-printed carbon electrode (SPCE), as depicted in figure 6.5(a). First, GO suspension was coated onto the SPCE, followed by electrochemical reduction to rGO by CV method. Onto this, Ni nanoparticles were electrodeposited employing the CA method. Next, the prepared Ni/rGO/space was transformed to NiO/rGO/SPCE using $Ni(NO_3)_2$ with the aid of the CV technique. Finally, $HAuCl_4$ solution was spotted on the NiO/rGO/SPCE, and CA was applied to obtain Au/NiO/rGO/SPCE-the—the proposed sensor depicted good conductivity, which is attributed to rGO's accelerated charge transfer process. The

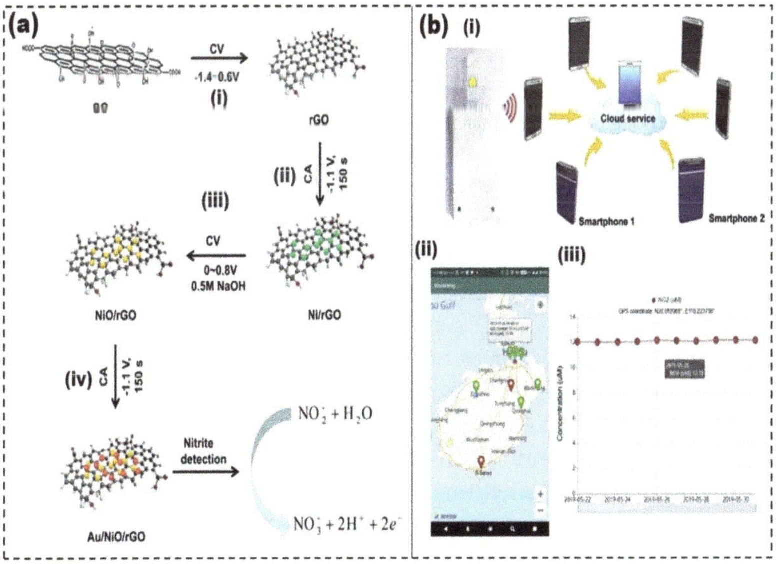

Figure 6.5. (a) Au/NiO/rGO composite preparation on SPCE via electrochemical deposition. (b) (i) Illustration of collecting nitrite contamination information from various locations to the Cloud server. (ii) Nitrite contamination details (spatiotemporal) aided by using Google Maps interface. (iii) Nitrite level tracking as a function of time per location. Reprinted from [69], Copyright (2020), with permission from Elsevier.

conductivity was attributed to the synergistic effects of the catalysts applied on SPCE. The sensor was employed in efficient water quality detection using a smartphone-based system employed DPV with a detection limit of 0.2μM, which is lower than the maximum allowable limit in drinking as per WHO. The smartphone operated the detector, displayed the detection results, and connected the device to the Cloud using a Home Mage Android application. The handheld detector, weighing around 42 g, was intended to stimulate signals to the altered SPCE and send the reaction data wirelessly to the smartphone using Bluetooth (figure 6.5(b)). It is possible to greatly increase participation in environmental monitoring programs by utilizing a smartphone-based platform.

6.4.2.4 3D nanocatalysts

Yue *et al* [70] produced porous carbon (PC) materials with a 3D structure through the pyrolysis of organic salts. These organic salts—sodium tartrate, sodium malate, and sodium succinate—had varying hydroxyl groups on their side chains. The researchers also studied the production process of these carbon materials with pores. For the purpose of detecting nitrite, electrochemical sensors were developed using three different carbon materials. The PC produced from sodium tartrate, or PC_{ST} for short, exhibited the best electrocatalytic performance for oxidizing nitrite among the three materials. This can be attributed to several factors. First, PC_{ST} possesses a high degree of graphitization, which promotes electron mobility and stabilizes reactive intermediates in radical-involved catalytic systems. Second, PC_{ST}/GCE boasts larger practical surface areas, facilitating electron transfer and enhancing electrocatalytic performance. In conclusion, PC_{ST}/GCE proved to be the most effective in terms of electrocatalytic performance. Finally, PC_{ST} exhibits mesoporous structures and abundant sp^3 C, which provide ample active sites for electrocatalytic reactions. The sensors created using PC_{ST} allowed for the swift detection of nitrite within a broad linear range of 0.1–100.0 μM, with a low detection limit of 0.043 μM. The sensor was applied to test nitrite levels in meat samples, and the results were consistent. However, Yue *et al* hypothesized that a correlation may exist between the hydroxyl group content in organic salt precursors' side chain and the morphology of PC, leading to consistent electrochemical catalytic activity. However, after conducting various experiments, they observed that while the hydroxyl groups impact the PC's morphology, their effect on electrochemical performance is not as significant as anticipated. This could be due to several other influencing factors that affect electrochemical catalytic activity, such as material type, geometry, 'surface, and energy factors. Further analysis of these factors is necessary to understand better their impact on electrochemical catalytic activity, which will be the focus of their future research efforts.

Wu *et al* [71] presented an amperometric sensor to detect nitrite. The sensor utilized a 3D network of Ni_7S_6 and MWCNTs to enhance sensitivity, with the large specific surface area of Ni_7S_6 and the good electrical conductivity of the MWCNTs playing a pivotal role. The synergy between Ni_7S_6 and the MWCNTs also contributed to the sensor's high sensitivity. Meanwhile, Zhu *et al* [72] proposed electrochemical nitrite sensing using carbon fiber paper (CFP) treated with air annealing (OCFP). The CFP underwent a process that resulted in an increase of defective edge/plane sites, oxygen-containing functional groups, surface roughness, and wettability. Electrochemical studies revealed that the OCFP exhibited outstanding nitrite sensitivity.

The other electrodes reported for nitrite are BDD electrodes that are highly sought-after in electroanalytical applications [73], which can be credited to their exceptional properties, such as a broad potential window and remarkably low background current. These characteristics crucially favored accurate electroanalysis of nitrite. Biochar, a carbon-rich material produced by biomass pyrolysis, has proven to be an excellent support for AuNPs. This is due to its unique properties, which include a high surface area, ample surface functional groups, superb electrical conductivity, and eco-friendliness. Zhang *et al* [74] developed an electrochemical sensor to detect nitrite, which is based on biochar immobilized gold nanoparticles (BC/Au).

6.4.3 Urea sensing

Urea is a vital component of modern agriculture that provides plants with a readily available source of nitrogen, which is necessary for their growth. It is a popular choice among farmers worldwide because it is cost-effective, versatile, and has a high nitrogen content. However, excessive fertilizer use can increase the environmental footprint and significantly threaten annual food production. Urea, a common type of fertilizer, can also negatively affect soil pH and natural fertility, ultimately reducing the productivity of food crops. Several methods are available to detect urea levels. In this section, we will discuss the electrochemical sensors that have been reported.

6.4.3.1 1D composite sensors

T H V Kumar and his team [75] synthesized silver nanoparticles decorated nitrogen-doped single-walled carbon nanotubes (Ag-N-SWCNTs) using melamine as the nitrogen source. They developed an electrochemical urea sensor by modifying GCE with Ag-N-SWCNTs and a layer of Nafion (Nf/Ag-N-SWCNTs/GCE) (figure 6.6(a)). The nitrogen-doping process significantly altered the properties of the SWCNT, making it more suitable for the attachment of Ag-NPs. The Ag-N-SWCNTs nanocomposite showed great catalytic activity due to the combination of the electrical properties and high surface area of N-SWCNTs with Ag-NPs. Therefore, the sensor could detect urea at concentrations as low as 4.7 nM. The researchers also tested the reliability of the sensor by successfully employing it to determine urea in milk and tap water samples. This sensor can help detect urea in food, fertilizer industries, and environmental fields.

Magar and colleagues [76] synthesized a nanocomposite of metal oxide nanostructures (CuO/Co_3O_4) and MWCNTs (CuO/Co_3O_4@MWCNTs), exhibiting synergetic electrocatalytic properties. This nanocomposite was used as an electrocatalyst for detecting urea, and a direct sensing platform was developed for impedimetric detection of urea in actual samples. Disposable SPEs modified with the nanocomposite showed a high sensitivity of 0.223 pM and selectivity towards urea,

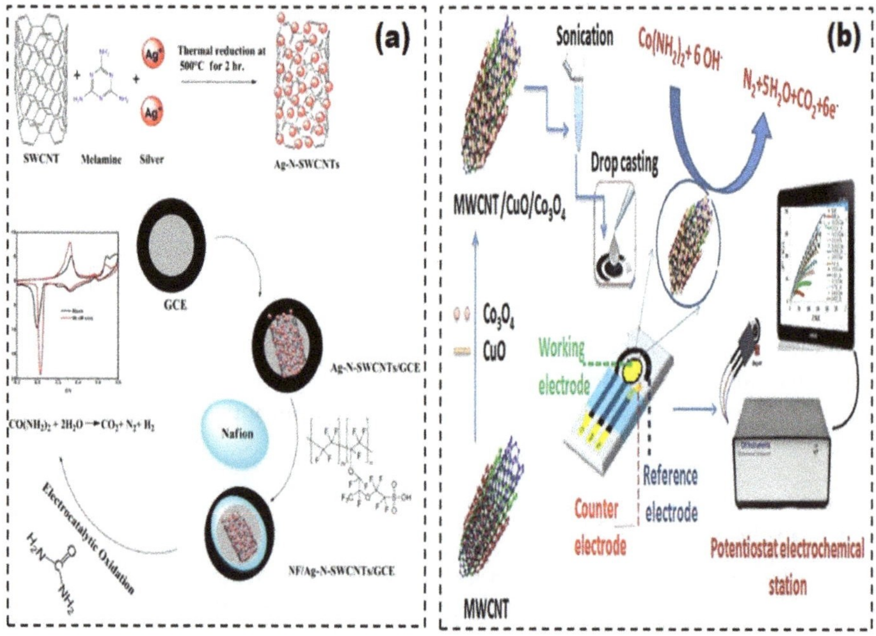

Figure 6.6. (a) Graphical representation of Ag-N-SWCNTs preparation and its subsequent application in urea sensing. Reproduced from [75]. CC BY 4.0. (b) Schematic illustration depicting the construction steps of CuO/Co_3O_4@MWCNTs sensor for urea oxidation. Reproduced from [76]. CC BY 4.0.

even when exposed to nontargeting molecules (figure 6.6(b)). The developed sensor was used for fast and direct urea determination in food and environmental samples for quality assurance.

6.4.3.2 2D composite sensors

In the field of electrochemical biosensors, Baabu *et al* [77] fabricated a urea biosensor by mixing manganese oxide (MnO_2) with rGO in a chitosan solution and subsequently adding a urease enzyme. This composite was coated on the Pt electrode (Pt/MnO_2/rGO/Urease), as shown in figure 6.7(a). The urea biosensor depicted an excellent linear range of detection, low detection limit, and selectivity. The sensor uses a novel mechanism involving an enzymatic-nanocomposite ensemble and Ni^{3+} ion center in the urease enzyme (figure 6.7(b)). This work could lead to real-time biosensors for detecting nitrogen fertilizers in plant roots to ensure healthy growth.

Dutta *et al* [78] developed a urea sensor that does not require enzymes, using a composite of SnO_2 quantum dots (QDs) and rGO (figure 6.7(c)). The SnO_2 QDs/rGO (SRGO) composite was found to be an excellent sensing probe due to its constituents' synergistic effect. The researchers developed a two-step method to synthesize the SRGO composite, which involves loading rGO sheets with SnO_2 QDs. The QDs prevent the restacking of graphene layers, which is a significant challenge fabricators face. Reduced restacking of graphene sheets results in a higher

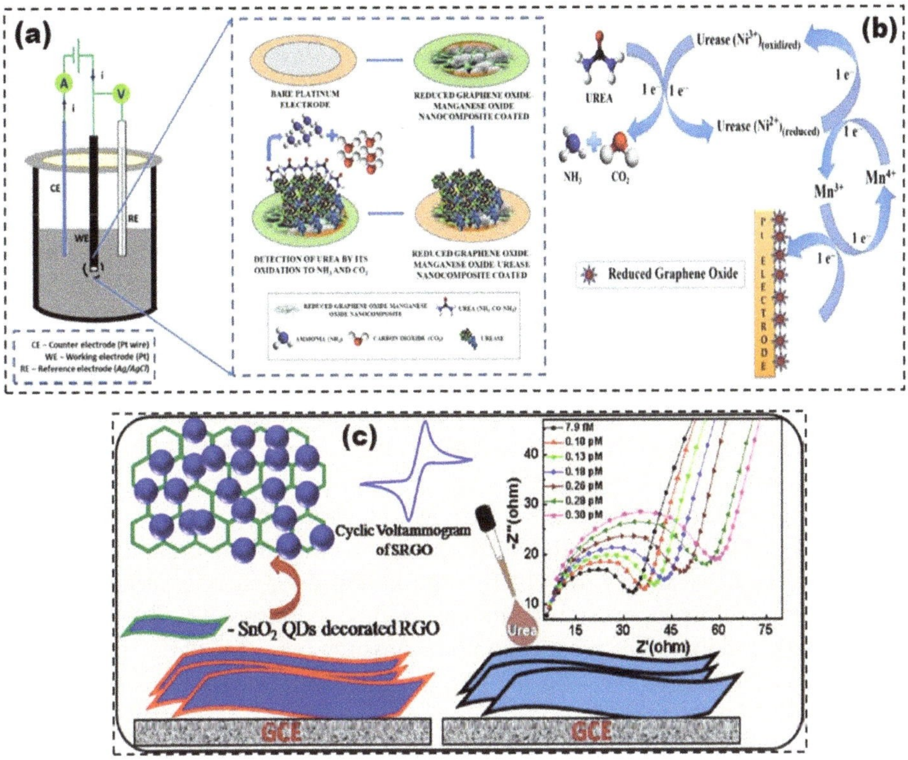

Figure 6.7. (a) Schematic illustration of a three-electrode setup along with sketches of surface immobilization by urease-MnO_2/rGO composite assembled over the chitosan matrix. (b) Schematic representation of urea detection. Reprinted from [77], Copyright (2020), with permission from Springer. (c) SnO_2 QDs/rGO (SRGO) composite. Reprinted with permission from [78]. Copyright (2014) American Chemical Society.

surface area for SRGO, which is a desirable characteristic for any suitable sensor. The SRGO-based enzyme-free sensor has been successfully used by amperometry to develop an efficient sensor for urea. The low detection limit of the sensor makes it promising for practical use in detecting urea in environmental samples with great ease.

Babitha and her colleagues [79] have prepared a composite material by reducing GO with nascent hydrogen using metallic zinc. The zinc was obtained as a waste by-product from an industry. The composite material comprises zinc oxide (ZnO) nanostructures and rGO nanosheets (ZnO@rGO). Combining these two materials' architecture on the electrode surface provided an excellent active surface area, improved immobilization of the target molecule urea, and a more efficient electron transfer.

6.4.4 Phosphate and potassium sensing

Phosphate-based fertilizers in agriculture are a significant source of water contamination, leading to eutrophication and algal blooms. These blooms harm aquatic life and limit microbial growth, damaging the aquatic ecosystem. Hence, Patella *et al* [80] constructed a working electrode using laser-scribed rGO on filter paper for phosphate determination. The process involved filtering a GO water suspension to produce a uniform film on the filter paper. Then, a CO_2 laser was employed to rGO in specific areas to create working, counter, and reference electrodes, forming a complete sensor system. Ag/AgCl reference electrodes were coated with a commercial Ag/AgCl conductive paste. This three-electrode system was used as an electrochemical sensor to detect phosphate ions in water using the molybdenum blue method. The sensor demonstrated high selectivity and sensitive detection of phosphate ions over a linear range, from 1.0 to 20.0 μM, with a detection limit of 0.4 μM. This work describes the development of a portable and fast in situ phosphate sensor for monitoring water quality, which is easy to use and biodegradable. A few other electrochemical carbon electrodes for phosphate detection have been reported in the literature, such as SPE-graphite macro electrodes, carbon black, rGO-ordered mesoporous carbon/SPE, pencil graphite electrodes, carbon paste-microelectrode [81–85]. Bhandari *et al* [86] reported a sensor based on SPC ink that has been modified with nafion. The ink has also been functionalized with 4-aminibenzo-18-crown-6 ether. The purpose of this sensor is to measure soil potassium levels. In terms of its functionality, it was discovered that 4-amino-benzo-18-crown-6 covalently attached to the nafion on a carbon surface possesses selective recognition properties for potassium ions, as opposed to sodium, ammonium, and calcium ions. The recognition of potassium occurs via host–guest binding of the crown ether derivative, and the straightforward fabrication protocol adds to the potential utility of these systems for soil analysis in real-time applications.

6.5 Conclusion

A significant aspect of excessive use of chemical fertilizers is their potential to contaminate water, soil, and food. Additionally, the influx of fertilizer nutrients fosters algae growth in water bodies. Therefore, in light of these environmental challenges, there is a pressing need to adopt sustainable agricultural practices that mitigate the hazards of fertilizers. Sustainable agriculture aims to optimize resource usage, maintain soil quality, and preserve the overall health of the biosphere. Organic farming is one way to achieve these goals by using crop rotation, natural compost, and biological pest control to minimize the need for synthetic fertilizers. This approach reduces the risks of nutrient leaching and water contamination, while promoting a healthy ecology. Another approach is precision farming, which uses advanced technologies such as electrochemical sensors to measure nutrient levels. This helps farmers apply fertilizers more precisely, reducing the amount of fertilizer needed and minimizing the potential for water pollution while optimizing crop yields. Additionally, the development of efficient monitoring techniques is paramount. Electrochemical sensors have emerged as promising tools for the on-field monitoring of pesticides due to their affordable instrumentation, rapid response times, sensitivity, selectivity, and real-time monitoring capabilities.

Carbon nanomaterials, including CNTs, graphene, and CNFs, possess exceptional electrical, mechanical, and chemical properties that make them ideal for sensor development. As a result, they have gained significant attention in the field and researchers are exploring their potential in various applications, from agriculture and environmental monitoring to food safety. These sensors were designed to detect fertilizers with high sensitivity, and researchers are working to optimize nanomaterial synthesis methods, explore new functionalization strategies, and integrate carbon nanomaterials with advanced signal transduction and data processing technologies to improve sensor performance further. Ultimately, the continued advancement of carbon nanomaterial-based sensors has the potential to enhance fertilizer detection sensitivity and contribute to the development of more sustainable agricultural practices and environmental protection.

The current electrochemical analysis has some limitations, such as the inability to detect other interfering species simultaneously as the target species. However, there is potential for improvement through advances in interdigitated planar electrode design, catalyst/nanomaterial selection, and various voltammetric detection techniques. These improvements will enhance the sensor's selectivity, sensitivity, portability, and reliability, making it ideal for field deployment applications. It is advantageous to have sensors that can detect, differentiate, and quantify the NPK nutrients and simultaneously detect soil pH, temperature, and moisture (figure 6.8). While real-time sensors exist, the ability to detect nitrate ion concentration in real-world settings provides instantaneous results. These sensors can be interfaced with an Internet of Things platform to monitor sensor data remotely. Furthermore, integrating electrochemical sensors with wireless communication technologies and data analytics platforms holds promise for establishing autonomous pesticides, herbicides, and fertilizer monitoring networks in agricultural landscapes.

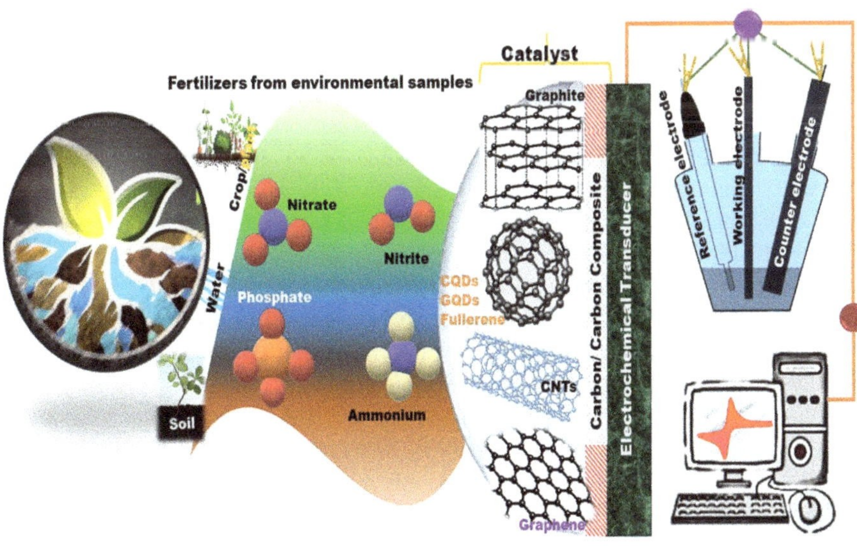

Figure 6.8. Summary of electrochemical sensing applications for nutrient detection from agricultural runoffs.

References

[1] Erenstein O, Jaleta M, Mottaleb K A, Sonder K, Donovan J and Braun H-J 2022 Global trends in wheat production, consumption and trade wheat improvement *Food Security in a Changing Climate* ed M P Reynolds and H-J Braun (Cham: Springer International Publishing) pp 47–66

[2] Grote U, Fasse A, Nguyen T T and Erenstein O 2021 Food security and the dynamics of wheat and maize value chains in Africa and Asia *Front. Sustain. Food Syst.* **4** 617009

[3] Bayabil H K, Teshome F T and Li Y C 2022 Emerging contaminants in soil and water *Front. Environ. Sci.* **10** 873499

[4] Galanakis C M 2023 The 'Vertigo' of the food sector within the triangle of climate change, the post-pandemic world, and the Russian–Ukrainian war *Foods* **12** 721

[5] Zia H, Harris N R, Merrett G V, Rivers M and Coles N 2013 The impact of agricultural activities on water quality: a case for collaborative catchment-scale management using integrated wireless sensor networks *Comput. Electron. Agric.* **96** 126–38

[6] Ingrao C, Strippoli R, Lagioia G and Huisingh D 2023 Water scarcity in agriculture: an overview of causes, impacts and approaches for reducing the risks *Heliyon* **9** e18507

[7] Trujillo-González J M, Mahecha-Pulido J D, Torres-Mora M A, Brevik E C, Keesstra S D and Jiménez-Ballesta R 2017 Impact of potentially contaminated river water on agricultural irrigated soils in an equatorial climate *Agriculture* **7** 52

[8] Moss B 2008 Water pollution by agriculture *Philos. Trans R. Soc. Lond. B. Bio.l Sci.* **363** 659–66

[9] Seijger C and Hellegers P 2023 How do societies reform their agricultural water management towards new priorities for water, agriculture, and the environment? *Agric. Water Manage.* **277** 108104

[10] Wyer K E, Kelleghan D B, Blanes-Vidal V, Schauberger G and Curran T P 2022 Ammonia emissions from agriculture and their contribution to fine particulate matter: a review of implications for human health *J. Environ. Manage.* **323** 116285

[11] Penuelas J, Coello F and Sardans J 2023 A better use of fertilizers is needed for global food security and environmental sustainability *Agri. Food Secur.* **12** 5

[12] Garg S 2018 The inorganic fertilizer as a pollutant in agriculture *J. Emerg. Technol. Innov. Res.* **5** J06048

[13] Shrestha J, Subedi S, Timsina K P, Subedi S, Pandey M, Shrestha A, Shrestha S and Hossain M A 2021 Sustainable intensification in agriculture: an approach for making agriculture greener and productive *J. Nepal Agric. Res. Council* **7** 133–50

[14] Fewtrell L 2004 Drinking-water nitrate, methemoglobinemia, and global burden of disease: a discussion *Environ. Health Perspect.* **112** 1371–4

[15] Li W, Liu H, Zhai L, Yen H, Hu W, Lei Q, Stewart R J, Guo S and Ren T 2019 Evaluation of concentration-discharge dynamics and nitrogen export on anthropogenic inputs and stormflow across alternative time-scales *Ecol. Indic.* **98** 879–87

[16] Fairbrother A, Purdy J, Anderson T and Fell R 2014 Risks of neonicotinoid insecticides to honeybees *Environ. Toxicol. Chem.* **33** 719–31

[17] Alegbeleye O O and Sant'Ana A S 2020 Manure-borne pathogens as an important source of water contamination: an update on the dynamics of pathogen survival/transport as well as practical risk mitigation strategies *Int. J. Hyg. Environ. Health* **227** 113524

[18] Rey-Romero D C, Domínguez I and Oviedo-Ocaña E R 2022 Effect of agricultural activities on surface water quality from páramo ecosystems *Environ. Sci. Pollut. Res.* **29** 83169–90

[19] Lynch J, Cain M, Frame D and Pierrehumbert R 2021 Agriculture's contribution to climate change and role in Mitigation is distinct from predominantly fossil CO_2-emitting sectors *Front. Sustain. Food Syst.* **4** 518039

[20] Zhai J, Luo B, Li A, Dong H, Jin X and Wang X 2022 Unlocking all-solid ion selective electrodes: prospects in crop detection *Sensors* **22** 5541

[21] Luna Juncal M J, Masino P, Bertone E and Stewart R A 2023 Towards nutrient neutrality: a review of agricultural runoff mitigation strategies and the development of a decision-making framework *Sci. Total Environ.* **874** 162408

[22] Yilong Z, Dean Z and Daoliang L 2015 Electrochemical and other methods for detection and determination of dissolved nitrite: a review *Int. J. Electrochem. Sci.* **10** 1144–68

[23] Amali R K A, Lim H N, Ibrahim I, Huang N M, Zainal Z and Ahmad S A A 2021 Significance of nanomaterials in electrochemical sensors for nitrate detection: a review *Trends Environ. Anal. Chem.* **31** e00135

[24] Manasa G, Bhakta A K, Bafna J, Mascarenhas R J, Malode S J and Shetti N P 2022 An amperometric sensor composed of carbon hybrid-structure for the degradation of amino-triazole herbicide *Environ. Res.* **212** 113541

[25] Manasa G, Bhakta A K, Mascarenhas R J and Shetti N P 2023 BaO-MWCNT composite material-based electrocatalytic amperometric sensor for the detection of environmentally hazardous Diuron *Microchem. J.* **191** 108778

[26] Manasa G, Bhakta A K, Mekhalif Z and Mascarenhas R J 2019 Voltammetric study and rapid quantification of resorcinol in hair dye and biological samples using ultrasensitive maghemite/MWCNT modified carbon paste electrode *Electroanalysis* **31** 1363–72

[27] Manasa G, Mascarenhas R J, Bhakta A K and Mekhalif Z 2020 MWCNT/Nileblue heterostructured composite electrode for flavanone Naringenin quantification in fruit juices *Electroanalysis* **32** 939–48

[28] Manasa G, Mascarenhas R J, Bhakta A K and Mekhalif Z 2021 Nano-graphene-platelet/brilliant-green composite coated carbon paste electrode interface for electrocatalytic oxidation of flavanone Hesperidin *Microchem. J.* **160** 105768

[29] Manasa G, Mascarenhas R J, Satpati A K, Basavaraja B M and Kumar S 2018 An electrochemical bisphenol F sensor based on ZnO/G nano composite and CTAB surface modified carbon paste electrode architecture *Colloids Surf.,* B **170** 144–51

[30] Baumbauer C L, Goodrich P J, Payne M E, Anthony T, Beckstoffer C, Toor A, Silver W and Arias A C 2022 Printed potentiometric nitrate sensors for use in soil *Sensors* **22** 4095

[31] Food and Agriculture Organization of the United Nations 2017 World fertilizer trends and outlook to 2020 https://openknowledge.fao.org/server/api/core/bitstreams/9ddf4aab-bc18-4d48-aeb6-ab14efaed1fd/content

[32] Food and Agriculture Organization of the United Nations 2020 World fertilizer trends and outlook to 2022 https://rowman.com/ISBN/9789251318942/World-Fertilizer-Trends-and-Outlook-to-2022

[33] Randive K, Raut T and Jawadand S 2021 An overview of the global fertilizer trends and India's position in 2020 *Miner. Econ.* **34** 371–84

[34] Naccarato A, Vommaro M L, Amico D, Sprovieri F, Pirrone N, Tagarelli A and Giglio A 2023 Triazine herbicide and NPK fertilizer exposure: accumulation of heavy metals and rare earth elements, effects on cuticle melanization, and immunocompetence in the model species tenebrio molitor *Toxics* **11** 499

[35] Simplício N, de C S, Muniz D H, de F, Rocha F R M, Martins D C, Dias Z M B, Farias B P, da C and Oliveira-Filho E C 2016 Comparative analysis between ecotoxicity of nitrogen-, phosphorus-, and potassium-based fertilizers and their active ingredients *Toxics* **5** 2
[36] Abouzeid A-Z M, Negm A T and Elgillani D A 2009 Upgrading of calcareous phosphate ores by flotation: effect of ore characteristics *Int. J. Miner. Process.* **1–4** 81–9
[37] Al-Shawi A W and Dahl R 1999 The determination of cadmium and six other heavy metals in nitrate/phosphate fertilizer solution by ion chromatography *Anal. Chim. Acta* **391** 35–42
[38] Pouyat R V and McDonnell M J 1991 Heavy metal accumulations in forest soils along an urban- rural gradient in Southeastern New York, USA *Water Air Soil Pollut.* **57** 797–807
[39] Cheraghi M, Lorestani B and Merrikhpour H 2012 Investigation of the effects of phosphate fertilizer application on the heavy metal content in agricultural soils with different cultivation patterns *Biol. Trace Elem. Res.* **145** 87–92
[40] Suciu N A, De Vivo R, Rizzati N and Capri E 2022 Cd content in phosphate fertilizer: which potential risk for the environment and human health? *Curr. Opin. Environ. Sci. Health* **30** 100392
[41] Mikkelsen R L and Roberts T L 2021 Inputs: potassium sources for agricultural systems *Improving Potassium Recommendations for Agricultural Crops* ed T S Murrell, R L Mikkelsen, G Sulewski, R Norton and M L Thompson (Cham: Springer International Publishing) pp 47–73
[42] Utz L R P and Bohrer M B C 2001 Acute and chronic toxicity of potassium chloride (KCl) and potassium acetate ($KC_2H_3O_2$) to *Daphnia similis* and *Ceriodaphnia dubia* (Crustacea; Cladocera) *Bull. Environ. Contam. Toxicol.* **66** 379–85
[43] Romano N and Zeng C 2007 Acute toxicity of sodium nitrate, potassium nitrate, and potassium chloride and their effects on the hemolymph composition and gill structure of early juvenile blue swimmer crabs (Portunus pelagicus Linnaeus, 1758) (Decapoda, Brachyura, Portunidae) *Environ. Toxicol. Chem.* **26** 1955–62
[44] Mahmoodi N M and Arami M 2010 Immobilized titania nanophotocatalysis: degradation, modeling and toxicity reduction of agricultural pollutants *J. Alloys Compd.* **506** 155–9
[45] Savci S 2012 An agricultural pollutant: chemical fertilizer *Int. J. Environ. Sci. Dev.* **3** 73–80
[46] Hyusein C and Tsakova V 2023 Nitrate detection at Pd–Cu-modified carbon screen printed electrodes *J. Electroanal. Chem.* **930** 117172
[47] Ali M A, Jiang H, Mahal N K, Weber R J, Kumar R, Castellano M J and Dong L 2017 Microfluidic impedimetric sensor for soil nitrate detection using graphene oxide and conductive nanofibers enabled sensing interface *Sensors Actuators* B **239** 1289–99
[48] Manasa G, Mascarenhas R J, Satpati A K, D'Souza O J and Dhason A 2017 Facile preparation of poly(methylene blue) modified carbon paste electrode for the detection and quantification of catechin *Mater. Sci. Eng.* C **73** 552–61
[49] Manasa G, Mascarenhas R J and Basavaraja B M 2019 Sensitively-selective determination of propyl paraben preservative based on synergistic effects of polyaniline-zinc-oxide nano-composite incorporated into graphite paste electrode *Coll. Surf.* B **184** 110529
[50] Feng X, Han G, Cai J and Wang X 2022 Au@carbon quantum Dots-MXene nanocomposite as an electrochemical sensor for sensitive detection of nitrite *J. Colloid Interface Sci.* **607** 1313–22
[51] Manasa G and Rout C S 2024 Versatile MXenes as electrochemical sensors for heavy metal ions and phenolic moiety-containing industrial chemicals: recent development and prospects *Mater. Adv.* **5** 83–122

[52] Mounesh K R, Reddy V, Pandith A, Eldesoky G E and Nagaraja B M 2023 Novel nitrogen-rich anchored nickel (II) phthalocyanine with composite of multiwalled carbon nanotubes on modified glassy carbon electrode: Sensitive and selective electrocatalytic activity of nitrite *Appl. Organometal. Chem.* **38** e7302
[53] Mounesh , Manriquez J M, Venugopala Reddy K R, Shilpa K G and Nagaraja B M 2023 Electrochemical, ultrasensitive, and selective detection of nitrite and H_2O_2: novel macrostructured phthalocyanine with composite MWCNTs on a modified GCE *Langmuir* **39** 1665–76
[54] Lu S, Hummel M, Kang S and Gu Z 2020 Selective voltammetric determination of nitrite using cobalt phthalocyanine modified on multiwalled carbon nanotubes *J. Electrochem. Soc.* **167** 046515
[55] Salhi O, Ez-zine T, Oularbi L and El Rhazi M 2022 Electrochemical sensing of nitrite ions using modified electrode by poly 1,8-diaminonaphthalene/functionalized multi-walled carbon nanotubes *Front. Chem.* **10** 870393
[56] Rajab N, Ibrahim H, Hassan R Y A and Youssef A F A 2023 Selective determination of nitrite in water and food samples using zirconium oxide (ZrO_2)@MWCNTs modified screen printed electrode *RSC Adv.* **13** 21259–70
[57] Nasraoui S, Al-Hamry A, Teixeira P R, Ameur S, Paterno L G, Ben Ali M and Kanoun O 2021 Electrochemical sensor for nitrite detection in water samples using flexible laser-induced graphene electrodes functionalized by CNT decorated by Au nanoparticles *J. Electroanal. Chem.* **880** 114893
[58] Zheng D, Hu C, Peng Y and Hu S 2009 A carbon nanotube/polyvanillin composite film as an electrocatalyst for the electrochemical oxidation of nitrite and its application as a nitrite sensor *Electrochim. Acta* **54** 4910–5
[59] Rajalakshmi K and John S A 2015 Highly sensitive determination of nitrite using FMWCNTs-conducting polymer composite modified electrode *Sens. Actuators* B **215** 119–24
[60] Huang X, Li Y, Chen Y and Wang L 2008 Electrochemical determination of nitrite and iodate by use of gold nanoparticles/poly(3-methylthiophene) composites coated glassy carbon electrode *Sens. Actuators* B **134** 780–6
[61] Arulraj A D, Sundaram E, Vasantha V S and Neppolian B 2018 Polypyrrole with a functionalized multi-walled carbon nanotube hybrid nanocomposite: a new and efficient nitrite sensor *New J. Chem.* **42** 3748–57
[62] Baciu A, Manea F, Pop A, Pode R and Schoonman J 2017 Simultaneous voltammetric detection of ammonium and nitrite from groundwater at silver-electrodecorated carbon nanotube electrode *Process Saf. Environ. Prot.* **108** 18–25
[63] Manoj D, Saravanan R, Santhanalakshmi J, Agarwal S, Gupta V K and Boukherroub R 2018 Towards green synthesis of monodisperse Cu nanoparticles: an efficient and high sensitive electrochemical nitrite sensor *Sensors Actuators* B **266** 873–82
[64] Valsalakumar V C and Vasudevan S 2023 Zirconium phosphate-incorporated polyaniline–graphene oxide composite modified electrodes for effective and selective detection of Nitrite *Langmuir* **39** 15730–9
[65] Li Y, Zhang X, Sun Y, Yang Z and Liu J 2023 Fabrication non-enzymatic electrochemical sensor based on methyl red and graphene oxide nanocomposite modified carbon paste electrode for determination of nitrite in food samples *Int. J. Electrochem. Sci.* **18** 100097
[66] Ezzat N, Hefnawy M A, Medany S S, El-Sharif R M and Fadallah S A 2023 Green synthesis of Ag nanoparticle supported on graphene oxide for efficient nitrite sensing in a water sample *Sci. Rep.* **13** 19441

[67] Ikhsan N I, Rameshkumar P, Pandilkumar A, Shahid M M, Huang N M, Kumar S V and Lim H N 2015 Facile synthesis of graphene oxide–silver nanocomposite and its modified electrode for enhanced electrochemical detection of nitrite ions *Talanta* **144** 908–14

[68] Guo X and Fan Y 2023 Determination of nitrite in food specimens using electrochemical sensor based on polyneutral red modified reduced graphene oxide paste electrode *Int. J. Electrochem. Sci.* **18** 100290

[69] Xu K, Chen Q, Zhao Y, Ge C, Lin S and Liao J 2020 Cost-effective, wireless, and portable smartphone-based electrochemical system for on-site monitoring and spatial mapping of the nitrite contamination in water *Sensors Actuators* B **319** 128221

[70] Yue X, Li Y, Li M, Luo X and Bai Y 2021 Three-dimensional porous carbon derived from different organic acid salts for application in electrochemical sensing *RSC Adv.* **11** 31834–44

[71] Wu W, Li Y, Jin J, Wu H, Wang S, Ding Y and Ou J 2016 Sensing nitrite with a glassy carbon electrode modified with a three-dimensional network consisting of Ni_7S_6 and multi-walled carbon nanotubes *Microchim. Acta* **183** 3159–66

[72] Zhu W, Zhang Y, Gong J, Ma Y, Sun J, Li T and Wang J 2019 Surface engineering of carbon fiber paper toward exceptionally high-performance and stable electrochemical nitrite sensing *ACS Sens.* **4** 2980–7

[73] Baciu A, Ardelean M, Pop A, Pode R and Manea F 2015 Simultaneous voltammetric/amperometric determination of sulfide and nitrite in water at BDD electrode *Sensors (Basel)* **15** 14526–38

[74] Zhang X and Sun R 2023 Construction of an electrochemical sensor for detection of nitrite by gold nanoparticles immobilized on biochar *Int. J. Electrochem. Sci.* **18** 100219

[75] Kumar T H V and Sundramoorthy A K 2018 Non-enzymatic electrochemical detection of Urea on silver nanoparticles anchored nitrogen-doped single-walled carbon nanotube modified electrode *J. Electrochem. Soc.* **165** B3006

[76] Magar H S, Hassan R Y A and Abbas M N 2023 Non-enzymatic disposable electrochemical sensors based on CuO/Co_3O_4@MWCNTs nanocomposite modified screen-printed electrode for the direct determination of urea *Sci. Rep.* **13** 2034

[77] Ramasami Sundhar Baabu P, Gumpu M B, Nesakumar N, Rayappan J B B and Kulandaisamy A J 2020 Electroactive manganese oxide–reduced graphene oxide interfaced electrochemical detection of urea *Water Air Soil Pollut.* **231** 545

[78] Dutta D, Chandra S, Swain A K and Bahadur D 2014 SnO_2 quantum dots-reduced graphene oxide composite for enzyme-free ultrasensitive electrochemical detection of urea *Anal. Chem.* **86** 5914–21

[79] Babitha K B, Soorya P S, Mohamed A P, Rakhi R B and Ananthakumar S 2020 Development of ZnO@rGO nanocomposites for the enzyme free electrochemical detection of urea and glucose *Mater. Adv.* **1** 1939–51

[80] Patella B, Parisi A, Moukri N, Gitto F, Busacca A, Aiello G, Russo M, O'Riordan A and Inguanta R 2023 Phosphate ions detection by using an electrochemical sensor based on laser-scribed graphene oxide on paper *Electrochim. Acta* **461** 142600

[81] Kolliopoulos A V, Kampouris D K and Banks C E 2015 Rapid and portable electrochemical quantification of phosphorus *Anal. Chem.* **87** 4269–74

[82] Cinti S, Talarico D, Palleschi G, Moscone D and Arduini F 2016 Novel reagentless paper-based screen-printed electrochemical sensor to detect phosphate *Anal. Chim. Acta* **919** 78–84

[83] Wei H, Pan D, Zhou Z, Han H and Zhu R 2021 On-site electrochemical determination of phosphate with high sensitivity and anti-interference ability in turbid coastal waters *Ecotoxicol. Environ. Saf.* **221** 112444
[84] Arvas M B, Gürsu H, Gençten M and Sahin Y 2018 Electrochemical formation of molybdenum phosphate on a pencil graphite electrode and its potential application for the detection of phosphate ions *Anal. Methods* **10** 4282–91
[85] Quintana J C, Idrissi L, Palleschi G, Albertano P, Amine A, El Rhazi M and Moscone D 2004 Investigation of amperometric detection of phosphate: application in seawater and cyanobacterial biofilm samples *Talanta* **63** 567–74
[86] Bhandari S, Singh U and Kumbhat S 2019 Nafion-modified carbon based sensor for soil potassium detection *Electroanalysis* **31** 813–9

Chapter 7

Carbon-based electrochemical sensors for the determination of pesticide residues from the environment

G Manasa, Pavithra Siddu and Chandra Sekhar Rout

Pesticides, such as insecticides, fungicides, and herbicides, are compounds that prevent, control, and reduce hazardous organisms affecting crops. Uncontrolled and prolonged use of pesticides is a significant concern that negatively impacts the environment and human health. Thus, ensuring human health, food safety, and sustainable agriculture requires environmental pesticides to be detected and ecosystems to be protected. Hence, developing efficient sensors to identify pesticides in varied samples will be discussed in this chapter. Carbon nanostructures have unique electrical, physical, chemical, and electrocatalytic properties that make them helpful modification agents for sensor designs. The most critical studies on the use of carbon-based sensors for the electroanalysis of pesticides (e.g., carbaryl, carbofuran, chlorpyrifos, malathion, methyl parathion (MP), metobromuron, cyanazine, paraquat, benzimidazoles, triazole, carbendazim) are reviewed in this chapter.

7.1 Introduction

The use of pesticides is known to increase crop yields significantly. These pesticides are classified into different types based on their intended use. The most prominent method of categorizing pesticides is based on their chemical composition and the nature of their active components [1]. The classification provides information about pesticide efficiency, composition, and physical characteristics. Understanding pesticide's physical and chemical features is particularly beneficial when deciding on the application method, safety measures to be taken when applying, and application rates. Figure 7.1 illustrates how various kinds of pesticides, including fungicides, herbicides, insecticides, and rodenticides, are separated based on their chemical

doi:10.1088/978-0-7503-5879-8ch7

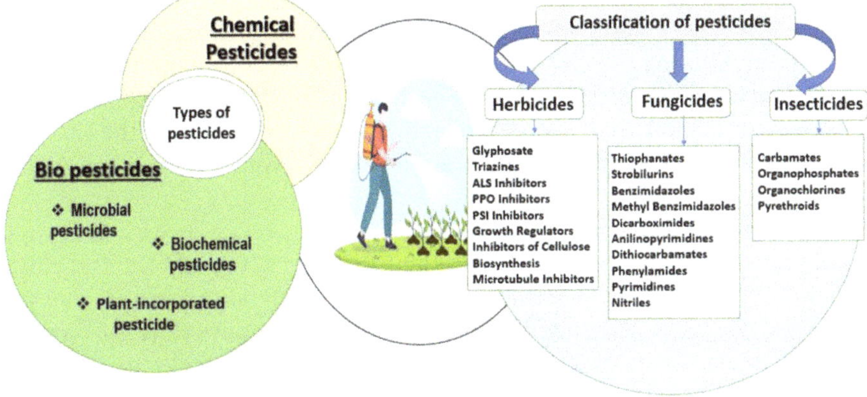

Figure 7.1. Types and classification of pesticides.

characteristics [2]. Excessive and prolonged usage of pesticides has detrimental effects on the environment, biological systems, and human health, with extreme use for agricultural purposes leading to food contamination and environmental pollution [3]. Pesticides can enter the body through various means, such as the skin, respiratory system, and injection. This can result in biotransformation of the substance, acute and chronic human poisoning, and air, soil, and water contamination [4]. The increased incidents of pesticide poisoning have led to severe health issues globally. To control their use and resolve cases in forensic science, it is necessary to monitor them [5].

Hence, researchers are keen on developing sensitive, accurate, and straightforward analytical techniques for detecting pesticide traces in ecological products such as soil, water, and food samples to safeguard and monitor their levels [6]. Traditional approaches such as high-performance liquid chromatography, gas chromatography, flow injection spectrometry, capillary electrophoresis, potentiometry, flow injection spectrometry, etc, have been widely used to detect pesticides. However, these methods have notable drawbacks, including expensive equipment, time-consuming preparation of samples, pretreatment procedures, and trained technicians to conduct analyses [7]. To address the current limitations, there is an urgent need for swift and precise pesticide detection methods that can bypass these constraints. Electrochemical sensors have emerged as a promising solution, offering superior performance compared to traditional techniques [8]. With their high sensitivity, selectivity, and speedy detection capabilities, electronics-based sensors are user-friendly for detecting pesticides and medicines. Additionally, electrochemical sensors offer numerous other benefits due to their lower detection limit and ease of construction [9]. Researchers are increasingly excited about employing electrochemical sensors for analyzing food, medicine, environment, and agriculture, thanks to their ability to measure the electrical behavior of biomolecules and the development of drugs [10]. Various voltammetry methods are available, such as CV, square wave voltammetry (SWV), ASV, CSV, LSV, differential pulse voltammetry (DPV), and others. These electrochemical methods offer lower detection and sensitivity thresholds, but they require design upgrades to increase the accuracy of pesticide determination. Altering the electrode surfaces with different materials can enhance their sensitivity and detection limits. The field of nanotechnology can meet the demand for equipment that can detect and degrade pesticides at the atomic and molecular scales. Carbon nanomaterials are the most commonly used nanomaterials for sensing applications [11].

Carbon nanomaterials possess unique characteristics such as excellent physical, chemical, and electrical conductivity, making them a top choice for electrode modification materials due to their superior electrocatalytic capabilities and perfect surface area. They are also highly beneficial for sensor devices [12]. To improve sensor performance, it is crucial to enhance the structural design of the material, utilizing structures such as nanotubes, nanolayers, and mesoporous spheres based on carbon nanomaterials. The most commonly used carbon-based compounds include carbon nanotubes, mesoporous carbon particles [13], graphene [14], and graphene oxide [15] and its derivatives. This chapter will delve into pesticides and their types, overuse pollution, and their long-term environmental impact. Furthermore, it will discuss the use of carbon-based electrochemical sensors to detect pesticide residues in the environment.

7.2 Carbon-based nanomaterials

The Earth's crust contains mostly carbon, an element whose presence has long been known. The concept of carbon-based materials has undergone a transformative journey, transitioning from the macroscale to the nanoscale. Materials with nanostructured carbon have frequently been employed for electrochemical applications, but presently carbon particles and the adaptive physical, chemical, and mechanical features of composite materials integrating carbon are required. Furthermore, the extraordinary benefits of carbon nanostructures' better electrical conductivity, catalytic abilities, and large surface areas are also apparent [16].

The concept of carbon-based materials has undergone a transformative journey, transitioning from the macroscale to the nanoscale. Carbon nanoparticles and adaptable mechanical, physical, and chemical characteristics of composite materials incorporating carbon are now necessary to apply electrochemical sensors. Electrochemical applications have frequently used materials with carbon nanostructures. Furthermore, the extraordinary benefits of carbon nanostructures' better electrical conductivity, catalytic abilities, and large surface areas are also apparent. Additionally, carbon nanoparticles interact strongly with other nanoscale substances. These interactions have attracted attention recently because they occur on surfaces or interfaces. In recent years, the structure of electrode materials has been one of the many domains in which carbon-based nanomaterials have increasingly been exploited. Carbon-based nanomaterials have exceptional qualities, such as high electrical conductivity and electrochemical activity, which makes them the optimal medium for transferring electrons. They also have a substantial surface area and excellent electrocatalytic performance, which broadens their applicability across

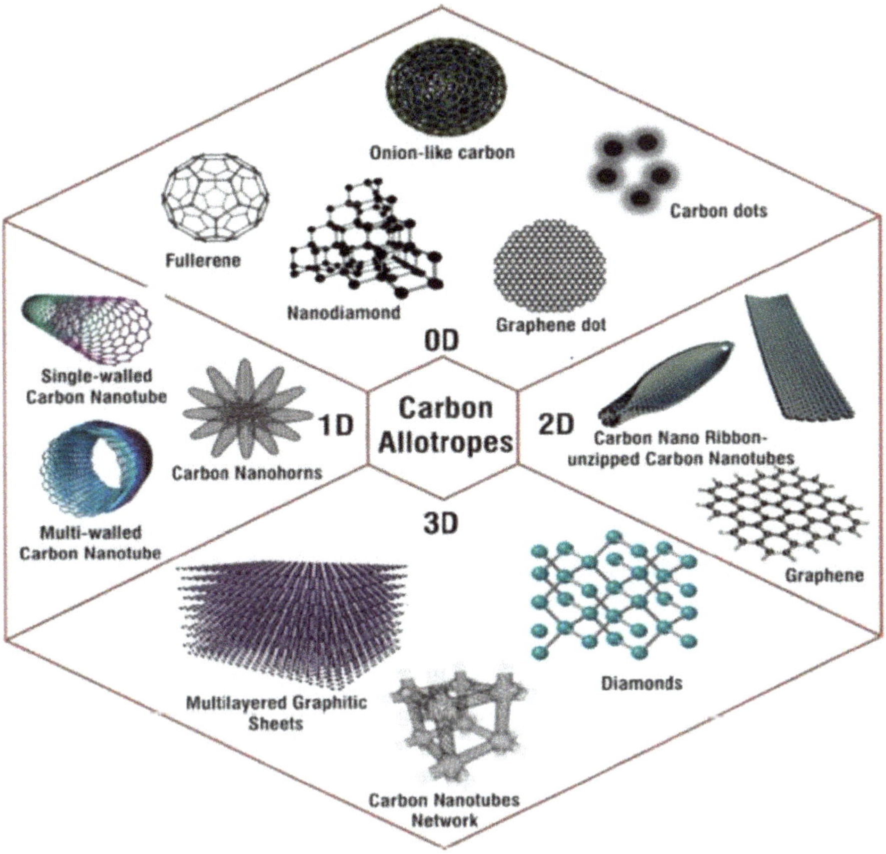

Figure 7.2. The molecular models of carbon nanostructures with varying sizes. Reproduced from [19].

diverse fields. For electrochemical research, various nanostructured carbon materials, including carbon dots, carbon nanotubes, carbon nanohorns, graphene, and carbon black (CB), are frequently preferred [17]. These carbon nanomaterials can be grouped and categorized according to their size, such as 0D: carbon dots, fullerene, nanotoroids, and graphene clusters; 1D: carbon nanotubes (CNTs) and helicoidal carbon nanotubes; 2D derivatives of graphene, 2D network nanoribbons, and Haeckelite surface; and 3D Schwarzite crystals, graphite, carbon nanofoams, and 3D nanotube networks [18]. The molecular models of many forms of carbon nanostructures with varying sizes are provided in figure 7.2.

7.2.1 0D carbon nanomaterials

Carbon dots are 0D carbon nanomaterials, which are tiny nanoparticles. Owing to their electro-optical and optical traits, and superior characteristics such as quantum confinement, carbon dots exhibit traits similar to those of quantum dots. Additionally, they have excellent biocompatibility, high light stability, environmental friendliness, low degree of toxicology, and efficiency, particularly in biosensors and catalysis. Carbon nanoparticles include quantum dots, nanohorns, nanotoroids, nanodiamonds, and graphene clusters [20]. Conical carbon nanostructures called carbon nanohorns measure 40–50 nm in length and 2–5 nm in diameter. Carbon nanohorns are known for their unique properties, including high electrical characteristics, significant porosity, and adsorption capacities, which make them suitable for electrochemical applications. Their conical form gives them electrical solid attributes, and when subjected to chemical or thermal treatments, oxidation may occur on their surface. The addition of nanopores increases their surface area, creating a porous structure. These distinguishing characteristics make carbon nanohorns ideal for sensors in electrochemical applications [21]. Carbon quantum dots (CQDs) and graphene quantum dots are significant carbon components. Amorphous CQDs are hemi-spherical particles with a diameter of less than 10 nm. Graphene quantum dots, on the other hand, have lateral dimensions under 20 nm and mimic the 2D plane of graphene. The primary difference between graphene quantum dots and CQDs is that graphene quantum dots are made up of polycyclic aromatic hydrocarbon molecules. In contrast, CQDs are made up of carbon atoms. Additionally, there is another critical 0D carbon material known as fullerene, which has a lattice structure. Fullerene is crucial for numerous applications because it is a carbon allotrope that accelerates electron transport due to its spherical shape. Its symmetric and closed cage structure shows unique properties that make it significant in various fields.

7.2.2 1D carbon nanomaterials

CNTs are a processed form of graphene and are 1D carbon nanomaterials that have been studied for many years. Since 1991, CNTs have attracted much attention in chemistry, physics, and materials due to their remarkable electrical conductivity. Based on the number of layers, CNTs with a cylindrical structure can be categorized as single or multiwalled (SWCNT or MWCNTs). A single wall has a 0.4–2 nm diameter and an empty internal area. Functionalizing their surfaces can provide crucial information regarding the optical, physical, and electrical properties of CNTs. CNTs are utilized as nanocarriers due to their primarily electrochemical capabilities. Additionally, CNTs have a more significant aspect ratio than CQDs as they join to form a conductive network. The surface of CNTs can also be modified through various functional groups to improve electrochemical sensor performance [22].

Halloysite nanotubes are clay minerals with a distinct chemical composition and a tubular shape. They are very helpful in various applications thanks to surface modification. This modification involves adding different functional substances to the nanotube's outer surface and inner lumen. Halloysite nanotubes have silica and aluminum groups on their inner and outer surfaces, which enhance the interfacial interaction between the nanotube and other functional agents. The most common form of Halloysite nanotubes is available in nanotubes, plates, or spheres. They can also be used to create sensors for various sensing applications. These nanotubes are an excellent substitute for carbon nanotubes because they are cost-effective, eco-friendly, and biocompatible. This makes them ideal for biological applications [23].

These materials have unique qualities that enable them to detect a range of agriculturally relevant analytes, including nutrients, insecticides, and soil components. Since they have large surface areas, they offer many active sites for catalytic reactions. This characteristic increases the sensitivity of electrochemical sensors, enabling the detection of traces of analytes. It is also corrosion-resistant, chemically inert, and biocompatible. Its high electrical conductivity guarantees effective electron transfer during electrochemical reactions, which is essential for quick and precise sensor responses [24].

7.2.3 2D and 3D carbon nanomaterials

2D nanomaterials, such as graphene, and their related materials, such as graphene oxide and graphene quantum dots, have unique properties. These materials have flat structures consisting of a single or a few layers of carbon atoms arranged in a planar lattice. The outstanding electrical conductivity, mechanical strength, and thermal properties of graphene make it a beneficial material. Graphene quantum dots are small fragments of graphene with lateral dimensions that are typically less than 20 nm. Their versatile electronic properties exhibit quantum confinement effects, making them highly promising for application in optoelectronics, catalysis, sensors, and biomedical devices [25].

The term 3D carbon nanomaterial refers to 3D structures such as graphitic crystals, carbon nanofoam, and nanotube networks. Black carbon is an amorphous carbon with a large surface area and is one of the commercial raw materials. Plastic, rubber, printer ink, and battery manufacturing sectors often employ CB. Due to its excellent electrical conductivity, it is crucial for electrocatalysis. The modified electrodes with black carbon offered a quick transfer of electrons when the most recent investigations were analyzed [26]. Electrochemical sensors made from 2D and 3D materials have several advantages over traditional sensors, including high sensitivity, excellent selectivity, ease of use, affordability, and efficiency in detecting analytes. They are increasingly used in agriculture and environmental applications, particularly for detecting heavy metal ions, pesticide residues, pathogenic bacteria, and more.

7.3 Electrochemical detection of herbicides

Herbicides can be categorized into major classes based on their chemical structure and mode of action. According to their chemical structure, the main classes of herbicides are classified as glyphosate, nonhormone herbicides, ALS inhibitors, PPO inhibitors, photosystem I (PSI) inhibitors, growth regulators (hormone mimics), glutamine synthetase inhibitors, inhibitors of cellulose biosynthesis, microtubule inhibitors, inhibitors of lipid synthesis, and so on.

Urea herbicides are agriculture's most commonly used pesticides and are used to control broadleaf weeds in various crops. These herbicides, including metobromuron (Mbn), inhibit photosynthesis by blocking the photosynthetic electron transport at photosystem two (PS II). Mbn is a selective, systemic, pre-emergence herbicide that protects crops such as common beans, potatoes, tomatoes, tobacco, maize, and sugar beet. Mbn is not readily biodegradable and has a high potential for bioaccumulation despite having modest mammalian toxicity. In addition, there have been reports linking Mbn to methemoglobinemia (MetHb), a blood disorder caused by the abnormal production of methemoglobin. Therefore, it is crucial to determine Mbn levels in crops [27].

Sipa *et al* [28] constructed a sensor for detecting Mbn in the presence of nanomaterials modified with graphene nano-platelets (GNP) and MWCNTs by the drop-casting method. The prepared electrodes were used to create the SWV method for determining the insecticide metobromuron. Comprehensive microscopic characterization using atomic force microscopy, electrochemical characterization with electrochemical impedance spectroscopy, and CV methods have been used to characterize the synthesized material. CV was supported by Britton–Robinson (B-R) buffer at pH 2.0 at a scan rate of 100 mV s^{-1} with the highest and most reproducible analytical signal of Mbn. Using GNP suspension at a concentration of 0.5 mg mL^{-1} produced the most robust and consistent analytical signal of Mbn ($n = 3$, RSD = 2.1%). In the oxidation signal of Mbn 4.8×10^{-5} mol L^{-1}, the impact of GNP suspension concentration in the 0.1–1.0 mg mL^{-1} range Mbn was determined electrochemically using the SWV method, and the detection limits were calculated using UTGE (0.13 μmol L^{-1}), UTGE-MWCNTs (0.11 μmol L^{-1}), and UTGE-GNPs (0.048 μmol L^{-1}). UTGE-GNPs represented the satisfactory limit of detection (LOD) of 4.8×10^{-8} mol L^{-1} readings and the broadest linearity range with excellent stability, reproducibility, sensitivity, and environmentally friendly.

For the accurate detection of fenuron (FU) and diuron (DU), Veerappan Mani *et al* [29] designed amperometric sensors using a composite composed of GO-MWCNT. A straightforward solution-based method was used to manufacture the GO-MWCNT composite. A glassy carbon electrode (GCE) modified with GO-MWCNT films demonstrated good electrocatalytic activity in the oxidation of DU and FU in terms of reduced overpotential and significantly increased peak currents. GO-MWCNT catalysts have demonstrated electrocatalytic performance that is noticeably better than DMF-dispersed MWCNTs. GO-MWCNT-based amperometric sensor with a wide linear range between 9.0 μM and 0.38 mM and a high sensitivity of 0.645 A M^{-1} cm^{-2} has been developed. The amperometric sensor could detect FU with a 1.20 μA μM^{-1} cm^{-2} sensitivity over a wide linear range of 0.9 and 47.0 μM. Additionally, the sensor has good repeatability with relative standard deviations (RSDs) of 3.87% and 3.25%, 3.96%, and 2.70% for reproducibility and stability, respectively. Amperometric tests were conducted at the GO-MWCNTs/GCE with a rotation speed of 2500 rpm and 1.0 mM DU. Even after 3600 s continuous use, just 8% of the initial I_p was reduced, demonstrating the electrode's strong operational stability in determining DIU. Additionally, the electrode has good operational stability to detect FU; even after 3600 s of nonstop operation, only 7% of the initial I_p was reduced. Various water samples from agricultural areas have been used to evaluate the practicability of the constructed amperometric sensor. In another work, Manasa *et al* [21] fabricated BaO-MWCNT/MCPE via a one-step bulk modification protocol shown in figure 7.3. FESEM, EDS, and EIS characterized the structural morphology of the modified composite.

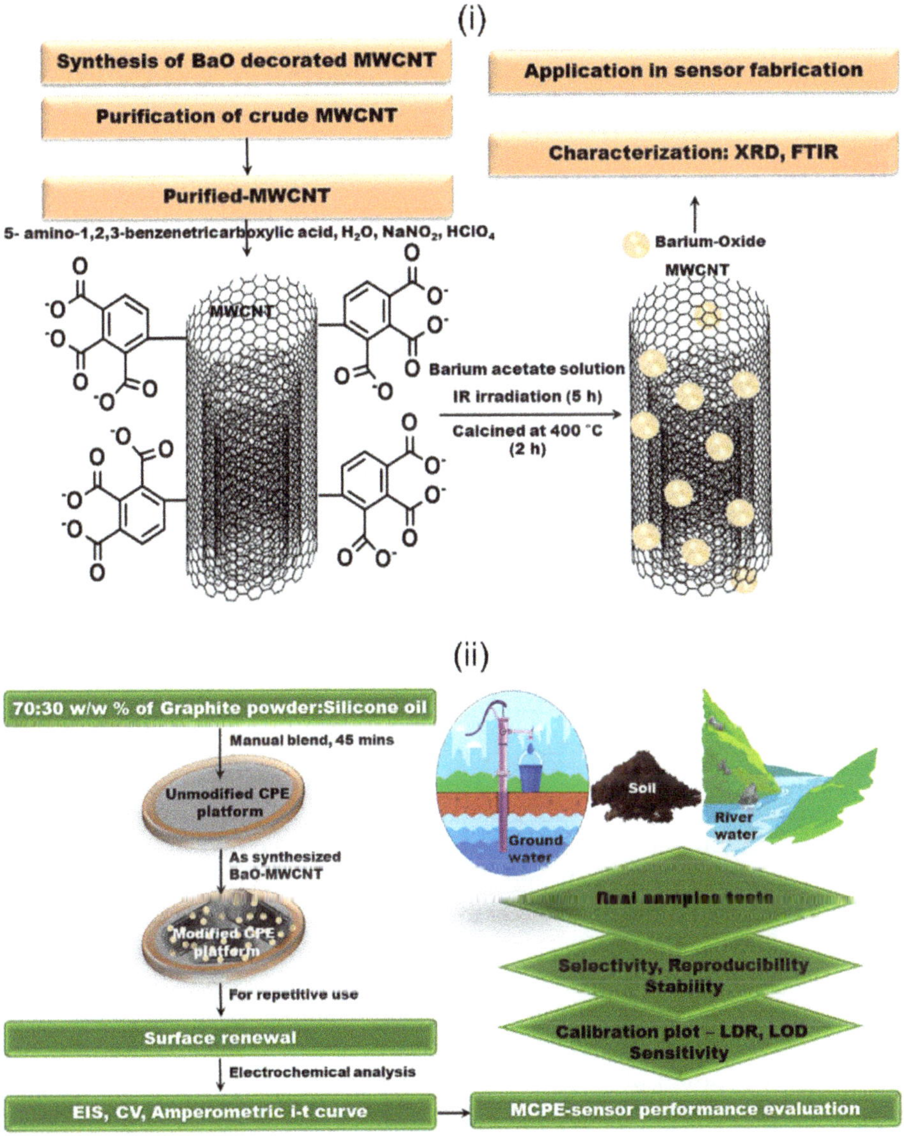

Figure 7.3. (i) A flow chart for the synthesis of BaO-MWCNT composite material and (ii) the preparation of bare and modified carbon paste electrode (CPE) for the electrochemical determination of diuron from environmental samples. Reprinted from [30], Copyright (2023), with permission from Elsevier.

The sensor confirmed the lowest charge transfer resistance and good electrocatalytic activity to identify the target analyte DIU. The sensor was devised to improve electrocatalytic performance and sensitivity at reduced activation energy by increasing the effective surface area on MCPE. The electrochemical analysis is carried out through CV with a low detection limit value of 0.31×10^{-6} mol L^{-1}, a LOQ of 1.06×10^{-6} mol L^{-1}, and good reproducibility. The developed sensor portrays good selectivity, sensitivity, and reliability for DIU determinations, and also displays quick response with portable and cost-effective potentiostats.

Furthermore, aminotriazole (ATZ) and linuron (LNR), another set of non-selective herbicides employed to manage several weeds in agriculture fields, have been combined with other active ingredients to safeguard crops. The environment is contaminated by their widespread and excessive use, particularly when combined with soil or water. In efforts to address these environmental issues and to detect trace quantities of the herbicides, g-C_3N_4 (carbon-rich graphitic carbon nitride) was synthesized through a high-temperature condensation process that was used to develop a new electrode material for the detection of ATZ and LNR at pH of 4.2 and 6.0, respectively, in the presence of a CTAB (cetyltrimethylammonium bromide) surfactant. The influence of accumulation time, pH variation, sweep rate, temperature, and changes in the concentrations of ATZ and LNR were studied. A linear relationship was detected between the concentrations of ATZ and LNR with the peak currents. The lowest LOD (ATZ—6.41×10^{-8} M and LNR—2.47×10^{-8} M) values had the maximum sensitivity and selectivity. This method developed has many advantages, e.g., it is simple and can efficiently detect minute quantities of the analytes from water and soil samples [31].

Bentazone is a type of herbicide that falls under the thiadiazine group. It controls post-emergent weeds that grow on beans, rice, maize, and peanuts. Since these herbicides are quickly released into the environment, it is essential to conduct extensive studies to evaluate the presence of bentazone. While chronic and high doses of bentazone did not increase significant tumors in rats and mice, it is still a concern for human health due to its potential carcinogenicity. Bentazone's high water solubility and low adsorption make it one of the most frequently detected contaminants in surface waters and groundwaters. Therefore, a modification of GCE by integrating MWCNT and b-cyclodextrin (β-CD) within a polyaniline coating for determining bentazone herbicide has been synthesized [32]. The chemical recognition of bentazone by CD is combined with the advantage of a faster electron transfer due to the negatively charged carboxylate functionalized MWCNT dispersed in the conducting polyaniline (PANI) matrix. The developed β-CD/MWCNT/GCE sensor has been examined via the CV method for the direct oxidative quantification of bentazone in pure and natural water samples, where a linear range of 10.0–80.0 mmol L^{-1}, with a LOD 1.6 mmol L^{-1}. The analyzed modified composite exhibited efficient electrochemical oxidation of bentazone with high sensitivity and stability. Table 7.1 summarizes the performance of the reported carbon-based sensors for herbicides.

7.4 Electrochemical detection of fungicides

Fungicides are commonly used in agriculture to prevent diseases and eliminate harmful fungi or spores. However, they can also harm soil functionality by killing or inhibiting beneficial microorganisms that help break down nutrients in the soil. Therefore, it is crucial to understand their impact and choose appropriate agro-chemicals to minimize adverse effects. Fungicides often target soil enzymes as their

Table 7.1. Electrochemical sensors reported for herbicides based on carbon nanomaterials.

Pesticide	Method	Electrode	Linear range	LOD	Real sample	References
Paraquat	SWV DPV	MWCNTs-DHP/GC	0.05–1.5 μmol L^{-1}	0.01 μmol L^{-1}	Water	[33]
Bentazone	CV	β-CD/MWCNT/GCE	10.0–80.0 μmol L^{-1}	1.6 μmol L^{-1}	Water	[32]
Isoproturon	SWV	GO-MWCNTs	0.30–15.0 μmol L^{-1}	0.1 μmol L^{-1}	Rice field water, tomato, lettuce	[34]
Bentazone	CV	MWCNT-IL/RGO/SiC/CILE	1.0–150.0 nM	0.25 nM	This study has not validated their sensor for practical applications	[35]
2,4-Dichlorophenoxy acetic acid	CV	AuNPs-PANABA-MWCNT	1.0–100.0 ppb	0.3 ppb	Tap water	[36]
Metobromuron	SWV	UTGE	0.8–2.0 μmol L^{-1}	0.13 μmol L^{-1}	Soil	[37]
Aminotriazole	CV	CuO-MWCNT@400	0.547 μmol L^{-1} and 0.165 μmol L^{-1}	0.165 μmol L^{-1}	Water	[38]

Abbreviations: MWCNTs-DHP/GC: Multiwalled carbon nanotube-Dihexadecylhydrogenphosphate, GR/GCE: polyaniline/graphene, β-CD/MWCNT/GCE: β-cyclodextrin multiwalled carbon nanotubes, GO-MWCNTs: graphene oxide-multiwalled carbon nanotubes, MWCNT-IL/RGO/SiC/CILE: multiwalled carbon nanotubes-ionic liquid/reduced graphene oxide/silicon carbide/carbon ionic liquid electrodes, 2,4-D: 2,4-dichlorophenoxy acetic acid.

primary mode of action, which can inhibit the growth of soil microorganisms responsible for producing these enzymes. As a result, fungicides can directly interact with the enzymes and hinder their functionality. There are several broad families of fungicides, including carbendazim, benzimidazoles, carbamic, quinone outside inhibitors, thiophenes, and others, which are formed based on the chemical composition and structure of the fungicides [39].

Carbendazim (CBZ) and thiabendazole (TBZ) are primary compounds of the benzimidazole fungicides. They are typically applied to crops to safeguard fruits and vegetables from pests and fungi, and to preserve their quality. Due to the difficulty in cleaving the benzimidazole's ring structure, most of these substances remain in the environment after use. Additionally, foods and water contain their remnants, which may be hazardous to human health because of their toxicity; hence, detection of CBZ is essential. To overcome this problem, Yuanyuan Dong *et al* [40] fabricated $ZnFe_2O_4$/SWCNTs nanohybrid through a facile one-step hydrothermal method for detecting CBZ and TBZ. The electrochemical behaviors of the prepared composite were investigated using CV and DPV. The developed sensors exhibit good performance, such as excellent sensitivity, a low detection limit of 0.09 and 0.05 μM, a more comprehensive linear range of 0.5–100.0 μM, and good stability and repeatability. CBZ and TBZ in various samples have been investigated, and the results were satisfactory.

Attributed to unique structural and electrical characteristics, transition-metal carbides (MXenes), a new class of 2D materials, show promise as electrochemical sensing materials. To improve the sensing capability of the electrode material employed for the electrochemical detection of CBZ, it was proposed to combine $Ti_3C_2T_x$–MXene and electrochemically reduced graphene oxide (MXene/ERGO). The MXene/ERGO was created using an easy-to-use, environmentally-friendly electrochemical process. Graphene oxide (GO) and MXene were first dropped on the electrode surface and then reduced electrochemically. The ERGO conductive networks closely coupled the divided $Ti_3C_2T_x$ layers and the separated particles of $Ti_3C_2T_x$. It improved the electrode materials' electrochemical reactivity, improved the electronic conductivity, and promoted electron transmission between the electrode and the detection molecules. As a result, the MXene/ERGO-based sensor demonstrated susceptible CBZ detection with a broad linear range of 2.0–10.0 nM and a low detection limit of 0.67 nM. Furthermore, the sensor showed extraordinary consistency and selectivity for CBZ recognition. The proposed sensor detected cucumber and orange juice samples with satisfactory recoveries [41]. Furthermore, Nevin *et al* [33] demonstrated the electroanalytical method for detecting a synthetic fungicide as a propamocarb (PM) pesticide belonging to the carbamic acid class of fungicides. The authors prepared reduced graphene oxide (rGO) via the green ultrasonic microwave-assisted method and studied rGO-based non-enzymatic electrochemical sensors. The modified non-enzymatic EC sensor exhibited high sensitivity, high selectivity, reproducibility, rapid response along rapid response within 1 min, a low detection limit of 0.6 μM and a linear range of 1.1–5.0 μM with a high of 101.1μA $\mu M^{-1} cm^{-2}$ for PM.

Ilager *et al* [42] have developed a GO and graphitic carbon nitride (g-C_3N_4) nanohybrid electrode assembly (GO/g-C_3N_4/GCE) for the detection of MP and carbendazim (CBZ). The synthesized materials were additionally characterized using TEM, AFM, and x-ray diffraction (XRD) techniques to reveal their purity, crystal structure, and shape. Using CV and square SWV methods, the entire voltammetric behavior of these analytes was examined. Linearity plots were obtained in the range of concentration from 8.0×10^{-8} M to 1.0×10^{-4} M with a limit of detection 0.824 nM for MP and 1.0×10^{-8} M to 2.5×10^{-4} M for CBZ with the detection limit of 2.82 nM. By monitoring MP and CBZ in water and soil samples, the significance of the developed method in the agricultural and environmental domains was successfully investigated. The results suggested the selectivity, stability, and reproducibility of the newly developed GO/g-C_3N_4/GCE electrode assembly. Using square wave voltammetry in Na_2HPO_4 0.1 mol L^{-1} as a supporting electrolyte, Franca and colleagues [43] have established electroanalytical determination of CBZ and fenamiphos (FNP) in natural and spiked water. The carbendazim detection calibration curve had a linearity of 0.998 and a sensitivity of 0.080 A mol^{-1} L, and it demonstrated high linearity in the concentration range of 0.50–15.0 μM. The dynamic range of concentration for fenamiphos oxidation on the boron-doped diamond electrode is 0.5–25.0 μM, with a corresponding sensibility of 0.14 A mol^{-1} L. The results of the recovery studies demonstrated that the electroanalytical technology is feasible for assessing FNP and CBZ in pure or natural waters, with values ranging from 70% to 100% for samples that had been spiked. Further high-sensitivity sensors were detected on the real cucumber sample. Table 7.2 shows the comparative performance of the reported sensors.

7.5 Electrochemical detection of insecticides

Insecticides are classified into four categories based on the chemicals they contain, i.e., carbamates, neonicotinoids, organophosphates, and organochlorines. It can be easier to understand how insecticides work and choose the appropriate pesticide for a specific weed management scenario by categorizing them according to their chemical activity. Given that pesticides are commonly used in both commercial and agricultural settings, it is essential to monitor their growth and impact on living things. As a result, electrochemical carbon-based sensors are critical for detecting insecticides in various sample types [45]. Although carbamates differ from organophosphates in their genesis, they share a similar structure. Carbamic acid is the source of carbamates; the working principle of these pesticides is that they affect the conduction of nerve signals, causing the pest's poisoning and death. Carbaryl, carbofuran, propoxur, and aminocarb are the most frequently utilized carbamates. Pegah Hashemi *et al* [46] synthesized a ternary nanocomposite Cu/CuO–Ag modified GCE (rGO/Cu/CuO-Ag/GCE) electrochemical sensor based on carbaryl (CA) and Fenamiphos (FEN) detection in fruit and vegetable samples. TEM, XRD, and FT-IR investigated the characterization of the proposed sensor, and CV and DPV techniques were used to study the electrochemical characteristics. The rGO/Cu/CuO-Ag/GCE was used in conjunction with a cost-effective for detecting low

Table 7.2. Comparison of electrochemical performance carbon-based materials for the detection of fungicides.

Pesticide	Method	Electrode	Liner range	LOD	Real sample	References
Carbendazim	DPV	MXene/ERGO/GCE	0.002–10.0 μM	0.67 nM	Cucumber, orange	[41]
MP and carbendazim	CV	GO/g-C_3N_4/GCE	8.0×10^{-8} M–1.0×10^{-4} M	0.824 nM for MP and 1.0×10^{-8} M to 2.5×10^{-4} M for CBZ	Water, soil	[42]
Carbendazim and fenamiphos (FNP)	SWV	Boron-doped diamond	0.50–15.0 μM	1.0×10^{-7} mol L^{-1}	Water	[43]
Carbamic	DPV	rGO-based non-enzymatic	1.0–5.0 μM	0.6 μM	Cucumber	[44]
Carbendazim	CV	$ZnFe_2O_4$/SWCNTs	0.5–100.0 μM	0.09 and 0.05 μM	This study has not validated their sensor for practical applications	[40]

levels of CA and FEN. The modified electrode displayed two separated oxidation signals with excellent sensitivity to determine carbaryl and fenamiphos simultaneously. The wide linear ranges of 0.05–20 and 0.01–30.0 μM and the detection limits were found as 0.005 and 0.003 μM for CA and FEN, respectively. Another work by Della Pelle *et al* [47] utilized nano CB in their study based on carbaryl, carbofuran, fenobucarb, and isoprocarb detection in durum wheat, soft wheat, and maize. The CB was used with a practical, repeatable, contamination-proof, low-cost, relocatable screen-printed sensor. SEM and FEM investigated the characterization of the proposed sensor, and its electrochemical properties were investigated using CV and EIS techniques. Using the DPV method, LOD values were found as 4.8×10^{-8} mol L^{-1}, 4.9×10^{-8} mol L^{-1}, 8.0×10^{-8} mol L^{-1}, and 7.9×10^{-8} mol L^{-1} for carbaryl, carbofuran, fenobucarb, and isoprocarb, respectively. The suggested method was successfully compared with a validated sample in real-world samples and the developed sensor can be used in delocalized analysis with fast, user-friendly, and reliable results.

Chemical pesticides typically include organophosphates as an active ingredient in killing pests. It inhibits the neuromuscular acetylcholinesterase enzyme, which is essential for numerous physiological processes in animals, insects, and humans. The neurotransmitter acetylcholine, which transmits messages to different nerve endings in the body, is broken down by the enzyme acetylcholinesterase. Parathion, malathion, MP, chlorpyrifos, diazinon, and dichlorvos are the most often utilized organophosphates. In fabricating carbon electrochemical sensors, a unique hybrid ferrocene-thiophene modified by carbon nanotube (FT@CNT) was developed as an electrochemical nanosensor to determine parathion and chlorantraniliprole pesticides [48]. As shown in figure 7.4, the DPV method was employed, and the working electrode was a GCE. For electrochemical determination, ideal circumstances such as pH and nanosensor concentration are investigated. The suggested nanosensor was used to electrochemically identify the chlorantraniliprole and parathion insecticides in soil, apple, and tomato samples. The optimal conditions at FT@CNT/GCE were used in this experiment to generate a linear relationship for chlorantraniliprole and parathion, and the LOD values were discovered to be 8.1 and 5.3 nmol L^{-1}, respectively. Electrochemical approaches are simple and quick to use, sensitive and selective for the instantaneous detection of parathion and chlorantraniliprole, according to an evaluation of the electrochemical methodology with further analytical methods for pesticide recognition.

2D MoS_2 has significant sensor usage due to its prominent physicochemical characteristics and ultrafine structure. Nevertheless, it has drawbacks, including simple collecting, surface area, poor electrical conductivity, or restacking. MoS_2 nanosheets doped with nitrogen and fluorine and coated with silver nanoparticles (Ag NPs-N-F-MoS_2) were synthesized by Dandan Song *et al* [49]. This displays excellent electroactive surface area, high conductivity, and exceptional electron mobility. Chlorpyrifos and monocrotophos were detected electrochemically using the enhanced AChE/CNTs-NH_2/Ag NPs-N-F-MoS_2/GCE sensor shown in figure 7.5. The proposed sensor is efficient in sensing chlorpyrifos and monocrotophos, with wide

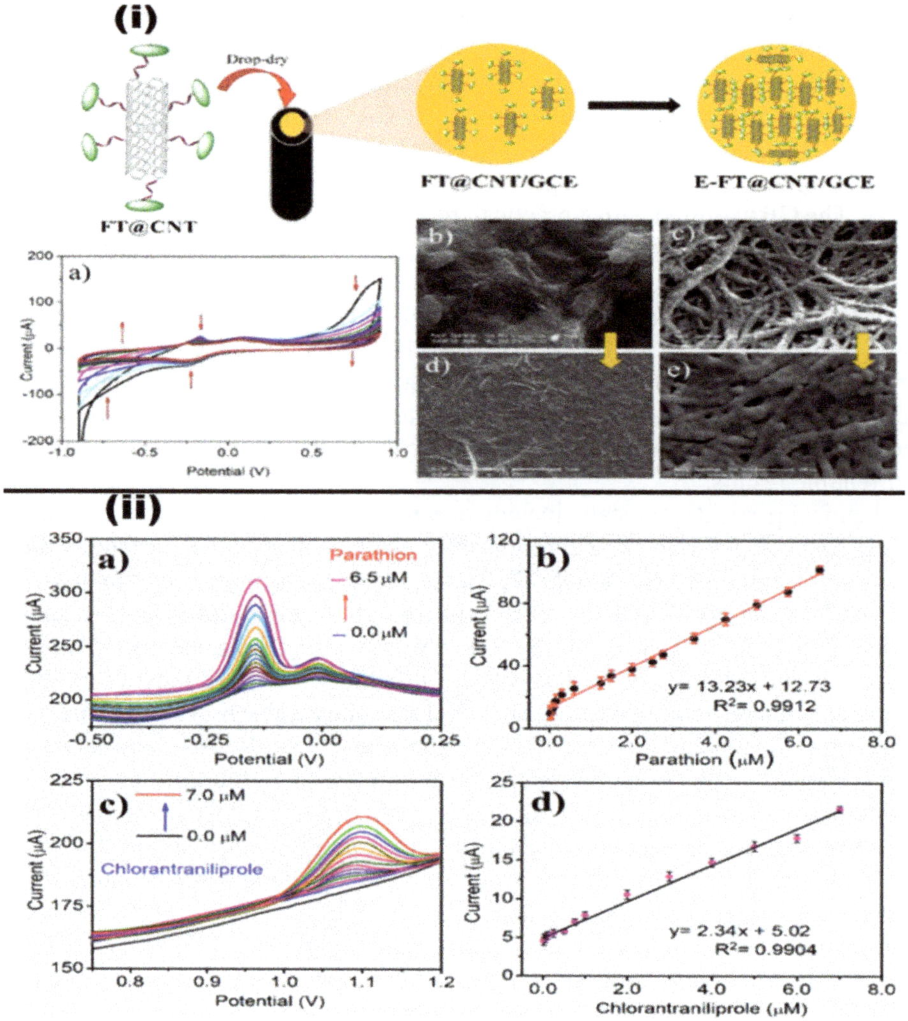

Figure 7.4. (i) Procedure for sensor assembly, electropolymerization of FT@CNT nanosensor with 25 cycles, (b, d, and c, e) SEM images of FT@CNT (ii) DPV responses on E-FT@CNT/GCE nanosensor systems at various concentrations of (a) parathion (b) linear response change of parathion concentration (c) chlorantraniliprole, (d) linear response change of chlorantraniliprole concentration. Reprinted from [48], Copyright (2021), with permission from Elsevier.

linear ranges of 5×10^{-8}–10^{-7} mg ml^{-1}, and 5×10^{-7}–10^{-4} mg ml^{-1} (chlorpyrifos), 5×10^{-10}–10^{-6} mg ml^{-1} (monocrotophos) minimal detection limits as 3.0 pM and 0.2 pM, correspondingly. The sensor's stability was demonstrated with a minimal variation of 2.8% after two weeks and 6.7% after 30 days, and its reproducibility is confirmed with a RSD of 2.6% through DPV measurements using six independently prepared and modified electrodes, along with maintaining outstanding sensitivity.

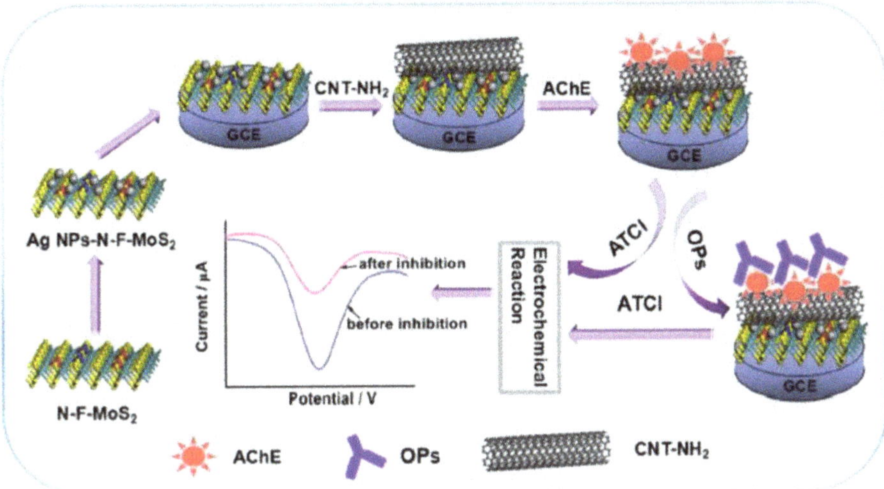

Figure 7.5. A schematic of the electrochemical biosensor fabrication process for chlorpyrifos and monocrotophos detection. Reprinted from [49], Copyright (2018), with permission from Elsevier.

Neonicotinoids are agonists that selectively bind to the nicotinic acetylcholine receptors in insects. This can prevent impulses from being transmitted, resulting in paralysis or even death. A novel form of nicotinamide insecticide is called nitenpyram (NIT). This is the primary substitute for pesticides that contain carbamates and organophosphorus. NIT has a hydrolytic half-life of 415 days, plays a crucial role in agricultural output, and degrades slowly in the environment. These characteristics suggest that an accumulation of NIT could significantly impact human health and cause significant environmental contamination. Interestingly, a study conducted by Hongwu Wang and coworkers [50] manufactured electrochemical sensors to monitor NIT utilizing a binary nanohybrid of hydroxylated multiwall carbon nanotubes/single-wall carbon nanohorns (HCNT/CNH). The geometries of binary nanohybrids that were investigated provided numerous active sites for the target analyte in the built electrochemical sensor, hence increasing the sensitivity of NIT determination. The prepared electrode was used to create the DPV method for determining nitenpyram. HCNT/CNH/GCE has good repeatability with a RSD of 5.19%. Similarly, we obtained DPV responses of six different HCNT/CNH/GCE in phosphate buffer solution (PBS) containing 1000 nM NIT. HCNT/CNH/GCE has satisfactory stability with an RSD of 5.0%. HCNT/CNH/GCE stability was further studied, and the current was reduced by 13.3% after 12 days. The results indicated that HCNT/CNH/GCE has good storage stability. NIT concentration in the range of 20.0–2000.0 nM was linearly linked with the peak current of NIT on HCNT/CNH/GCE. NIT had a detection limit of 4.0 nM. The suggested sensor effectively tracked NIT in a precise corn sample.

DDT, lindane, endosulfan, aldrin, dieldrin, and chlordane are the most widely utilized organochlorine chemicals. Environmental pollutants, such as gamma-lindane (γ-LND), are hazardous and often found in organochlorine chemicals. Canan Pelin Boke *et al* [51]. have developed a novel molecular imprinted electrochemical sensor on polyoxometalate (POM, $H_3PW_{12}O_{40}$)/carbon nitride nanotubes (C_3N_4 NTs) composite prepared for γ-LND detection. The morphology structure of a synthesized composite was studied. Its electrochemical analysis was carried out using the CV method. LOD values are 2.0×10^{-11} M and Liner range 1.0×10^{-10}–1.0×10^{-8}. The γ-LND imprinted electrode was synthesized with 100.0 mM pyrrole containing 25.0 mM γ-LND. The POM, $H_3PW_{12}O_{40}/C_3N_4$ NTs were observed regarding reproducibility, repeatability, stability, and reusability. Additionally, real samples were subjected to the sensor, such as orange juice, to monitor γ-LND. Furthermore, electrochemical sensing applications for detecting insecticides are reported in table 7.3.

7.6 Conclusion

Overusing and prolonged pesticide use to safeguard crop yields and agricultural products is a severe problem that damages the environment and food supply. These groups have different toxicity and contamination profiles; hence, monitoring the environment to maintain human health is crucial, and detecting the pesticides in the environment is an important aspect of this.

This chapter overviews the significance of carbon and its derivatives, and their hybrid nanomaterials for sensor devices to determine herbicide, fungicide, and insecticide residues in the environment. Some of the developed carbon-based electrochemical sensors have been explained. Electrodes of carbon allotrope and their hybrid materials and electrochemical sensors technique have a great future (figure 7.6). The theoretical and experimental approaches that can be used to detect herbicides, fungicides, and insecticides are highlighted in this chapter. Various techniques are available to investigate pesticides among different sensing methods; electrochemical sensing contributes significantly due to its advantages, including being eco-friendly, very efficient, and low cost. The analyte has pentazocine, isoprocarb, nitenpyram, organophosphates, carbamates, carbendazim, triazole, benzimidazoles, and metobromuron detected by carbon-hybrid composite as an effective electrode in the electrochemical method. Carbon nanomaterials, such as CNTs, graphene, and carbon dots, are excellent materials for enhancing sensor performance in various applications. They offer a range of advantages, including high surface area, excellent electrical conductivity, chemical stability, and biocompatibility. These properties make them effective in sensor design. In summary, the unique properties of carbon nanomaterials, including high surface area, excellent electrical conductivity, chemical stability, biocompatibility, tunable surface properties, miniaturization, flexibility, and cost-effectiveness, collectively enhance sensor performance. The development of simple, new, and efficient synthesis and fabrication processes that allow precise control over the size and morphology of the resulting products can further improve the performance of carbon material in electrochemical sensor applications.

Table 7.3. Electrochemical sensors reported for insecticides based on carbon nanomaterials.

Pesticide	Method	Electrode	Liner range	LOD	Real sample	References
Carbaryl	DPV	rGO/Cu/CuO-Ag/GCE	0.05–20.0 μM	0.005–0.003 μM	Vegetable, fruits	[46]
Chlorantraniliprole	DPV	FT@CNT/GCE	0.0[illegible]–7.00 μmol L^{-1}	8.1 nmol L^{-1}	Food, soil	[48]
MP	DPV	HCP5 @AuNPs–ERGO/GCE	0.005–30.0 μM	0.001 μM	Water sample	[52]
Isoprocarb	DPV	CB-SPE	1.0×10^{-7}–1.0×10^{-4} mol L^{-1}	0.79 μM	Grains	[47]
Chlorpyrifos	DPV	AChE/ATO/OMC/SPE	0.01–105 mg L^{-1}	0.01 μg L^{-1}	Fresh vegetables	[53]
Fenitrothion	CV	CNT/GCE	0.54–6.84 μM	0.090 μM	Pistachio extract	[54]
Nitenpyram	DPV	HCNT/CNH/GCE	20.0–2000.0 nM	4.0 nM	Corn	[50]
Dichlorvos	DPV	AChE/CS@TiO2m–CSm/rGO/GC	0.036–22.6 μM	29.0 nM	Cabbage juice	[55]

Abbreviations: HCP5 @AuNPs–ERGO/GCE—hydroxylatopillar [5] arene@gold nanoparticles and electrochemical reduced graphene oxide, AChE/ATO/OMC/SPE—acetylcholinesterase/antimony tin oxide/ordered mesoporous carbon/screen-printed carbon electrodes, CNT/GCE—glassy carbon electrode modified with carbon nanotubes and AChE/CS@TiO2m–CSm/rGO/GC—acetylcholinesterase/multi-layered immobilization matrix/glassy carbon electrode.

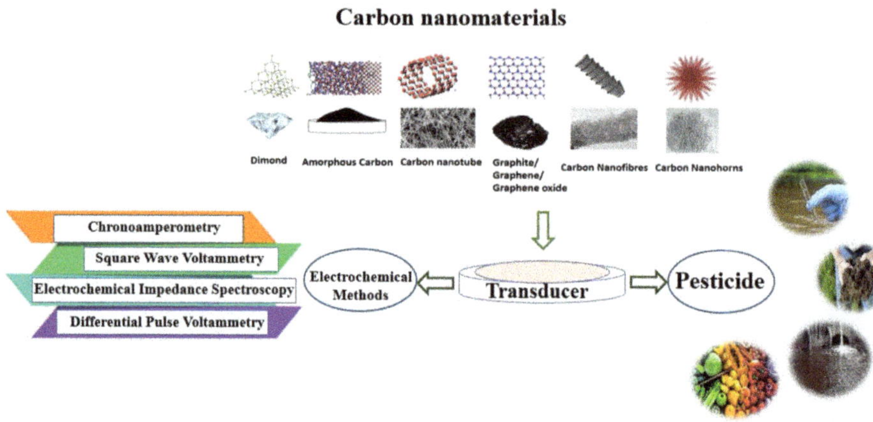

Figure 7.6. Carbon nanomaterial-based electrochemical sensors for pesticide detection from environmental samples.

References

[1] Kaur R, Mavi G K, Raghav S and Khan I 2019 Pesticides classification and its impact on environment *Int. J. Curr. Microbiol. App. Sci.* **8** 1889–97

[2] Manasa G, Mascarenhas R J, Satpati A K, Basavaraja B M and Kumar S 2018 An electrochemical bisphenol F sensor based on ZnO/G nano composite and CTAB surface modified carbon paste electrode architecture *Colloids Surf.* B **170** 144–51

[3] Khanal S, Kc K, Fulton J P, Shearer S and Ozkan E 2020 Remote sensing in agriculture—accomplishments, limitations, and opportunities *Remote Sens* **12** 3783

[4] Manasa G, Bhakta A K, Mekhalif Z and Mascarenhas R J 2019 Voltammetric study and rapid quantification of resorcinol in hair dye and biological samples using ultrasensitive maghemite/MWCNT modified carbon paste electrode *Electroanalysis* **31** 1363–72

[5] Shanmugapriya P, Rathika S, Ramesh T and Janaki P 2019 Applications of remote sensing in agriculture—a review *Int. J. Curr. Microbiol. Appl. Sci.* **8** 2270–83

[6] Manasa G, Mascarenhas R J, Bhakta A K and Mekhalif Z 2020 MWCNT/Nileblue heterostructured composite electrode for flavanone Naringenin quantification in fruit juices *Electroanalysis* **32** 939–48

[7] Manasa G, Mascarenhas R J, Bhakta A K and Mekhalif Z 2021 Nano-graphene-platelet/brilliant-green composite coated carbon paste electrode interface for electrocatalytic oxidation of flavanone Hesperidin *Microchem. J.* **160** 105768

[8] Kim H-J, Sudduth K A and Hummel J W 2009 Soil macronutrient sensing for precision agriculture *J. Environ. Monit.* **11** 1810

[9] Beck M L, Freihaut B, Henry R, Pierce S and Bayer W L 1975 A serum haemagglutinating property dependent upon polycarboxyl groups *Br. J. Haematol.* **29** 149–56

[10] Srivastava A K, Dev A and Karmakar S 2018 Nanosensors and nanobiosensors in food and agriculture *Environ. Chem. Lett.* **16** 161–82

[11] Madhusudhana , Manasa G, Bhakta A K, Mekhalif Z and Mascarenhas R J 2020 Bismuth-nanoparticles decorated multi-wall-carbon-nanotubes cast-coated on carbon paste electrode; an electrochemical sensor for sensitive determination of gallic acid at neutral pH *Mater. Sci. Energy Technol.* **3** 174–82

[12] Oliveira T M B F, Ribeiro F W P, Sousa C P, Salazar-Banda G R, De Lima-Neto P, Correia A N and Morais S 2020 Current overview and perspectives on carbon-based (bio)sensors for carbamate pesticides electroanalysis *TrAC, Trends Anal. Chem.* **124** 115779

[13] Ndamanisha J C and Guo L 2012 Ordered mesoporous carbon for electrochemical sensing: a review *Anal. Chim. Acta* **747** 19–28

[14] Da Silva A D, Paschoalino W J, Damasceno J P V and Kubota L T 2020 Structure, properties, and electrochemical sensing applications of graphene-based materials *ChemElectroChem.* **7** 4508–25

[15] Roy S, Soin N, Bajpai R, Misra D S, McLaughlin J A and Roy S S 2011 Graphene oxide for electrochemical sensing applications *J. Mater. Chem.* **21** 14725

[16] Mukherjee A, Majumdar S, Servin A D, Pagano L, Dhankher O P and White J C 2016 Carbon nanomaterials in agriculture: a critical review *Front. Plant Sci.* **7** 168246

[17] Mauter M S and Elimelech M 2008 Environmental applications of carbon-based nanomaterials *Environ. Sci. Technol.* **42** 5843–59

[18] Ni J and Li Y 2016 Carbon nanomaterials in different dimensions for electrochemical energy storage *Adv. Energy Mater.* **6** 1600278

[19] Gaur M, Misra C, Yadav A B, Swaroop S, Maolmhuaidh F Ó, Bechelany M and Barhoum A 2021 Biomedical applications of carbon nanomaterials: fullerenes, quantum dots, nanotubes, nanofibers, and graphene *Materials* **14** 5978

[20] Mostofizadeh A, Li Y, Song B and Huang Y 2011 Synthesis, properties, and applications of low-dimensional carbon-related nanomaterials *J. Nanomater.* **2011** 1–21

[21] Baptista F R, Belhout S A, Giordani S and Quinn S J 2015 Recent developments in carbon nanomaterial sensors *Chem. Soc. Rev.* **44** 4433–53

[22] Capek I 2009 Dispersions, novel nanomaterial sensors and nanoconjugates based on carbon nanotubes *Adv. Colloid Interface Sci.* **150** 63–89

[23] Chopra N, Gavalas V G, Bachas L G, Hinds B J and Bachas L G 2007 Functional One-dimensional nanomaterials: applications in nanoscale biosensors *Anal. Lett.* **40** 2067–96

[24] Knihnicki P, Skrzypek A, Jakubowska M, Porada R, Rokicińska A, Kuśtrowski P, Kościelniak P and Kochana J 2022 Electrochemical sensing of Pb^{2+} and Cd^{2+} ions with the use of electrode modified with carbon-covered halloysite and carbon nanotubes *Molecules* **27** 4608

[25] Su C C, Liu T, Chang N K, Wang B R and Chang S H 2012 Two dimensional carbon nanotube based strain sensor *Sensors Actuators* A **176** 124–9

[26] Arduini F, Di Nardo F, Amine A, Micheli L, Palleschi G and Moscone D 2012 Carbon black-modified screen-printed electrodes as electroanalytical tools *Electroanalysis* **24** 743–51

[27] Battaglino B, Grinzato A and Pagliano C 2021 Binding properties of photosynthetic herbicides with the QB site of the D1 protein in plant photosystem II: a combined functional and molecular docking study *Plants* **10** 1501

[28] Sipa K, Brycht M, Leniart A, Nosal–Wiercińska A and Skrzypek S 2018 Improved electroanalytical characteristics for the determination of pesticide metobromuron in the presence of nanomaterials *Anal. Chim. Acta* **1030** 61–9

[29] Mani V, Devasenathipathy R, Chen S-M, Wu T-Y and Kohilarani K 2015 High-performance electrochemical amperometric sensors for the sensitive determination of phenyl urea herbicides diuron and fenuron *Ionics* **21** 2675–83

[30] Manasa G, Bhakta A K, Mascarenhas R J and Shetti N P 2023 BaO-MWCNT composite material-based electrocatalytic amperometric sensor for the detection of environmentally hazardous Diuron *Microchem. J.* **191** 108778
[31] Ilager D, Shetti N P, Reddy K R, Tuwar S M and Aminabhavi T M 2022 Nanostructured graphitic carbon nitride (g-C_3N_4)-CTAB modified electrode for the highly sensitive detection of amino-triazole and linuron herbicides *Environ. Res.* **204** 111856
[32] Rahemi V, Garrido J M P J, Borges F, Brett C M A and Garrido E M P J 2013 Electrochemical determination of the herbicide bentazone using a carbon nanotube β-cyclodextrin modified electrode *Electroanalysis* **25** 2360–6
[33] Garcia L L C, Figueiredo-Filho L C S, Oliveira G G, Fatibello-Filho O and Banks C E 2013 Square-wave voltammetric determination of paraquat using a glassy carbon electrode modified with multiwalled carbon nanotubes within a dihexadecylhydrogenphosphate (DHP) film *Sensors Actuators* B **181** 306–11
[34] Zhou Y, Cheng F, Hong Y, Huang J, Zhang X and Liao X 2020 Rapid and sensitive detection of isoproturon via an electrochemical sensor based on highly water-dispersed carbon hybrid material *Food Anal. Methods* **13** 839–49
[35] Ganjali M R N P 2014 A novel method for ultra trace measurement of bentazon based on nanocomposite electrode and continuous coulometric FFT cyclicvoltammetry *Int. J. Environ. Res.* **9** 101–8
[36] Fusco G, Gallo F, Tortolini C, Bollella P, Ietto F, De Mico A, D'Annibale A, Antiochia R, Favero G and Mazzei F 2017 AuNPs-functionalized PANABA–MWCNTs nanocomposite-based impedimetric immunosensor for 2,4-dichlorophenoxy acetic acid detection *Biosens. Bioelectron.* **93** 52–6
[37] Wei X-P, Zhang R-Q, Wang L-B, Luo Y-L, Xu F and Chen Y-S 2019 Novel multi-walled carbon nanotubes decorated with gold nanoparticles with poly(2-methacryloyloxyethyl ferrocenecarboxylate) grafted on to form organic–inorganic nanohybrids: preparation, characterization, and electrochemical sensing applications *J. Mater. Chem.* C **7** 119–32
[38] Manasa G, Bhakta A K, Bafna J, Mascarenhas R J, Malode S J and Shetti N P 2022 An amperometric sensor composed of carbon hybrid-structure for the degradation of amino-triazole herbicide *Environ. Res.* **212** 113541
[39] Klittich C J 2008 Milestones in fungicide discovery: chemistry that changed agriculture *Plant Health Progress* **9** 31
[40] Dong Y, Yang L and Zhang L 2017 Simultaneous electrochemical detection of benzimidazole fungicides carbendazim and thiabendazole using a novel nanohybrid material-modified electrode *J. Agric. Food Chem.* **65** 727–36
[41] Xie Y, Gao F, Tu X, Ma X, Xu Q, Dai R, Huang X, Yu Y and Lu L 2019 Facile synthesis of MXene/electrochemically reduced graphene oxide composites and their application for electrochemical sensing of carbendazim *J. Electrochem. Soc.* **166** B1673–80
[42] Ilager D, Shetti N P, Foucaud Y, Badawi M and Aminabhavi T M 2022 Graphene/g-carbon nitride (GO/g-C_3N_4) nanohybrids as a sensor material for the detection of methyl parathion and carbendazim *Chemosphere* **292** 133450
[43] França R F, De Oliveira H P M, Pedrosa V A and Codognoto L 2012 Electroanalytical determination of carbendazim and fenamiphos in natural waters using a diamond electrode *Diam. Relat. Mater.* **27–28** 54–9

[44] Taşaltın N, Karakuş S, Taşaltın C and Baytemir G 2022 Highly sensitive and selective rGO based non-enzymatic electrochemical sensor for propamocarb fungicide pesticide detection *Food Chem.* **372** 131267

[45] Sparks T C 2013 Insecticide discovery: an evaluation and analysis *Pestic. Biochem. Physiol.* **107** 8–17

[46] Hashemi P, Karimian N, Khoshsafar H, Arduini F, Mesri M, Afkhami A and Bagheri H 2019 Reduced graphene oxide decorated on Cu/CuO–Ag nanocomposite as a high-performance material for the construction of a non-enzymatic sensor: Application to the determination of carbaryl and fenamiphos pesticides *Mater. Sci. Eng.* C **102** 764–72

[47] Della Pelle F, Angelini C, Sergi M, Del Carlo M, Pepe A and Compagnone D 2018 Nano carbon black-based screen printed sensor for carbofuran, isoprocarb, carbaryl and fenobucarb detection: application to grain samples *Talanta* **186** 389–96

[48] Tümay S O, Şenocak A, Sarı E, Şanko V, Durmuş M and Demirbas E 2021 A new perspective for electrochemical determination of parathion and chlorantraniliprole pesticides via carbon nanotube-based thiophene-ferrocene appended hybrid nanosensor *Sensors Actuators* B **345** 130344

[49] Song D, Wang Y, Lu X, Gao Y, Li Y and Gao F 2018 Ag nanoparticles-decorated nitrogen-fluorine co-doped monolayer MoS_2 nanosheet for highly sensitive electrochemical sensing of organophosphorus pesticides *Sensors Actuators* B **267** 5–13

[50] Wang H, Pan L, Liu Y, Ye Y and Yao S 2020 Electrochemical sensing of nitenpyram based on the binary nanohybrid of hydroxylated multiwall carbon nanotubes/single-wall carbon nanohorns *J. Electroanal. Chem.* **862** 113955

[51] Pelin Böke C, Karaman O, Medetalibeyoglu H, Karaman C, Atar N and Lütfi Yola M 2020 A new approach for electrochemical detection of organochlorine compound lindane: development of molecular imprinting polymer with polyoxometalate/carbon nitride nanotubes composite and validation *Microchem. J.* **157** 105012

[52] Hou X, Liu X, Li Z, Zhang J, Du G, Ran X and Yang L 2019 Electrochemical determination of methyl parathion based on pillar[5]arene@AuNPs@reduced graphene oxide hybrid nanomaterials *New J. Chem.* **43** 13048–57

[53] Hou W, Zhang Q, Dong H, Li F, Zhang Y, Guo Y and Sun X 2019 Acetylcholinesterase biosensor modified with ATO/OMC for detecting organophosphorus pesticides *New J. Chem.* **43** 946–52

[54] Soltani-Sarvestani M, Shamspur T, Mostafavi A, Falahati-Pour S K, Mohamadi M and Saljooqi A 2020 A novel preconcentration/extraction method for fenitrothion residues and its electrochemical sensing in pistachio kernels *J. Mater. Sci: Mater. Electron.* **31** 11268–75

[55] Cui H-F, Wu W-W, Li M-M, Song X, Lv Y and Zhang T-T 2018 A highly stable acetylcholinesterase biosensor based on chitosan–TiO_2–graphene nanocomposites for detection of organophosphate pesticides *Biosens. Bioelectron.* **99** 223–9

Chapter 8

Carbon-based electrochemical sensors for the detection of heavy metal ions from agricultural contamination

G Manasa, Mansi Pathak and Chandra Sekhar Rout

As environmental contamination worsens, it is essential to identify heavy metal ions (HMIs) because they are retrieved in various water supplies and pose a severe threat to human health. Toxic chemicals generated from human activities have polluted numerous water bodies worldwide, and many of these pollutants have found their way into the drinking water supply chain. Due to their toxicity, biological accumulation potential in ecological systems, and lack of biodegradability, HMIs represent the greatest threat to human health in natural and agricultural systems. Compared to other traditional methods, the electrochemical technique is straightforward, sensitive, and quick to respond. The crucial factor in the electrochemical sensor performance is determination and detection. Reliable, highly specific, and selective electrochemical detection methods are needed to enable the quick identification of hazardous pollutants to successfully address this problem. Thus, the unique abilities of carbon nanomaterials present the possibility of creating valuable instruments for regular sensing and biosensing uses. High specific surface area and good electrical conductivity are two benefits of carbon-based nanomaterial with exceptional performance. The harmful effects of HMI are specifically outlined. This chapter highlights recent developments in creating carbon-based nanomaterials for effective electrochemical HMI detection. Herein, we highlighted the usage of carbon-based nanomaterials in the electrochemical detection of HMIs. In addition, based on recent advances in research and experimental techniques, potential difficulties and future opportunities for applying carbon-based nanomaterials in the electrochemical detection of HMIs are discussed.

doi:10.1088/978-0-7503-5879-8ch8

8.1 Introduction

The growing population, human actions, hasty industrialization, and untrained utilization of natural water possessions have negatively impacted water quality. Water contamination is caused by the by-products of rapid industrialization and improper farming methods, such as hazardous heavy metals, drugs, pesticides, and chemicals [1–4]. Since many people live in densely populated cities, there is a growing need to supply them with uncontaminated potable water. Given the increasing need for uncontaminated water, it is crucial to discover suitable methods for water purification and guarantee its recyclability [4–7]. HMIs are a prominent category of pollutants in water contamination, adversely affecting both land and aquatic ecosystems. Pharmaceuticals, agricultural contamination, and their by-products are the primary origin of these HMIs.

Although industrial and pharmaceutical by-products are the primary source of HMIs, synthetic pesticides have also contributed significantly to their contamination, are widely dispersed, and cannot be broken down. The primary sources of HMI are agricultural fertilizer applications [8–12]. Chromium (Cr), copper (Cu), lead (Pb), arsenic (As), cadmium (Cd), and mercury (Hg) are poisonous and carcinogenic heavy metals present in the environment. Even minor quantities of exposure to these metals can significantly risk human well-being and the natural surroundings [13–16]. These HMIs pose a threat to human health, even at low levels of concentration. This is because these metal ions interact with the thiol group of proteins and subsequently pass into cells, altering the metabolic processes. In addition, elevated levels of silver and copper might also have harmful consequences [17–19]. These HMIs are very hazardous pollutants, classified among the top 10 on the 'Priority List of Hazardous Substances of Toxic Substances and Disease Registry' [20]. Prominent global institutions, including the World Health Organization (WHO), the US Environmental Protection Agency, the Centers for Disease Control, and the European Union, have identified heavy metals as necessary chemicals and set specific thresholds for their permissible concentrations [20, 21].

Considering the risks posed by ions of heavy metals to both the ecosystem and human health, it is crucial to have precise and effective detection methods. Several techniques have been devised to identify HMIs, including atomic absorption spectroscopy, neutron activation analysis, inductively coupled plasma-mass spectroscopy, x-ray-based spectrometric techniques, and inductively coupled plasma-optical emission spectrometry [22–29]. Although these technologies have good sensitivity in detecting metal ions and can test numerous ions concurrently, they pose a few setbacks. The other prior techniques applied to heavy metal detection include inductively coupled plasma-Mass spectrometry (ICP-MS), UV–Vis spectrometry, liquid chromatography, atomic emission spectrometry (AES), atomic absorption spectroscopy, atomic fluorescence spectrometry, capillary electrophoresis (CE), cold vapor atomic fluorescence spectrometry, and laser-induced breakdown spectroscopy (LIBS) [30–35]. Despite the excellent sensitivity and selectivity of these approaches, they still have significant problems in heavy metal detection [31]. The challenges associated with this include the considerable expense, intricate operating protocols, the extended time required for detection, and difficulty accomplishing detection in real-world circumstances [32, 33]. Nevertheless, spectroscopic approaches are costly. Proficient experts are needed to operate the instruments necessary for these approaches, which include intricate sample preparation and analysis procedures. While optical approaches effectively detect HMIs, they need expensive equipment and complex procedures. Furthermore, these approaches are not ideal for detecting on-site [20, 36]. Hence, developing cost-effective, uncomplicated, and precise detection technology is crucial for the on-site detection of metal ions.

Electrochemical technologies are increasingly acknowledged for their effectiveness in detecting heavy metals. These approaches provide equivalent sensitivity at a reduced cost, simplified operating processes, and rapid on-site detection. The limitations of previous methods can be overcome by employing electrochemical detection. Electrochemical approaches are characterized by their user-friendly nature, low cost, and high reliability [35, 36]. Various electrochemical systems have been devised to detect heavy metals. Nanomaterials have brought numerous advances due to their exclusive electronic, chemical, and mechanical properties. Consequently, many electrochemical sensors utilizing nanoparticles have been developed to detect heavy metals. Moreover, electrochemical detection may be utilized in the field, providing mobility and quick answers for the on-site examination of contaminated materials. Nevertheless, pristine/bare working electrode (sensor) exhibits reduced sensitivity and limits of detection (LOD) related to spectroscopic and optical methods. Thus, electrochemical sensor performance can be enhanced by selectively modifying them with specific elements [37, 38]. Enhancements in design are necessary to strengthen the efficacy of electrochemical techniques in detecting HMIs. Multiple electrochemical methodologies with diverse biosensing electrodes are used to amplify their sensitivity and improve their detection limits by modifying the electrode material [36, 37].

Advanced sensing techniques and portable devices have been made more accessible to design and develop through recent developments in nanotechnology and novel pathways for synthesizing nanomaterials. Specifically, several categories of nanomaterials, such as carbon nanomaterials, metal oxide nanoparticles, metal nanoparticles, 2D materials, and different nanocomposites, have been used to alter the working electrode. Through deposition and drop casting, nanomaterials can alter the electrode surface, allowing for nanoscale control over the desired material's structure and form [37]. The remarkable qualities of carbon-based nanomaterials, including their high electrical conductivity, substantial definite surface area, strong chemical stability, many adsorption-active sites, repeatability, and selectivity, make them ideal for electrochemical detection of HMIs. Due to their exceptional mechanical, chemical, electrical, and thermal properties, carbon nanomaterials such as graphene, graphene oxide (GO), reduced GO (rGO), carbon nanotubes (CNTs), multiwalled CNTs (MWCNTs), single-walled CNTs (SWCNTs), activated carbon, nanoporous carbon, and carbon nanofibers (CNFs) have been widely used in the sensitive and selective electrochemical sensing of a wide range of electroactive targets, including HMIs [14–18]. Carbon nanoparticles are crucial in electrocatalytic processes due to their large specific surface area and outstanding biological suitability. The material's extensive surface area and strong surface reactivity result in increased adsorption capacity, enhanced surface activity, and improved catalytic efficiency. Carbon nanomaterial-based sensors provide superior characteristics, including reduced size and enhanced rapidity, as well as improved accuracy and enhanced consistency. This chapter introduces the design, structure, mechanism analysis, and experimental performance of the electrochemical sensors modified with carbon-based materials and their derivatives for detecting HMIs from agricultural pollutants.

8.2 Heavy metal ions: agricultural sources and toxicity

Heavy metals such as Pb and Hg generally contaminate water, soil, and plants due to synthetic fertilizers, untreated sewage disposal, and fossil fuel combustion. One factor contributing to the Pb contamination in soil is using pesticides and fertilizers in agricultural activities. Industrial discharge, phosphate fertilizers, and sewage sludge additives are the main causes of lead contamination in soils [38]. The selected food items consisted of very high Pb concentrations within cereals, which include rice, wheat, and maize. Of these, wheat had the highest concentration (4.04 $\mu g\ g^{-1}$), while the concentrations in rice and maize were 2.22 and 1.43 $\mu g\ g^{-1}$, respectively, above the maximum acceptable concentration (MAC, 0.20 $\mu g\ g^{-1}$) for cereals. All vegetables except mushrooms, green bananas, cauliflower, and arum had Pb concentrations more significant than the maximum acceptable concentration of 0.01 $\mu g\ g^{-1}$ [39]. This is highly hazardous and detrimental to human health, especially to the developing brain and bones of young children. Pb may harm the immune system and kidneys, as well as induce anemia, high blood pressure, dyspepsia, indigestion, and endocrine issues. It can also cross the blood–brain barrier, which provides protection, and it has been shown to increase the risk of developing Alzheimer's disease [38, 39].

The kind and location of the source of contamination might affect the concentration of Cd in herbal species growing on contaminated soils, which can reach high levels [38]. Cadmium (Cd) is an element of trace amount commonly present in the environment but not necessarily. Human and geogenic sources can increase the levels of Cd in soils and groundwater, which is crucial for preserving a wholesome food supply and clean drinking water. Individuals can develop cancer from high levels of mercury. A recommended level of Cd is 3.0 $\mu g\ l^{-1}$ according to the WHO Guidelines for drinking water quality. Anthropogenic sources of Pb include mining, fertilizer usage containing Cd, and combustion emissions that are dumped into the atmosphere [40]. Cd readily accumulates in the kidneys and liver when entering the body via the bloodstream and is a potent carcinogen that hinders the function of enzymes responsible for DNA error repair (hence intensifying cellular mistakes and genetic mutations, ultimately resulting in the development of cancer). Prolonged use of spacers can harm the renal tubules and glomeruli, leading to the presence of protein and amino acids in the urine, which can lead to the development of diabetes [41].

Furthermore, mercury is the primary pollutant in water contaminated by heavy metals [43]. Mercury pollution is still a significant concern and can lead to various health issues if the consumption of fish is not appropriately controlled, even though fish is a relatively common dietary source. The public may readily get national standards for fish consumption and regional cautions regarding the safety of fish collected in the surrounding waterways. The worldwide mercury cycle depends heavily on soil, a necessary medium that connects the atmosphere and water [42, 43]. In addition to being a mercury reservoir, soil releases mercury into the atmosphere, water, and plants when it absorbs mercury from the surrounding environment. The WHO's International Intervention for Research on Cancer has classified organic and inorganic mercury compounds as carcinogenic. Mercury, which is soluble in water and eventually found its way into human bodies through the food chain, is absorbed by fish and shellfish. Mercury has a significant affinity for sulfur and may readily bind to thiol-containing molecules in the human body, including cysteine, glutathione reductase, and superoxide dismutase. This inhibits many enzymes and the tricarboxylic acid cycle [44]. Mercury can also result in oxidative stress and interfere with the mitochondria's regular function. These effects can lead to hypertension, hypotonia, acrodynia, increased salivation, Minamata illness, and harm to the human neurological system, gastrointestinal system, immunological system, lungs, skin, kidneys, and eyes. The most hazardous organic mercury compound is dimethylmercury [45]. Should a few microliters come into direct touch with the skin, it can be fatal. As a result, mercury monitoring and detection have long been of importance.

Silver and copper have extensive applications in our everyday existence. Silver has been utilized in a range of industrial items, including filters, textiles, and food storage. On the other hand, copper is commonly found in sectors such as fertilizers, tanners, and solar power systems. Ag(I) and Cu(II) toxicities are comparatively lower than previously listed HMIs. Nevertheless, at elevated quantities, Ag(I) and Cu(II) can potentially pose a threat to human health [38]. Silver ions (Ag(I)) have the potential to cause gastroenteritis, neurological disorders, cognitive tiredness, rheumatism, cartilage nodules, and several other ailments. Copper (II) can be a causative factor in conditions such as hair loss, allergies, anemia, arthritis, adrenal hyperfunction, autism, cystic fibrosis, and other disorders [46, 47].

8.3 Various electrochemical techniques to detect heavy metal ions

Electrochemical sensors operate based on output transducer signals and potentiostat-based potential difference detection. The electrochemical sensor's sense signal is gathered via a conducting wire, enabling the integration of several sensors into a small device. Moreover, bare electrode sensing is made possible by the specified redox potential of HMIs, which does away with the need for molecule-specific probes employed in optical sensors [48]. Based on the various electrical signals that HMIs produce in the solution, electrochemical techniques for identifying HMIs in an aqueous solution are categorized. Changes in current, voltage, charge, electrochemical impedance, and electroluminescence can all be brought about by the presence of HMIs. As depicted in figure 8.1, the amperometric, voltammetric,

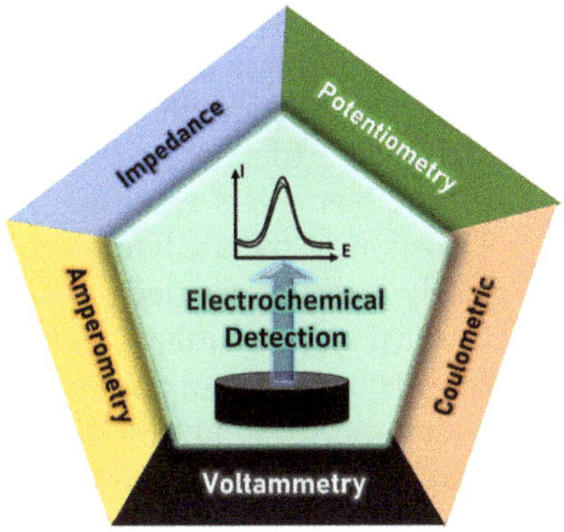

Figure 8.1. Schematic of various electrochemical techniques for the detection of HMIs.

potentiometric, impedance measuring, coulometric, and electrochemiluminescent techniques are several categories into which electrochemical techniques are divided based on different electrical signals [48, 49]. Most of these methods assess changes in one parameter by controlling the potential or the current. The lack of a process to regulate current and voltage concurrently serves as an initial basis for measuring techniques that are either potentiostatic or galvanostatic. Additionally, alternative methods exist in which there is no influence signal, i.e., there is zero current and potential across the electrodes. For example, methods such as potentiometry determine the potential to identify the kind of HMI [50–54].

Certain HMIs in water may be quantitatively determined with extreme selectivity using potentiometric techniques. The electric field (*E*) at zero current is measured using this method. This implies that no current is used for this specific type of measurement. Using selected electrodes, potentiometric methods are mostly used to quantify the ions in solutions. Unlike other electroanalytical methods, they assess a solution's conductivity instead of its concentration for qualitative and quantitative examination. Because of their quick reaction time, low cost, good selectivity, and wide series of responses, these approaches have been widely employed in detecting HMIs in complicated environmental matrices [55, 56]. The high concentration range detection limits, low sensitivity, and challenges with electrode reduction of these approaches are some of the shortcomings. With carbon nanotubes and metal nanoparticles being the most commonly used categories, applying nanomaterials as the interface material for working electrodes in conjunction with these approaches is a promising field of study [57].

Amperometry is another form of regulated potential technology that uses a working electrode made of non-mercury to regulate and measure minuscule currents at a fixed voltage. This method typically provides a potential step indicator between the reference electrode and working electrodes in solutions containing electroactive molecules. Large current flows result from the subsequent decrease at the electrode surface, and this current flow is proportionate to the gradient of concentrations at the electrode surface. These investigations, which track the current as a function of time, are known as amperometric methods [48]. The constant voltage of the working electrode enables this approach to determine only one specific component from an electrochemically accessible molecule. At a specific applied potential magnitude and polarity, the analyte to be detected experiences a faradaic response. However, considering the working electrode has a less extensive surface area, the faradaic reaction is partial and only a portion of the analyte responds [56, 57].

Voltammetry is a particularly widely reported electrochemical technique for detecting HMIs. All electrochemical systems utilizing potential-dependent measurements of current are frequently defined by voltammetry. A working electrode, a reference electrode, and a counter electrode are the usual components of a three-electrode electrochemical setup. Though the current is monitored between the working and counter electrodes, the voltage is delivered between the working and reference electrodes. When one modifies the perspective change strategy, they arrive at distinct approaches. The four main forms of voltammetry are linear sweep voltammetry (LSV), differential pulse voltammetry (DPV), anodic stripping voltammetry (ASV), and cyclic voltammetry (CV) [36, 37]. The main distinction between these technologies is the time waveform produced by the corresponding functional applications. Prior concentration, the initial stage in ASV detection, implies electro-reducing (depositing) the metal ion components in the solution to coordinate zero-valent metal on the outermost surface of the working electrode at a constant voltage. The analyte deposited on the electrode's surface is stripped (dissolved) at a certain potential in the second stage, which involves applying a sweep of voltage in the anode direction to re-oxidize the zero-valent metal [58]. Based on the unique oxidation potential of each metal, this technique may achieve the particular detection of various metal ions. The simplest method for sweeping the potential linearly with time is LSV [36]. The process of CV involves reversing the potential of a working electrode after linearly scanning the potential in one direction. Stated differently, one or more triangular potential waveforms are involved. The fundamental concept underlying pulsed voltammetry is the use of a voltage signal pulse. Different forms of pulsed voltammetry are possible by adjusting the amplitude and shape of the pulses [58]. A linear potential ramp is overlaid with fixed magnitude pulses. Square wave voltammetry (SWV) applies a symmetric square waveform to the functioning electrode by superimposing it on a base staircase potential [36].

Electrochemical impedance spectroscopy (EIS) and AC voltammetry measurement are the most used impedance measuring methods for figuring out the analyte's concentration in an aqueous solution. Among these two methods, researchers have used EIS to identify metal ions in diverse biological and environmental materials. The EIS method is frequently used to investigate the interfacial characteristics of changed electrodes, particularly in multiple-layer substrates [59]. The circuit's reaction to a voltage or alternating current as a function of frequency is described by the well-developed field of electrical and electronic systems theory, or EIS [60]. Compared to other electroanalytical methods, this method provides sensitive and affordable detection of hazardous metal ions in biological and chemical matrices. An electrical equivalent circuit is used in EIS to depict an electrochemical reaction in an electrolytic cell. Both faradaic and non-faradaic components are subsequently produced by charge transfer over an electrical contact brought through the result of an electrochemical reaction in the current channel. Chemiluminescence is produced by a few homogeneous electron transfer processes in chemical solutions containing radical ions. Electrochemical processes typically produce free radicals by electrolysis, a process known as electrochemiluminescence that initiates this chemiluminescence. These procedures are frequently used to identify a particular metal ion in a solution using fluorescence detection, which is informal, affordable, and relatively sensitive (parts per billion or trillion) [60]. The recent developments in voltammetric, amperometric, and impedance methods for electrochemical identification of HMIs in water samples, such as Cd(II), As(III), Pb(II), Hg(II), Ag(I), Cu(II), etc, are addressed below, along with advances in a range of interface materials that modify the electrodes which these approaches implement.

8.4 Carbon-based electrode materials for the electrochemical detection of heavy metal ions

Carbon nanostructures' unique electrical, magnetic, and optical properties, including graphene, carbon nanoparticles, and carbon nanotubes, have led to their extensive synthesis and study. Researchers are now looking into further carbon nanomaterials due to their remarkable qualities, which include strong electrical conductivity, mechanical robustness, structural and chemical stability, and the surface-to-volume ratio. Numerous carbon allotropes with various functional properties and dimensions, including 0D, 1D, and 2D, have been formed by the capacity of carbon atoms to bond together in diverse ways [60–63]. These materials are well-known for their remarkable qualities and capacity to act as electrodes or electrode modifiers. The ability of carbon materials to operate as both a detection system and an adsorbent/pre-concentrator agent is a significant benefit. Remarkable optical attributes, increased biodegradation, robust resistance to corrosion, high repeatability, better directionality, higher electrical conductivity, nontoxicity, and modifiability are some of these assets. The vast definite surface area, broad potential window, outstanding physicochemical features, and mechanical toughness of carbon nanomaterials make them particularly suitable for detecting HMIs. In addition, strong covalent bonds between carbon nanoparticles and other materials allow for the construction of materials of exceptional strength, hardness, and density. Changes in the density and structure of the material can also be used to modify the surface functional groups of these nanoparticles, improving the sensitivity of HMI detection [58–63]. Since they improve the electrochemical sensor's overall performance (i.e., oxidation and reduction) and sensitivity while reducing the adverse effects of selective identification and interference, carbon nanomaterials are essential to the research and design of electrochemical sensors (figure 8.2).

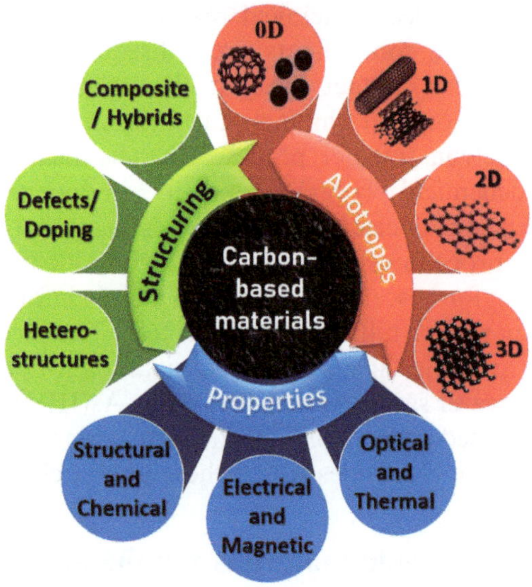

Figure 8.2. The beneficial features of carbon-based electrode materials.

8.4.1 Graphene-based sensors for heavy metal ions

The physical characteristics of graphene include a large specific surface area, flexibility, superior electrical conductivity, a substantial ratio of surface to volume, higher chemical, mechanical strength, and thermal resilience, and exceptional transparency, which are only a few of its outstanding chemical and structural qualities. Graphene exhibits exceptional optical, electrical, and morphological properties that have rendered it beneficial for a wide range of applied sciences and technological uses, such as electrochemical biosensors, energy storage devices, fuel cells, electromagnetic shielding, aerospace, photonics, electronic components, organic light-emitting diode barrier coatings, sensors with transducers integrated circuits, and biomedical devices. Graphene and its analogs comprising oxygen, such as GO and rGO, represent a significant category of nanomaterials in the sensing field [64–66]. Although GO nanosheets feature oxidized functional groups, they are also relatively hydrophilic, facilitating chemical functionalization. Graphene-based nanocomposites that increase the sensitivity of sensor applications can be made by simply combining graphene, GO, and rGO nanosheets with different kinds of inorganic nanoparticles, such as metals, metal oxides, organic polymer compounds, semiconductor nanoparticles, quantum dots, and biomolecules.

Direct electrode modification using graphene has made significant improvements. For instance, Tan *et al* [67] integrated gold nanoparticles with cysteine to develop the gold nanoparticle–cysteine composite (Au-GN–Cys). By using ultrasonic treatment alongside rapid stirring, uniform AU-GN–Cys-dispersion was produced. Evaporative deposition was then used to modify it on a bismuth sheet glassy carbon electrode. Applying square wave anodic stripping voltammetry (SWASV), a highly sensitive framework for the instantaneous electrochemical detection of Cd(II) and

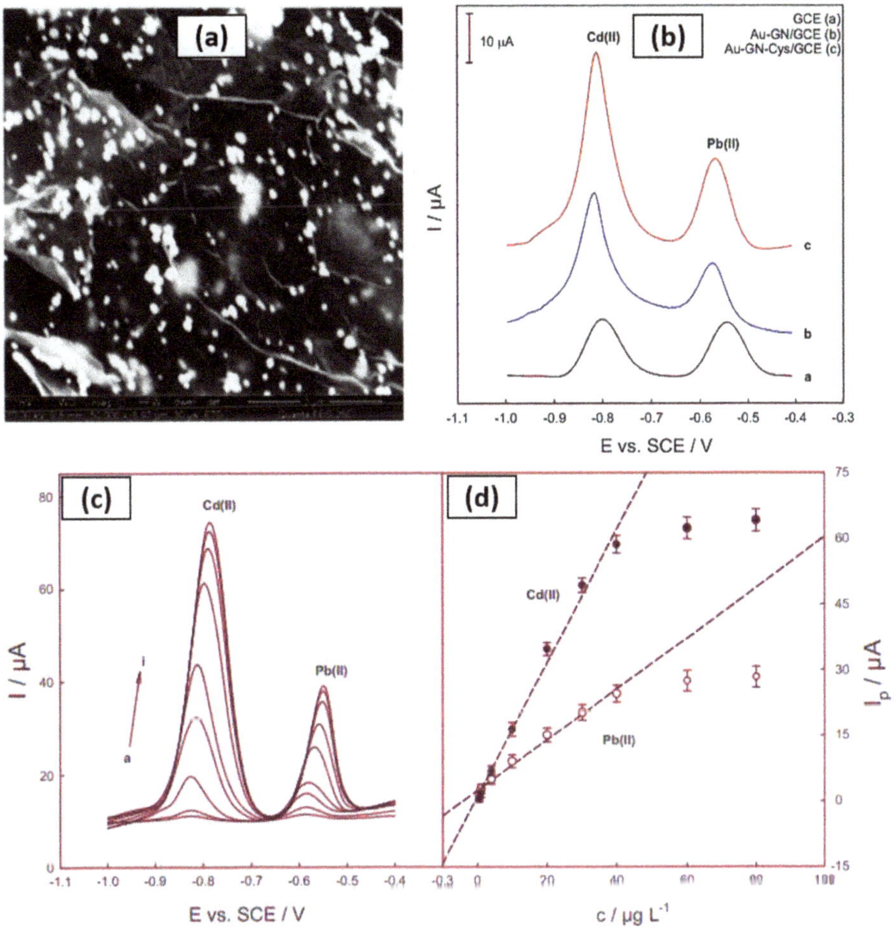

Figure 8.3. (a) Scanning electron microscope (SEM) micrographs of Au-GN–Cys/GCE surface. (b) SWASV curves at GCE (a), Au-GN/GCE (b), Au-GN–Cys/GCE (c) in 0.1 mol l^{-1} pH 4.5 ABS comprising 20 $\mu g\ l^{-1}$ Cd^{-1}(II), 20 $\mu g\ l^{-1}$ Pb(II) and 300 $\mu g\ l^{-1}$ Bi(III). (c) SWASV curvatures at Au-GN–Cys/GCE in 0.1 mol l^{-1} pH 4.5 ABS with 300 $\mu g\ l^{-1}$ Bi(III), Cd(II), and Pb(II) at varying concentrations, [0.5, 1, 4, 10, 20, 30, 40, 60, 80 $\mu g\ l^{-1}$] from a to i. Amplitude: 0.025 V, increment potential: 0.004 V, deposition time: 800 s, and deposition potential: −1.2 V. (d) Plots showing the stripping peak current against Pb(II) and Cd(II) concentrations. The mean ± SD (error bar) of the three experiments is displayed. Reprinted from [67], Copyright (2014), with permission from Elsevier.

Pb(II) in an aquatic solution has been constructed on the modified bismuth film glassy carbon electrode (GCE) with gold nanoparticle-graphene–cysteine composite (Au-GN–Cys), as shown in figure 8.3(a). From figure 8.3(b), the deposition of Pb(II) and Cd(II) on the electrode surface was facilitated by the synergistic impact of cysteine, in addition to the larger, active surface, and excellent electrical conduction of gold nanoparticles and graphene. The currents and the concentrations of Pb(II) and Cd(II) were linearly related by detection limits of 0.05 $\mu g\ l^{-1}$ and 0.10 $\mu g\ l^{-1}$ for Pb(II) and Cd(II), respectively (figures 8.3(c) and (d)). According to the interference experiments, certain metal cations did not significantly affect the SWASV signals of Pb(II) and Cd(II). The Au-GN–Cys/GCE electrode has a highly promising metal detection capability, owing to the apparent synergistic interaction between cysteine and Au-GN on metal deposition. Measuring Cd(II) and Pb(II) in an aqueous solution offers a high-performance platform.

By employing doping and additional methods, graphene may maintain its inherent chemical characteristics while preserving the exceptional qualities of composite materials. Aicheng *et al* [68] employed functionalization and doping techniques to enhance the electrochemical capabilities of graphene derivatives. A fluorinated graphene oxide material (FGO) was produced via a one-pot procedure. Their characterization approaches unveiled nanosheets and a layered structure with an approximate fluorine content of 1.0 atomic percent, figures 8.4(g) and (h). This fluorine content enhanced the material's capacitance compared to GO material. The electrochemical detection experiment yields a notable enhancement in the detection efficacy. Figures 8.4(a)–(f) display the characterization diagram and detection findings of FGO. The carbon bonded to F displayed semi-ionic bonding properties, resulting in a notable increase in the capacitance of FGO related to GO. In addition,

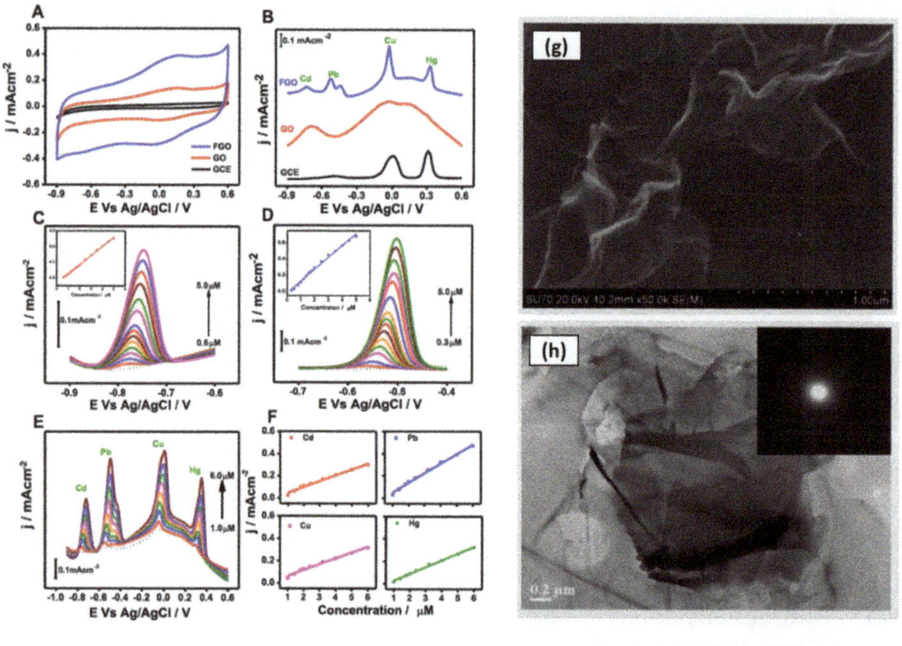

Figure 8.4. (A) CVs of a modified GCE electrode composed of GO and FGO in an acetate buffer. (B) SWASVs on GO (red line), FGO (blue line), and GCE (black line) for 2.0 μM analytes of each of Cd(II), Pb(II), Cu(II), and Hg(II). (C) The calibration curve is inset for FGO SWASVs for Cd(II) sensing. (D) The compatible calibration curve is inset, along with the SWASVs of FGO for Pb(II) sensing. (E) FGO's SWASVs for the instantaneous detection of Hg(II), Pb(II), Cu(II), and Cd(II). (F) Calibration plots showing the ions of Cu(II), Cd(II), Pb(II), and Hg(II) electrochemical detection. (g) SEM images of (GO) and (FGO). (h) Transmission electron microscope (TEM) image of FGO and selected area electron diffraction pattern (inset). Reprinted from [68], Copyright (2017), with permission from Elsevier.

the FGO has been utilized for the concurrent identification of HMIs Cu^{2+}, Cd^{2+}, Pb^{2+}, and Hg^{2+} by SWASV. This technique has resulted in a significant enhancement in the electrochemical sensing capabilities compared to GO.

As reported by Huang *et al* [69], HMIs, including Cd(II) and Pb(II), can be detected electrochemically by using a unique nanohybrid catalyst made of 1D MWCNTs and 2D GR sheets (called G-MWCNTs), figure 8.5(a). Owing to the G-MWCNT nanocomposite's dissolution in water and strong electrochemical conductivity, HMIs were detected. For bismuth and Nafion-modified G-MWCNTs, the differential pulse anodized stripping voltammetry (DPASV) peak current rose linearly across 0.5–30 μg l^{-1} in response to Pb(II) and Cd(II) ion concentrations. LOD values for Cd(II) and Pb(II) remained at 0.1 and 0.1 μg l^{-1}, respectively. By using ASV to measure Pb^{2+} and Cd^{2+} ions concurrently, the electrochemical findings show that G-MWCNTs nanocomposites can function as an example of beneficial sensing material, as shown in figure 8.5(d). The Pb^{2+} and Cd^{2+} linear calibration plots varied in magnitude from 0.5 to 30 μg l^{-1}. For Pb^{2+} and Cd^{2+}, the detection limits were 0.2 μg l^{-1} (S/N = 3) and 0.1 μg l^{-1} (S/N = 3), respectively, when considering a 180-second deposition period. Notably, the modified electrodes with G-MWCNTs effectively detected Cd^{2+} and Pb^{2+} ions simultaneously in actual electroplating effluent specimens with a high concentration of surface-active impurities. This indicates a promising application in detecting trace amounts of heavy metals.

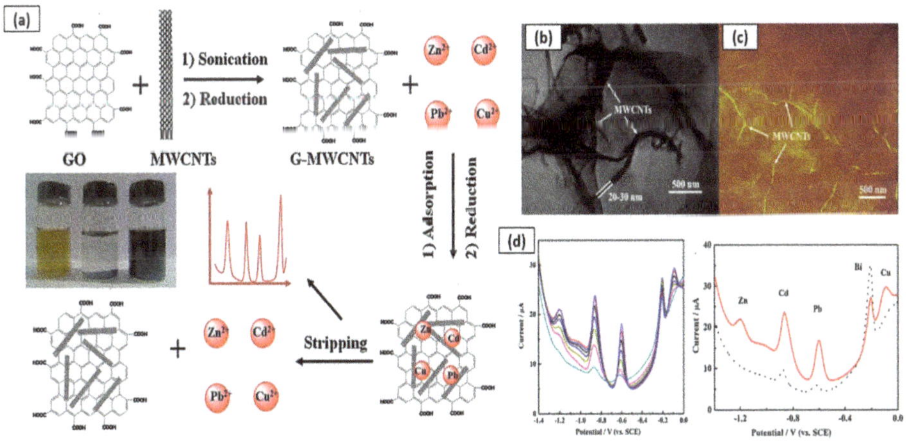

Figure 8.5. (a) Schematic illustrating the production of hybrid nanomaterials GO-MWCNTs and their use as new electrode materials for the ASV technique of electrochemically detecting HMIs. The GO, MWCNTs, and GO-MWCNTs solutions are digital representations in the inset. (b) Low magnification TEM image, and (c) atomic force microscopy images of the nanocomposites composed of GO-MWCNTs. Arrows highlight the MWCNTs and (d) DPASV stripping signals on bismuth and Nafion films modified G/MWCNTs/GCE for Zn^{2+}, Cd^{2+}, Pb^{2+}, and Cu^{2+} ions at varying concentrations (0.5, 5.0, 7.0, 10, 15, 25, and 30 μg l^{-1} from bottom to top). DPASV stripping signals on bismuth film modified bare GCE and G/MWCNTs/GCE for Zn^{2+}, Cd^{2+}, Pb^{2+}, and Cu^{2+} ions at a similar concentration (15 μg l^{-1}). Reprinted from [69], Copyright (2014), with permission from Elsevier.

8.4.2 Carbon nanotube-based sensors for heavy metal ions

CNTs have been employed as an electrode material for several devices, such as biosensors, batteries, supercapacitors, transistors, membranes, electrochemical sensors, electrocatalysis, and electrochemical water splitting [70]. CNTs have been utilized for many different biosensor applications because of their large surface expanse, strong mechanical and electric properties, outstanding chemical steadiness, and ability to bond with different nanomaterials [71]. Owing to their great superficial surface areas and electrocatalytic activity, which is attributed to the function of the edge-plane-alike graphite sites located on the ends, CNTs, SWCNT, or MWCNT are the most commonly employed carbon-based material for heavy metals detection. CNTs are carbon allotropes made from graphite with an outside diameter ranging from 3 to 30 nm and a tubular structure [72]. These narrow tubes have several layers that were subjected to sp^2 hybridization. In addition to their tiny size, low weight, high aspect ratio, superior electrical conductivity, and high tensile strength, CNTs have been employed as fillers for various materials, including metals, polymers, and ceramics [70–72]. With a particular focus on sensitive voltammetric Pb^{2+} and Cu^{2+} detection, Morton and colleagues [73] achieved 8.9 and 23.0 nM detection boundaries, respectively. The suggested accretion and voltammetric mechanisms, including the complex development between the metal ion and cysteine (A), the reduction of the accumulated M^{2+} (B), and the final stripping phase (C), are depicted in figure 8.6(a). Figure 8.6(b) displays the differential pulse anodic stripping voltage measurements of GCE-MWNT-CO–Cys following accumulation in 20.0 ppm of Cu^{2+} solution. As estimated, the oxidation of Cu was responsible for a peak at around −0.02 V. Modified carbon nanotubes on electrode exhibit distinctive voltammograms at 1.4 μM of Pb^{2+} and 3.9 μM of Cu^{2+}. The primary flaw of these systems is the lengthy accumulation duration (up to 30 min) employed in the detection process. The concentrations of the metal ions were directly correlated with the peak currents that resulted. The reduction potential, accumulation time, and reduction time of the procedure were all optimized. Pb^{2+} and Cu^{2+} were found to have detection limits of 1 ppb and 15 ppb, respectively. The Pb^{2+} and Cu^{2+} in spiked lake water were found using this method. With corresponding relative standard deviations of 8.43% and 7.53%, the average recoveries of Pb^{2+} and Cu^{2+} were 96.2% and 94.5%. It was also shown that the modified CNTs can detect HMIs simultaneously. A screen-printed electrode (SPE) with a carbon black (CB) film modification was developed by Arduini *et al* [74]. CB is a nanostructured material with a large amount of defect sites. They present an indirect technique employing the detection of thiols as a first step toward mercury detection. Thiols are easily recognized by CV because they are oxidized when mercury is not present. The thiol–Hg^{2+} complex that forms when mercury is present cannot be oxidized at the electrode surface, which lowers the oxidation current. A 5 mM Hg^{2+} detection limit is reached. Figure 8.6(c) illustrates the CB dispersion made in the DMF/H_2O combination results in a well-defined drip on the working electrode surface that leaves a CB 'film'. After that, the solvent disintegrated. Different concentrations of CB 5% and 10% (wt%) were added to the graphite ink employed to print the SPE.

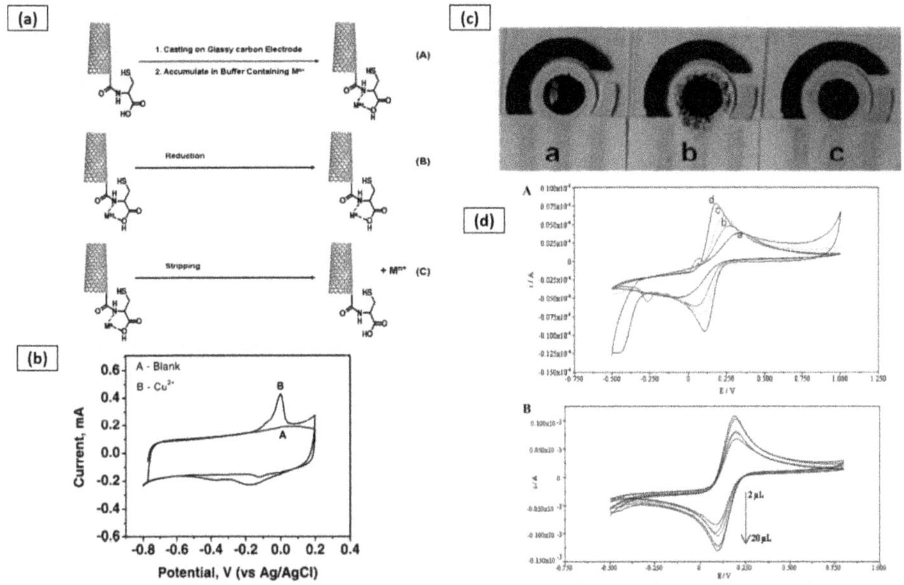

Figure 8.6. (a) Schematic representation of voltammetric mechanism and accumulation were proposed, (b) CV of GCE-MWNT-CO–Cys electrode in 0.1 M acetate buffer (5 ppm Cu^{2+}) before A and after B accumulation. 50 mV s^{-1}. [73] John Wiley & Sons. Copyright © 2009 WILEY-VCH Verlag GmbH & Co. KGaA, Weinheim. (c) Photograph of SPE altered by adding 2 ml of CB dispersion (1 mg ml^{-1}) to a combination of ethanol—c, acetonitrile—b, and DMF/H_2O—a. (d) CV of 1 mM ferricyanide in 0.1 M KCl at a scan rate of 50 mV s^{-1} using a bare SPE—a, CB5%-SPE—b, CB10%-SPE—c, and CB-SPE—d. (B) By modifying CB-SPE with 2, 4, 6, 10, and 20 μl of CB dispersion, CV of 10 mM ferricyanide in 0.1 M KCl was performed at a scan rate of 50 mV s^{-1}. [74] John Wiley & Sons. Copyright © 2012 WILEY-VCH Verlag GmbH & Co. KGaA, Weinheim.

CV was used to examine the SPE types generated in a 1×10^{-3} M ferricyanide solution made in 0.1 M KCl. Figure 8.6(d) shows that the addition of CB results in an increase in anodic and cathodic peak current as well as a decrease in peak-to-peak separation.

Aragay, Pons, and Merkoçi have investigated the use of carbon nanoparticles (CNP)-based SPE for the detection of heavy metals [75]. They compared the outcomes with a commercial carbon microparticle-based SPE and showed how temperature affects the electrochemical removal of HMIs. With a temperature rise, both sensors were susceptible to an enhanced yield of heavy metal deposition; however, the CNP-based electrode exhibited a more significant impact because of its larger accessible surface area and more edge planes, facilitating a higher electron transfer. Images taken by SEM of the working electrode surface recorded the deposition of many heavy metals (Cd^{2+}, Pb^{2+}, Cu^{2+}, and Hg^{2+}) utilizing two distinct interfaces (CNP and carbon-microparticles-based SPE) at two different temperatures (room temperature and 40 °C) are displayed in figures 8.7(a1) and (b2). Figures 8.7(a1) and (b1) show that distinct deposition patterns are observed at room temperature for every heavy metal deposited employing both SPEs. Nevertheless, it was discovered that a uniform layer formed when the temperature was raised due to

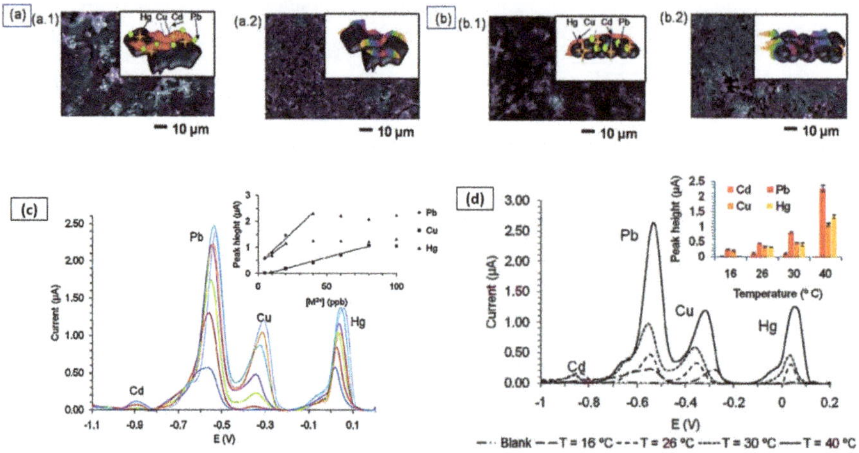

Figure 8.7. Electrodes constructed via screen printing using carbon nanoparticles. (a, b) SEM descriptions of the working electrode external surface of a carbon nanoparticle-based SPE at room temperature (a1) and at 40 °C (a2) and for a carbon nanoparticle-based SPE at room temperature working electrode surface (b1) and 40 °C (b2) following the deposition of heavy metals (Cd^{2+}, Pb^{2+}, Cu^{2+}, and Hg^{2+}). The schematic method of heavy metal deposition at particle-based surfaces, both micro (a1 and a2) and nano (b1 and b2), is depicted in the insets. Reproduced from [75] with permission from the Royal Society of Chemistry.

the more homogenous metal deposition (see figures 8.7(a2) and (b2)). Figure 8.7(c) illustrates how the temperature and the degree of the metallic ion's voltammetric signals increase. Figure 8.7(d) shows typical square wave voltammograms and the matching linear relationship for the multi-detection of heavy metals at 40 °C. Because of its non-linear behavior at this temperature, cadmium is not considered for the linear correlation.

Additionally, modified MWCNTs have demonstrated impressive electrochemical activity for detecting HMIs. When b-cyclodextrin (β-CD) was covalently modified with MWCNTs and coated on a SPE (figure 8.8(a)), for instance, the resultant MWCNT-β-CD(Phys/SE)/SPE showed increased sensor activity used for HMIs detection [76]. With a LOD of 0.03 μM, DPASV was utilized to detect Pb(II) in the range of 0.015–1.5 μM (figure 8.8(b)). After four iterations of the experiment in Pb (II) solution, the electrode showed a comparable electrochemical response, indicating that the sensor was relatively robust. Pb(II) ions were also found in actual water samples using the standard addition procedure, yielding a 90% recovery rate (figure 8.8(c)). The covalently modified MWCNT-β-CD proved more reliable and reusable than the physically changed composite. The combination of organic compounds and the active sites of MWCNTs led to metal coordination with Pb (II) ions, which boosted sensor performance and allowed for both the selective and sensitive detection of Pb(II) in actual samples [76].

For the electrochemical detection of As(III) in water tasters, Baghayeri *et al* [77] recently created a new catalyst with a mix of magnetic MWCNTs and polyamidoamine (PAMAM) dendrimers (MMWCNTs-D-NH_2). This catalyst was deposited on a GCE using a straightforward drop-casting approach (figure 8.9(a)).

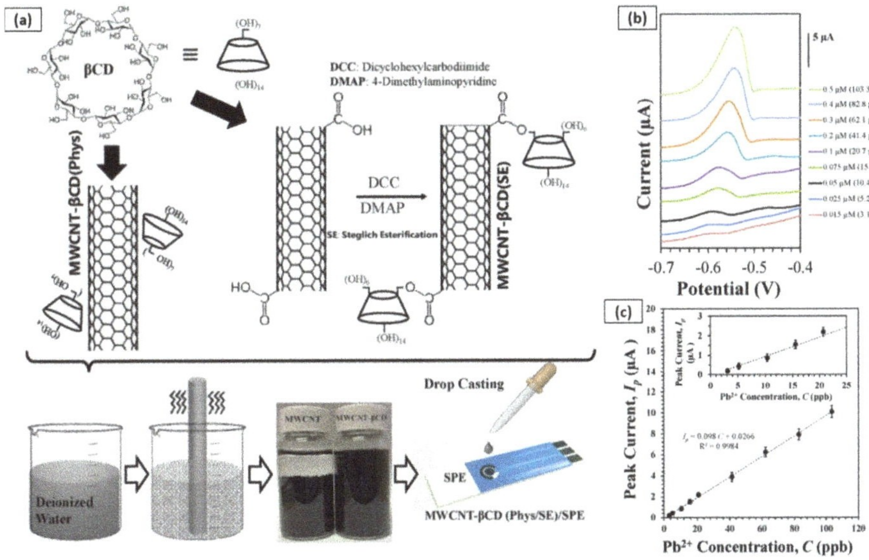

Figure 8.8. (a) A schematic representation of the MWCNT-βCD(Phys/SE)/SPE electrode procedure for manufacture, (b) MWCNT-βCD(Phys)/SPE DPASV in 0.1 M acetate buffer (pH 5) with 0.025–20.0 μM (3.1–103.3 ppb) Pb^{2+} present and (c) The calibration curve for MWCNT-βCD(Phys)/SPE, which shows peak current vs Pb^{2+} concentration. Before measurements, all tests were conducted with a deposition potential of −0.8 V for 600 s while magnetic churning was in place. Reprinted from [77], Copyright (2019), with permission from Elsevier.

Using TEM examination, the morphological characterization of the MMWCNTs-D-NH_2 nanocomposite was investigated (figures 8.9(b) and (c)). TEM pictures demonstrate very evenly distributed Fe_3O_4 nanoparticles on the MWCNT wall. When interfering metal ions are present, such as Hg(II), Pb(II), Cd(II), and Cu(II), the MMWCNT-D-NH2 modified GCE preferentially recognized As(III) within the scope of 1–50 μg l^{-1} (figure 8.9(d)), with a LOD of 0.46 μg l^{-1} obtained under optimal circumstances. The prior concentration of As(III) by hydrogen bonding at the pH of the acetate buffer solution was identified as the cause of the sensor's extraordinary sensitivity for As(III) detection. SWASV also quantified the As(III) levels in drinking, mineral, and laboratory tap water samples. A 99.1%–105.6% recovery was attained, and the results agreed with ICP-AES. The electrochemical detection of HMIs by electroanalytical techniques achieved by MWCNT-based composites showed a lot of possibilities for the sensitive and specific verification of HMIs in water and food samples.

A molybdenum disulfide MWCNT (Au/MoS_2-MWCNT) nanocomposite, coated with AuNP, was created by Mohammadi *et al* [78] as an electrochemically active material for the autosensing of solvated mercuric ions. The mechanism behind the detection of Hg(II) ions was the reduction in the peak current of the redox mediator (ferro/ferrocyanide). In contrast to an immobilized aptamer composite (aptamer/Au/MoS_2-MWCNT), in a ferri/ferrocyanide solution, the Au/MoS_2-MWCNT nanocomposite's redox peak current displayed a strong and distinct peak. The interaction of the aptamer/Au/MoS_2-MWCNT composite and Hg(II) with one other caused the redox peak current

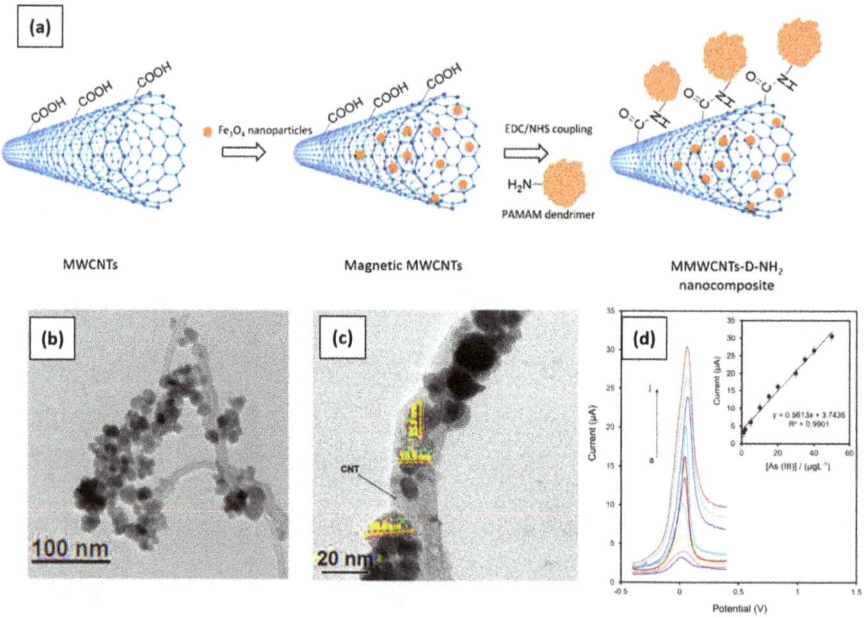

Figure 8.9. (a) Diagrammatic illustration of the glassy carbon electrodes-MMWCNTs-D-NH_2 nanocomposite (sensor's fabrication), (b and c) TEM images of the nanocomposite made of MMWCNTs-D-NH_2 and (d) Anodic stripping voltammograms of MMWCNTs-D-NH_2/GCE were recorded in acetate buffer (0.1 M, pH 5.0) with varying concentrations of As(III): (curve a) 1.0, (curve b) 2.0, (curve c) 5.0, (curve d) 10.0, (curve e) 15.0, (curve f) 20.0, (curve g) 30.0, (curve h) 35.0, (curve i) 40.0, and (curve j) 50.0 μg l^{-1}. A similar calibration plot is shown in the inset. Reprinted from [76], Copyright (2021), with permission from Elsevier.

to drop even further. Furthermore, a linear drop in the redox peak current was verified by DPV analysis following the sequential accumulation of Hg(II) ions throughout a broad range of 0.1 nM–1.0 μM with an LOD of 0.05 nM. In a 10.0 nM Hg(II) ion solution, the sensor showed 90% of its original activity and remained stable for up to 30 days. Real wastewater, river water, and tap water samples likewise produced impressive findings, with recovery rates ranging from 93.0% to 103.7%. The significant number of active sites on the MWCNT's surface and the high electrical conductivity of AuNPs and MWCNTs were credited with the efficient and specific detection of Hg(II) [78]. An alternative platform for the electrochemical detection of Pb(II) ions was created by Alizadeh *et al* [79] using an electrochemical nanostructured materials ion-imprinted polymer (IIP) coated with MWCNTs (IIP/MWCNTs). Pb(II) was successfully determined by this approach with a LOD of 3.8 pmol l^{-1} (S/N = 3) throughout a broad range of 1.0×10^{-11} to 8.0×10^{-8} mol l^{-1}. With an average recovery of 95.4%–102.4%, the manufactured sensor yielded great results for samples of rivers and oceans. This approach proved very sensitive and selective for Pb(II) in real samples. Modified MWCNTs have also demonstrated significant electrochemical activity for the detection of HMIs.

For application in several electrical, mechanical, thermal, and optical applications, SWCNTs have been one of the materials that have been explored the most. With an exceptional structure consisting of sp^2 hybridized carbon atoms organized in hexagons,

SWCNTs are the cylindrical version of mono-layered graphene. SWCNTs have excellent mechanical strength, strong electrical conductivity, high thermal conductivity (about 3500 W m^{-1} K^{-1}), and a chiral index-driven structure [80–82]. These characteristics have promoted the application of SWCNTs in several fields. These characteristics have promoted the use of SWCNTs in many different applications, including drug delivery systems, electrocatalysis, batteries, transistors, biosensors (including sensors for malignant cells), DNA analysis, glucose sensors, and virus sensors [83, 84]. A stainless-steel (SS) electrode modified with a nanocomposite consisting of the chelating ligand ethylenediaminetetraacetic acid (EDTA), polyaniline (PANI), and SWCNTs (EDTA-PANI/SWNCT) has demonstrated strong catalytic activity towards Cu(II), Pb(II), and Hg(II) ions currently [85]. Cu(II) in the range of 1.2 μM to 2.0 mM, Pb(II) from 2.0 to 37.0 μM, and Hg(II) from 2.0 μM to 2.0 mM increased linearly with the addition of the DPV current of the EDTA-PANI/SWNCT-modified SS electrode in acetate buffer solution (pH 4.5. During the HMI addition, the DPV current was enhanced by the EDTA, PANI, and SWCNTs (figure 8.10(a)). The PANI made the SWCNTs less

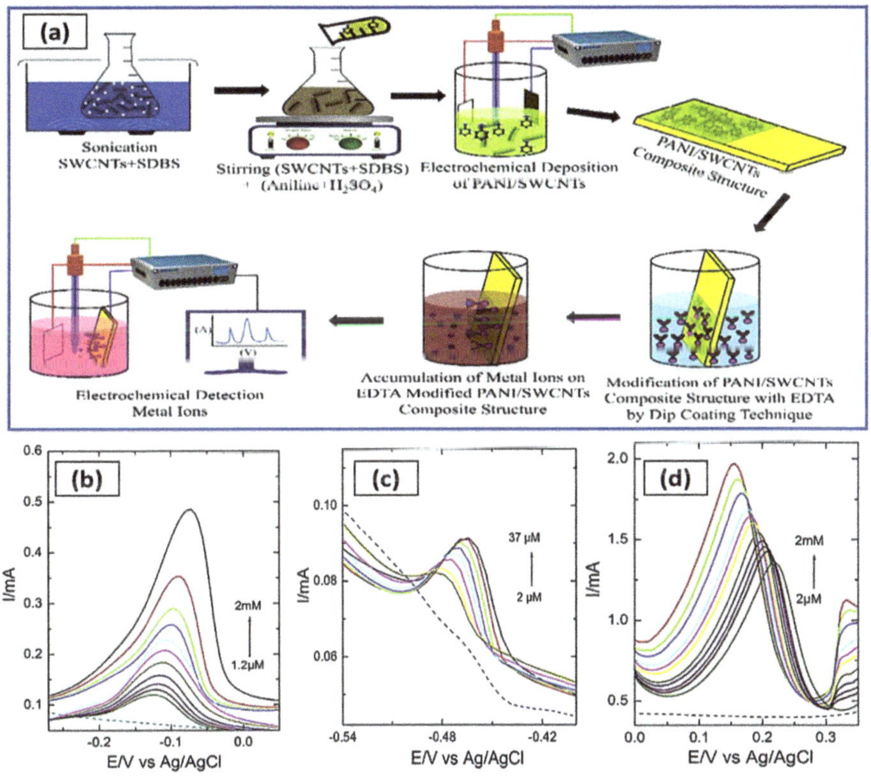

Figure 8.10. (a) schematic illustration of EDTA_PANI/SWCNTs nanostructure is formed on an SS electrode and used to determine HMIs using the DPV approach. The DPV response of the EDTA_PANI/SWCNTs nanocomposite was examined for each of the following three concentration ranges: (b) Cu(II) over 2–1.2 mM, (c) Pb(II) over 37–2 mM, and (d) Hg(II) over 2.0–2.0 mM. Reprinted from [85], Copyright (2017), with permission from Elsevier.

hydrophobic and increased their electrical conductivity. The quicker electron transfer and higher sensor sensitivity were caused by the p-p contact that existed between PANI and SWCNTs. Following the addition of the HMIs, the DPV current was enhanced by the EDTA, PANI, and SWCNTs. The PANI decreased the hydrophobicity and increased the electrical conductivity of the SWCNTs. The increased sensor sensitivity and more rapid electron transfer were caused by the π-π interaction that occurred between PANI and SWCNTs. Due to its ring-like shape, EDTA preferentially bonds with specific metallic ions in electrolytic solutions. Therefore, the sensor's selectivity was enhanced by the presence of EDTA. The LODs for Cu(II), Pb(II), and Hg(II) obtained with this suggested approach were 0.08, 1.65, and 0.68 μM, respectively (figures 8.10(b)–(d)). Thus, the previously outlined features of materials derived from carbon are responsible for the accurate and focused identification of HMIs. SWCNTs were used as the basis material in the experiment conducted by Fu *et al* [86] on the electrochemical detection of Hg(II) in water. They presented a new nanohybrid material, electro-polymerized ion-imprinting poly (2-mercaptobenzothiazole) film, on a GCE that was modified with SWCNT and gold nanoparticles (AuNP) (PMBT/AuNP/SWCNT/GCE). Even after the homogeneous deposition of AuNPs on the surface of SWCNTs, the morphology of the SWCNTs was preserved. This enhanced the electrical conductivity of the AuNP/SWCNT/GCE composite because of its larger active area of surface and roughness at the surface. Hg(II) sensors were developed using Hg(II)-imprinted PMBT/AuNP/SWCNT/GCE, imprinted PMBT/AuNP/SWCNT/GCE, and non-imprinted PMBT/AuNP/SWCNT/GCE. The DPASV current measured for the Hg(II)-imprinted PMBT/AuNP/SWCNT/GCE was about 3.7 and 10.5 times more than that of the non-imprinted PMBT/AuNP/SWCNT/GCE and imprinted PMBT/AuNP/SWCNT/GCE, respectively. In the presence of a 20-fold excess of Ag(I) and a 100-fold molar surplus of Cd(II), Pb(II), Zn(II), and Cu(II), the imprinted PMBT/AuNP/SWCNT/GCE showed good selectivity. Throughout a broad linear range of 0.4–96.0 nM, with a LOD of 0.08 nM, the DPASV's highest current was correlated with the Hg (II) concentration. This technique had a sensitivity of 0.749 $\mu A\ nM^{-1}$ and good repeatability in general. Real river and tap water specimens were also evaluated for Hg (II) detection, and the results showed a fantastic recovery of 93.1%–108.7%. After 10 and 30 days, respectively, the sensor effectiveness of the imprinted PMBT/AuNP/SWCNT/GCE dropped to 96% and 80% of the initial current response. As a result, the new method for finding traces of Hg(II) in water samples showed excellent selectivity and exceptional sensitivity.

8.5 Conclusion

HMIs significantly threaten both individuals and the environment because of their high toxicity and low pathogenic concentration. Electrochemical sensors based on carbon nanomaterial modification have advanced considerably in detecting HMIs because of the development of nanomaterial technologies in recent years. Several electrochemical techniques for tracking HMIs in water were covered in the present study. Electrochemical detection provides several noteworthy benefits when compared to conventional detection techniques. In particular, electrochemical detection is rapid,

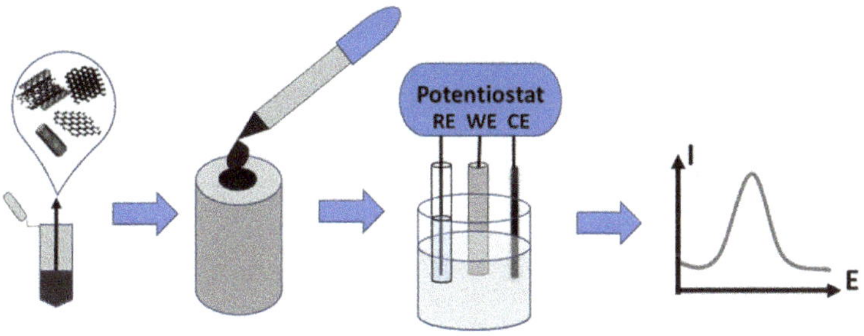

Figure 8.11. Electrochemical detection of HMIs from environment samples.

sensitive, and somewhat portable. It may be used for on-site testing in a variety of settings. As previously mentioned, the best techniques, including a porous carbon sensor, a carbon-based nanocomposite matrix, and a nanostructured sensor, for detecting various metal ions such as As(III), Cr(VI), Ag(I), Pb(II), Hg(II), Cd(II), and Cu(II) in water, soil, and plants due to the usage of synthetic fertilizers, untreated sewage disposal, and fossil fuel combustion. There are various electrochemical approaches, including DPV, SWV, CV, and the current approach. There are also several options for detecting HMIs (figure 8.11). ASV is the most sensitive and accurate approach for detecting man-machine interaction. HMI detection using electrochemical techniques has demonstrated significant promise. The remarkable performance of modified carbon-based nanocomposites has drawn much attention, but many development issues still need to be resolved. For instance, it is challenging to identify HMIs in solid media and suspended materials using the modified electrode intended to detect them in an aqueous medium. Furthermore, before deploying the interface material to actual water specimens, it is essential to consider its toxicity. Further preconfigured electrodes for reusable evaluation strips may be developed, allowing for more sanitary and efficient drinking and residential water testing. This chapter addresses the development of innovative carbon nanomaterial-modified electrochemical electrodes for electrochemical sensors. Due to their exceptional electrical qualities and unique structural characteristics, carbon-based materials and their derivatives are frequently utilized to form electrochemical sensors. New derivative materials, such as graphene aerogels and graphene quantum dots, have opened up new avenues for advancement in electrochemical sensing technology. This has dramatically expanded the range of materials used to modify electrochemical sensors and enhanced their detection capabilities. Most existing investigations are still restricted to laboratory examination of samples, and using the combination of embedded innovative technology to accomplish the miniaturization of apparatus is also a worthy direction of study. In addition, detecting HMIs should attempt to meet the requirements for on-site monitoring.

References

[1] García-Miranda Ferrari A, Carrington P, Rowley-Neale S J and Banks C E 2020 Recent advances in portable heavy metal electrochemical sensing platforms *Environ. Sci.: water Res. Technol.* **6** 2676–90

[2] Gumpu M B, Sethuraman S, Krishnan U M and Rayappan J B B 2015 A review on detecting heavy metal ions in water—an electrochemical approach *Sensors Actuators* B **213** 515–33

[3] Singh A, Sharma R K, Agrawal M and Marshall F M 2010 Health risk assessment of heavy metals via dietary intake of foodstuffs from the wastewater irrigated site of a dry tropical area of India *Food Chem. Toxicol.* **48** 611–9

[4] Álvarez-Torrellas S, Peres J A, Gil-Álvarez V, Ovejero G and García J 2017 Effective adsorption of non-biodegradable pharmaceuticals from hospital wastewater with different carbon materials *Chem. Eng. J.* **320** 319–29

[5] Deo R P and Halden R U 2013 Pharmaceuticals in the built and natural water environment of the United States *Water* **5** 1346–65

[6] Heberer T 2002 Occurrence, fate, and removal of pharmaceutical residues in the aquatic environment: a review of recent research data *Toxicol. Lett.* **131** 5–17

[7] GracePavithra K, Jaikumar V, Kumar P S and SundarRajan P 2019 A review on cleaner strategies for chromium industrial wastewater: present research and future perspective *J. Clean. Prod.* **228** 580–93

[8] Bixio D, Thoeye C, Wintgens T, Ravazzini A, Miska V, Muston M, Chikurel H, Aharoni A, Joksimovic D and Melin T 2008 Water reclamation and reuse: implementation and management issues *Desalination* **218** 13–23

[9] Siyal A A, Shamsuddin M R, Khan M, Rabat N E, Zulfiqar M, Man Z, Siame J and Azizli K A 2018 A review on geopolymers as emerging materials for the adsorption of heavy metals and dyes *J. Environ. Manage.* **224** 327–39

[10] Srivastava N K and Majumder C B 2008 Novel biofiltration methods for the treatment of heavy metals from industrial wastewater *J. Hazard. Mater.* **151** 1–8

[11] Wang L, Ma W, Xu L, Chen W, Zhu Y, Xu C and Kotov N A 2010 Nanoparticle-based environmental sensors *Mater. Sci. Eng.: R: Rep.* **70** 265–74

[12] Pradeep T and Anshup 2009 Noble metal nanoparticles for water purification: a critical review *Thin Solid Films* **517** 6441–78

[13] Hu H, Hu Y, Xie B and Zhu J 2023 High sensitivity electrochemical as (III) sensor based on Fe_3O_4/MoS_2 nanocomposites *Nanomaterials* **13** 16

[14] Male K B, Hrapovic S, Santini J M and Luong J H T 2007 Biosensor for arsenite using arsenite oxidase and multiwalled carbon nanotube modified electrodes *Anal. Chem.* **79** 7831–7

[15] Aragay G, Pons J and Merkoçi A 2011 Recent trends in macro-, micro-, and nanomaterial-based tools and strategies for heavy-metal detection *Chem. Rev.* **111** 3433–58

[16] Barvin R K B, Prakash P, Ganesh V and Jeyaprabha B 2019 Highly selective and sensitive sensing of toxic mercury ions utilizing carbon quantum dot-modified glassy carbon electrode *Int. J. Environ. Res.* **13** 1015–23

[17] Torrinha Á, Oliveira T M B F, Islam S ul and Morais S 2023 Green carbon (nano)materials-based sensors for analysis of hazardous metal ions *Green Carbon Materials for Environmental Analysis: Emerging Research and Future Opportunities* vol 1441 (Washington, DC: American Chemical Society) pp 5–91

[18] Veerakumar P, Veeramani V, Chen S-M, Madhu R and Liu S-B 2016 Palladium nano-particle incorporated porous activated Carbon: electrochemical detection of toxic metal ions *ACS Appl. Mater. Interfaces* **8** 1319–26

[19] Waheed A, Mansha M and Ullah N 2018 Nanomaterials-based electrochemical detection of heavy metals in water: current status, challenges and future direction *TrAC, Trends Anal. Chem.* **105** 37–51

[20] Sawan S, Maalouf R, Errachid A and Jaffrezic-Renault N 2020 Metal and metal oxide nanoparticles in the voltammetric detection of heavy metals: a review *TrAC, Trends Anal. Chem.* **131** 116014
[21] Lu L, Zhou L, Chen J, Yan F, Liu J, Dong X, Xi F and Chen P 2018 Nanochannel-confined graphene quantum dots for ultrasensitive electrochemical analysis of complex samples *ACS Nano* **12** 12673–81
[22] Wang L, Peng X, Fu H, Huang C, Li Y and Liu Z 2020 Recent advances in the development of electrochemical aptasensors for detection of heavy metals in food *Biosens. Bioelectron.* **147** 111777
[23] Shirani M, Habibollahi S and Akbari A 2019 Centrifuge-less deep eutectic solvent based magnetic nanofluid-linked air-agitated liquid–liquid microextraction coupled with electrothermal atomic absorption spectrometry for simultaneous determination of cadmium, lead, copper, and arsenic in food samples and non-alcoholic beverages *Food Chem.* **281** 304–11
[24] Olsen T A, Huang T H, Kanissery R and Hudson R J M 2015 Mercury–thiourea complex ion chromatography: advances in system chemistry and applications to environmental mercury speciation analysis *Trace Materials in Air, Soil, and Water* vol 1210 (Washington, DC: American Chemical Society) pp 115–51 SE–6
[25] Kong L, Hu X, Peng X and Wang X 2020 Specific H_2S release from thiosulfate promoted by UV irradiation for removal of arsenic and heavy metals from strongly acidic wastewater *Environ. Sci. Technol.* **54** 14076–84
[26] Jackson B, Taylor V, Baker R A and Miller E 2009 Low-level mercury speciation in freshwaters by isotope dilution GC-ICP-MS *Environ. Sci. Technol.* **43** 2463–9
[27] Hong A *et al* 2021 Identification and speciation of nanoscale silver in complex solid matrices by sequential extraction coupled with inductively coupled plasma optical emission spectrometry *Anal. Chem.* **93** 1962–8
[28] Lin J, Chen N, Feng R, Nilges M J, Jia Y, Wang S and Pan Y 2020 Sequestration of selenite and selenate in gypsum ($CaSO_4{\cdot}2H_2O$): insights from the single-crystal electron paramagnetic resonance spectroscopy and synchrotron x-ray absorption spectroscopy study *Environ. Sci. Technol.* **54** 3169–80
[29] Umegaki I *et al* 2020 Nondestructive high-sensitivity detections of metallic lithium deposited on a battery anode using muonic x-rays *Anal. Chem.* **92** 8194–200
[30] Qian J, Gao X and Pan B 2020 Nanoconfinement-mediated water treatment: from fundamental to application *Environ. Sci. Technol.* **54** 8509–26
[31] Yin C, Iqbal J, Hu H, Liu B, Zhang L, Zhu B and Du Y 2012 Sensitive determination of trace mercury by UV–visible diffuse reflectance spectroscopy after complexation and membrane filtration-enrichment *J. Hazard. Mater.* **233–4** 207–12
[32] Pohl P 2009 Determination of metal content in honey by atomic absorption and emission spectrometries *TrAC, Trends Anal. Chem.* **28** 117–28
[33] Gómez-Ariza J L, Lorenzo F and García-Barrera T 2005 Comparative study of atomic fluorescence spectroscopy and inductively coupled plasma mass spectrometry for mercury and arsenic multispeciation *Anal. Bioanal. Chem.* **382** 485–92
[34] Aranda P R, Pacheco P H, Olsina R A, Martinez L D and Gil R A 2009 Total and inorganic mercury determination in biodiesel by emulsion sample introduction and FI-CV-AFS after multivariate optimization *J. Anal. At. Spectrom.* **24** 1441–5
[35] Ma S, Cao F, Wen X, Xu F, Tian H, Fu X and Dong D 2023 Detection of heavy metal ions using laser-induced breakdown spectroscopy combined with filter paper modified with PtAg bimetallic nanoparticles *J. Hazard. Mater.* **443** 130188

[36] Lu Y, Liang X, Niyungeko C, Zhou J, Xu J and Tian G 2018 A review of the identification and detection of heavy metal ions in the environment by voltammetry *Talanta* **178** 324–38
[37] Aragay G and Merkoçi A 2012 Nanomaterials application in electrochemical detection of heavy metals *Electrochim. Acta* **84** 49–61
[38] Ding Q, Li C, Wang H, Xu C and Kuang H 2021 Electrochemical detection of heavy metal ions in water *Chem. Commun.* **57** 7215–31
[39] Kumar S, Islam R, Akash P B, Khan M H R, Proshad R, Karmoker J and MacFarlane G R 2022 Lead (Pb) contamination in agricultural products and human health risk assessment in Bangladesh *Water Air Soil Pollut.* **233** 257
[40] Kubier A, Wilkin R T and Pichler T 2019 Cadmium in soils and groundwater: a review *Appl. Geochem.* **108** 104388
[41] Krishnamurti G S R, McArthur D F E, Wang M K, Kozak L M and Huang P M 2005 Biogeochemistry of soil cadmium and the impact on terrestrial food chain contamination ed P M Huang and G R Gobran *Biogeochemistry of Trace Elements in the Rhizosphere* (Amsterdam: Elsevier) ch 7 pp 197–257
[42] Qu R, Han G, Liu M and Li X 2019 The mercury behavior and contamination in soil profiles in Mun river Basin, Northeast Thailand *Int. J. Environ. Res. Public Health* **16** 4131
[43] Li P, Feng X B, Qiu G L, Shang L H and Li Z G 2009 Mercury pollution in Asia: a review of the contaminated sites *J. Hazard. Mater.* **168** 591–601
[44] Johansson K, Bergbäck B and Tyler G 2001 Impact of atmospheric long range transport of lead, mercury, and cadmium on the Swedish forest environment *Water, Air and Soil Pollution: Focus* **1** 279–97
[45] Driscoll C T, Mason R P, Chan H M, Jacob D J and Pirrone N 2013 Mercury as a global pollutant: sources, pathways, and effects *Environ. Sci. Technol.* **47** 4967–83
[46] Li Y, Gou X, Wang G, Zhang Q, Su Q and Xiao G 2008 Heavy metal contamination and source in arid agricultural soil in central Gansu Province, China *J. Environ. Sci.* **20** 607–12
[47] Tripathi R M, Raghunath R and Krishnamoorthy T M 1997 Dietary intake of heavy metals in Bombay city, India *Sci. Total Environ.* **208** 149–59
[48] Bansod B, Kumar T, Thakur R, Rana S and Singh I 2017 A review on various electrochemical techniques for heavy metal ions detection with different sensing platforms *Biosens. Bioelectron.* **94** 443–55
[49] Cui L, Wu J and Ju H 2015 Electrochemical sensing of heavy metal ions with inorganic, organic and bio-materials *Biosens. Bioelectron.* **63** 276–86
[50] Locatelli C and Melucci D 2013 Voltammetric method for ultra-trace determination of total mercury and toxic metals in vegetables. Comparison with spectroscopy *Cent. Eur. J. Chem.* **11** 790–800
[51] Nejdl L *et al* 2014 Remote-controlled robotic platform ORPHEUS as a new tool for detection of bacteria in the environment *Electrophoresis* **35** 2333–45
[52] Pan D, Wang Y, Chen Z, Lou T and Qin W 2009 Nanomaterial/ionophore-based electrode for anodic stripping voltammetric determination of lead: an electrochemical sensing platform toward heavy metals *Anal. Chem.* **81** 5088–94
[53] Umapathi R, Sonwal S, Lee M J, Mohana Rani G, Lee E-S, Jeon T-J, Kang S-M, Oh M-H and Huh Y S 2021 Colorimetric based on-site sensing strategies for the rapid detection of pesticides in agricultural foods: new horizons, perspectives, and challenges *Coord. Chem. Rev.* **446** 214061

[54] Umapathi R, Ghoreishian S M, Sonwal S, Rani G M and Huh Y S 2022 Portable electrochemical sensing methodologies for on-site detection of pesticide residues in fruits and vegetables *Coord. Chem. Rev.* **453** 214305
[55] Chaudhary V, Kaushik A, Furukawa H and Khosla A 2022 Review—towards 5th generation AI and IoT driven sustainable intelligent sensors based on 2D MXenes and borophene *ECS Sens. Plus* **1** 13601
[56] Mohammadi H, Amine A, Cosnier S and Mousty C 2005 Mercury–enzyme inhibition assays with an amperometric sucrose biosensor based on a trienzymatic-clay matrix *Anal. Chim. Acta* **543** 143–9
[57] Arduini F, Majorani C, Amine A, Moscone D and Palleschi G 2011 Hg^{2+} detection by measuring thiol groups with a highly sensitive screen-printed electrode modified with a nanostructured carbon black film *Electrochim. Acta* **56** 4209–15
[58] Borrill A J, Reily N E and Macpherson J 2019 Addressing the practicalities of anodic stripping voltammetry for heavy metal detection: a tutorial review *Analyst* **144** 6834–49
[59] Orazem M and Tribollet B 2008 *Electrochemical Impedance Spectroscopy* (New York: Wiley-Interscience)
[60] Djurdjevic Z, Buica G-O, Miskovic-Stankovic V, Ungureanu E-M and Amarandei C 2013 Electrochemical impedance spectroscopy investigations on glassy carbon electrodes modified with poly(4-azulen-1-yl-2,6-bis(2-thienyl)pyridine) *UPB Sci. Bull. B: Chem. Mater. Sci.* **75** 125
[61] Li G, Qi X, Wu J, Xu L, Wan X, Liu Y, Chen Y and Li Q 2022 Ultrasensitive, label-free voltammetric determination of norfloxacin based on molecularly imprinted polymers and Au nanoparticle-functionalized black phosphorus nanosheet nanocomposite *J. Hazard. Mater.* **436** 129107
[62] Thue P S, Lima D R, Naushad M, Lima E C, de Albuquerque Y R T, Dias S L P, Cunha M R, Dotto G L and de Brum I A S 2021 High removal of emerging contaminants from wastewater by activated carbons derived from the shell of cashew of para *Carbon Lett.* **31** 13–28
[63] Yan Y, Shin W, Chen H, Lee S-M, Manickam S, Hanson S, Zhao H, Lester E, Wu T and Pang C H 2021 A recent trend: application of graphene in catalysis *Carbon Lett.* **31** 177–99
[64] Zhou A, Bai J, Hong W and Bai H 2022 Electrochemically reduced graphene oxide: preparation, composites, and applications *Carbon* **191** 301–32
[65] Thakur K and Kandasubramanian B 2019 Graphene and graphene oxide-based composites for removal of organic pollutants: a review *J. Chem. Eng. Data* **64** 833–67
[66] Aykut Y and Yurtcan A B 2022 Electrocatalysts based on graphene and its composites *Noble Metal-Free Electrocatalysts: Fundamentals and Recent Advances in Electrocatalysts for Energy Applications. Volume 1* vol 1431 (Washington, DC: American Chemical Society) pp 165–99 SE–7
[67] Zhu L, Xu L, Huang B, Jia N, Tan L and Yao S 2014 Simultaneous determination of Cd(II) and Pb(II) using square wave anodic stripping voltammetry at a gold nanoparticle-graphene–cysteine composite modified bismuth film electrode *Electrochim. Acta* **115** 471–7
[68] Thiruppathi A R, Sidhureddy B, Keeler W and Chen A 2017 Facile one-pot synthesis of fluorinated graphene oxide for electrochemical sensing of heavy metal ions *Electrochem. Commun.* **76** 42–6

[69] Huang H, Chen T, Liu X and Ma H 2014 Ultrasensitive and simultaneous detection of heavy metal ions based on three-dimensional graphene-carbon nanotubes hybrid electrode materials *Anal. Chim. Acta* **852** 45–54
[70] Saeed K and Khan I 2013 Carbon nanotubes–properties and applications: a review *Carbon Lett.* **14** 131–44
[71] Vashist S K, Zheng D, Al-Rubeaan K, Luong J H T and Sheu F-S 2011 Advances in carbon nanotube based electrochemical sensors for bioanalytical applications *Biotechnol. Adv.* **29** 169–88
[72] Agüí L, Yáñez-Sedeño P and Pingarrón J M 2008 Role of carbon nanotubes in electroanalytical chemistry: a review *Anal. Chim. Acta* **622** 11–47
[73] Morton J, Havens N, Mugweru A and Wanekaya A K 2009 Detection of trace heavy metal ions using carbon nanotube-modified electrodes *Electroanalysis* **21** 1597–603
[74] Arduini F, Di Nardo F, Amine A, Micheli L, Palleschi G and Moscone D 2012 Carbon black-modified screen-printed electrodes as electroanalytical tools *Electroanalysis* **24** 743–51
[75] Aragay G, Pons J and Merkoçi A 2011 Enhanced electrochemical detection of heavy metals at heated graphite nanoparticle-based screen-printed electrodes *J. Mater. Chem.* **21** 4326–31
[76] Baghayeri M, Amiri A, Karimabadi F, Di Masi S, Maleki B, Adibian F, Pourali A R and Malitesta C 2021 Magnetic MWCNTs-dendrimer: a potential modifier for electrochemical evaluation of As (III) ions in real water samples *J. Electroanal. Chem.* **888** 115059
[77] Alam A U, Howlader M M R, Hu N-X and Deen M J 2019 Electrochemical sensing of lead in drinking water using β-cyclodextrin-modified MWCNTs *Sensors Actuators* B **296** 126632
[78] Mohammadi A, Heydari-Bafrooei E, Foroughi M M and Mohammadi M 2020 Heterostructured Au/MoS_2-MWCNT nanoflowers: a highly efficient support for the electrochemical aptasensing of solvated mercuric ion *Microchem. J.* **158** 105154
[79] Alizadeh T, Hamidi N, Ganjali M R and Rafiei F 2017 An extraordinarily sensitive voltammetric sensor with picomolar detection limit for Pb^{2+} determination based on carbon paste electrode impregnated with nano-sized imprinted polymer and multi-walled carbon nanotubes *J. Environ. Chem. Eng.* **5** 4327–36
[80] Rao R *et al* 2018 Carbon nanotubes and related nanomaterials: critical advances and challenges for synthesis toward mainstream commercial applications *ACS Nano* **12** 11756–84
[81] Yang F, Wang M, Zhang D, Yang J, Zheng M and Li Y 2020 Chirality pure carbon nanotubes: growth, sorting, and characterization *Chem. Rev.* **120** 2693–758
[82] Li Y 2017 The quarter-century anniversary of carbon nanotube research *ACS Nano* **11** 1–2
[83] Rasheed T, Hassan A A, Kausar F, Sher F, Bilal M and Iqbal H M N 2020 Carbon nanotubes assisted analytical detection—sensing/delivery cues for environmental and biomedical monitoring *TrAC, Trends Anal. Chem.* **132** 116066
[84] Trojanowicz M 2006 Analytical applications of carbon nanotubes: a review *TrAC, Trends Anal. Chem.* **25** 480–9
[85] Deshmukh M A, Celiesiute R, Ramanaviciene A, Shirsat M D and Ramanavicius A 2018 EDTA_PANI/SWCNTs nanocomposite modified electrode for electrochemical determination of copper (II), lead (II) and mercury (II) ions *Electrochim. Acta* **259** 930–8
[86] Fu X-C, Wu J, Nie L, Xie C-G, Liu J-H and Huang X-J 2012 Electropolymerized surface ion imprinting films on a gold nanoparticles/single-wall carbon nanotube nanohybrids modified glassy carbon electrode for electrochemical detection of trace mercury(II) in water *Anal. Chim. Acta* **720** 29–37

IOP Publishing

Electrochemical Interfaces for the Detection of Agricultural Pollutants

Chandra Sekhar Rout

Chapter 9

Application of carbon-based biosensors for contaminants from modern agricultural practices

G Manasa, Vishwanath Ankalgi and Chandra Sekhar Rout

With the increasing concern surrounding the threats of harmful chemicals to human health and aquatic and agricultural ecosystems caused by modern agricultural practices, the need for effective and efficient detection methods has never been more crucial. While conventional analytical methods such as gas chromatography/liquid chromatography-mass spectroscopy (GC/LC-MS) and atomic adsorption spectroscopy (AAS) offer precision and sensitivity, they are costly, labor intensive, and impractical for on-site monitoring, demanding intricate sample preparation before analysis. Moreover, these techniques fall short of furnishing vital toxicity data essential for assessing the influence of multiple toxicants in agricultural and aquatic environments. This chapter delves into the advances in the existing electrochemical biosensors designed to detect environmental toxicants, specifically pesticides and heavy metals. The detection and analysis of agricultural contaminants in soil, water, and food is not just important, but it is a matter of ensuring the safety of our environment and food supply. Biosensors and carbon-based biosensors are commonly used for this purpose, employing various active functional materials and material compositions to achieve optimal sensitivity, selectivity, linear dynamic range, and limits of detection (LODs). Electrochemical techniques are often utilized as a transducer to convert the signal for further processing. The forefront of this biosensor array is electrochemical carbon-based biosensors, demonstrating exceptional efficacy. Their compact, portable, and user-friendly attributes, coupled with cost-effectiveness, position them as the optimal selection for detecting environmental contamination.

doi:10.1088/978-0-7503-5879-8ch9

9.1 Introduction

Recent decades have witnessed a dramatic shift in modern agriculture, characterized by the introduction of novel techniques, greater efficiency, and technological breakthroughs. Although these breakthroughs have many benefits, there are drawbacks, particularly agricultural pollutants that can potentially harm the environment and human health [1]. With the help of technology, modern agricultural methods have raised crop yields and overall production. Genetic engineering, mechanized equipment, and precision farming all help to maximize resource efficiency [2]. Modern tools, such as data analytics, GPS tracking, and drones, as well as the integration of advanced sensing technologies in agriculture, have significantly favored crop yield and production by providing real-time data on soil health, moisture levels, and crop conditions, allowing farmers to make informed decisions for optimized cultivation practices [3]. This results in better resource management, less waste, and better agricultural results. A more excellent range of crops, frequently adapted to particular environmental circumstances, may be grown thanks to modern agriculture. Resilient agricultural systems are aided by this diversification [4]. The effectiveness of current methods of agriculture is essential for resolving issues related to global food security. Modern agricultural practices, including agricultural chemicals, biosolids, and animal manures, have led to significant environmental contaminations [5]. Intensive agrarian methods may contribute to contamination of water supplies, biodiversity loss, and soil erosion, among other environmental problems. Using chemical fertilizers and pesticides containing chemicals may harm ecosystems [6]. Due to the emphasis it places on non-renewable resources, such as synthetic fertilizers and fossil fuels for machinery, modern agriculture can lead to resource depletion and unsustainable methods of agriculture [7]. The high initial expenses associated with modern agricultural technology might affect farmer income inequality. Small-scale and subsistence farmers may face challenges adopting these technologies [8]. The ability of the Earth's ecosystem to operate has typically been disrupted by the deposition of various toxins in agricultural products, soil, water, air, and even higher food chain trophic levels [9] (figure 9.1).

Multiple research investigations have demonstrated the importance of monitoring toxins for maintaining a good environment and human health. They highlight the importance of identifying and looking for possible environmental contaminants to safeguard people, animals, and plants. This stresses the need for accurate data and monitoring efforts to offer a better overview of human exposure to chemical pollutants in agriculture. Modern agriculture uses pesticides and herbicides to protect crops, but there are worries that the residues in the soil and water might harm ecosystems and even pose health hazards [11]. Excessive fertilizers and pesticides can cause nutrient runoff, contaminating water. Nitrogen and phosphorus from this runoff lead to toxic algal blooms and oxygen-depleted 'dead zones' [12]. The intended outcome of fertilizer and pesticide application is that plants can absorb it. However, unintentional processes include volatilization, deterioration, runoff, leaching, and photodecomposition [13]. These procedures draw attention to the intricate relationships between fertilizers, pesticides, and the environment, and the possibility of

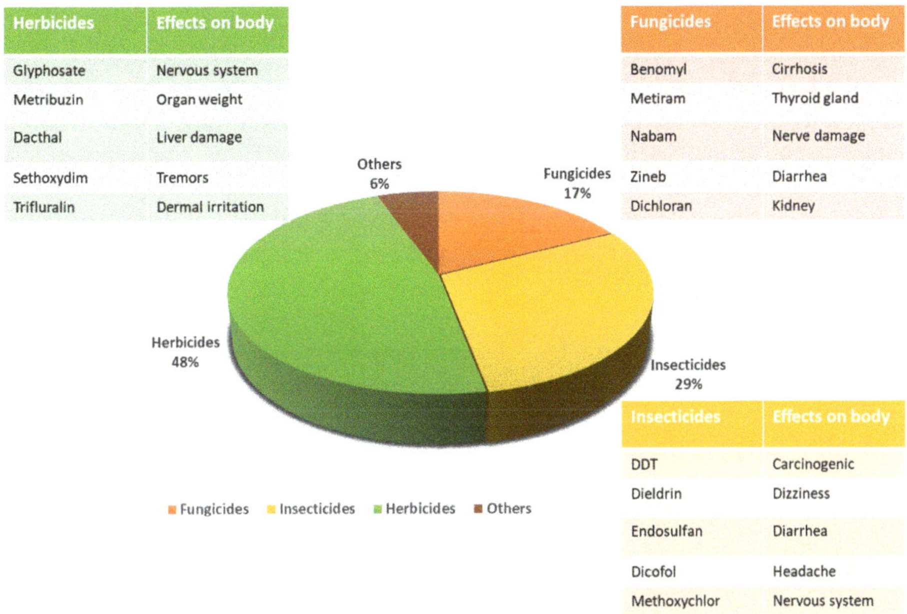

Figure 9.1. Pie chart of the percentage distribution of pesticides.

unforeseen repercussions beyond plant nourishment. Insecticides used in agricultural practices may also affect the soil and ecosystem, where contamination can be carried through different phenomena. There are natural insecticides, and there are synthetic insecticides. In agriculture, insecticides are frequently used with fungicides and herbicides to manage pests. Insecticides help crops, but they can significantly affect the ecosystem. The overuse of pesticides has the potential to wipe out biodiversity. They can join the food chain and bioaccumulate at a more elevated tropical level [14]. Chemical pesticides are highly effective, but there are concerns about their effects on soil, the environment, and the residue they leave in food items [14]. Because of their biocide activity and possible consumer danger, pesticides are becoming a bigger worry for the environment and the general public. Other commonly used agrochemicals in contemporary agricultural techniques are organophosphates, herbicides, and fungicides [15]. They are essential for managing diseases and controlling weeds and pests. However, their extensive usage prompts questions about how they affect the environment as pollutants [16]. A type of pesticide known as organophosphates inhibits the enzyme acetylcholinesterase, which is necessary for the proper operation of the nervous system of pests. Organophosphate residues have the potential to contaminate nontarget species by seeping into soil and water [17]. Water bodies may get contaminated by runoff from treated fields, negatively impacting aquatic ecosystems and possibly harming human health. Chemicals called herbicides are intended to suppress or eradicate undesirable plants, sometimes referred to as weeds [18]. When herbicides move beyond their intended region or get into water sources, they can contribute to environmental damage. Herbicide-resistant weeds might emerge due to the long environmental half-lives of certain herbicides, which affect nontarget plants [19].

Chemicals called fungicides are used to stop or manage fungal infections in crops. When fungicides are used excessively or without the necessary safety measures, residues may end up in the soil and water [20]. This may cause nontarget species, such as helpful soil microbes, to suffer negative consequences and result in resistant fungi. By incorporating several control techniques, including cultural control, the use of resistant genotypes, and physico-mechanical control, in addition to chemical control, integrated pest management can help reduce the quantity and number of pesticide, herbicide, fertilizer, and organophosphates treatments applied [21]. In particular, they emphasize the need for fundamental agricultural contamination monitoring and evaluation programs and the necessity of long-term monitoring of metals, plastic waste, and persistent organic pollutants, especially in developing nations [22].

Several approaches have been developed to detect agricultural contaminants in a sensitive, effective, and selective manner. So, several existing methods, such as high-performance liquid chromatography (HPLC), colorimetry, gas chromatography (GC), and electrochemical (EC) biosensors, are advantageous thanks to their sensitivity, selectivity, etc. EC biosensors have several benefits compared to other methods, such as colorimetry, GC, and HPLC [23]. Because biological recognition components (such as enzymes and antibodies) are particular, EC biosensors frequently offer excellent sensitivity and selectivity. In contrast to specific conventional methods, this enables the identification of target analytes at lower concentrations. EC biosensors make real-time analyte monitoring possible, and provide quick and continuous data. This is especially useful for dynamic processes and systems, enabling prompt interventions and data-driven decision-making. Compact and portable designs are possible for EC biosensors [24]. While HPLC and GC are frequently large and necessitate laboratory settings, the mobility of EC biosensors is helpful for on-site and point-of-care applications, making them appropriate for field use and decentralized testing [25]. The reaction times of EC biosensors are usually fast. Unlike the more time-consuming analytical periods involved with HPLC and GC, directly translating biological processes into electrical signals enables prompt detection [26]. When detecting trace quantities of analytes is required, EC biosensors are an excellent choice because of their ability to attain lower detection limits. For environmental monitoring and biological diagnostics, this is especially pertinent. Compared to methods such as HPLC and GC, EC biosensors frequently require smaller sample quantities [23]. Sample consumption is reduced, which is helpful when working with scarce or valuable sample quantities. In terms of reagent and equipment expenses, EC biosensors can be economical. Compared to specific conventional methods, the total cost-effectiveness is enhanced by the instrumentation's simplicity and possibility for miniaturization [27]. Most EC biosensors are easy to use and do not require any training to operate. Because of their simplicity, they are usable by a wider variety of users, including nonspecialized staff.

Biosensors, utilizing biological components to detect contaminants, offer rapid and sensitive detection methods. They have been used to identify soil and water contaminants, such as fertilizers and pesticides [28]. Even though technology has transformed the sector, the effects of pollutants on the environment and human health must be carefully considered. Sustainable agricultural practices and effective detection techniques are essential for reducing the adverse consequences of modern agriculture, and maintaining a balance between environmental responsibility and production [29].

In 1950, American scientist 'L L Clark' created the first biosensor. The electrode utilized in this sensor is known as the Clark electrode or oxygen electrode, and it is used to measure blood oxygen levels. A gel containing the enzyme glucose oxidization was placed on the oxygen electrode to calculate blood sugar. The urease enzyme was used to measure the amount of urea in body fluids, including blood and urine, by combining it with an electrode for NH_4^+ ions [30]. After this attempt, biosensors have become a viable choice for biological and medical analysis in applications related to agriculture, food security, biomedical research, and the environment. Taking this into account, biosensors are used to identify agricultural pollutants. However, we must be aware of the present state of affairs about the development of biosensor technology and the varieties of biosensors that currently exist in the market. There are now three types of biosensors on the market (table 9.1): the first produces an electrical response when the product's reaction spreads to the sensor, the second type of sensor manipulates the response using specific mediators to get a better response, and in the third type the reaction is sparked by the response rather than a direct mediator [31] (figure 9.2).

A biosensor is an analytical instrument that integrates transducer and sensor systems with additional biological detection elements. These sensors are superior in terms of both sensitivity and selectivity when compared to any other diagnostic tool currently on the market [33]. The primary uses of these biosensors are in the food and agricultural industries, and also in monitoring ecological pollution control. Stability, affordability, sensitivity, and repeatability are the primary characteristics of biosensors [32]. A signal processor, a detecting component, and a recognizing component are the three primary parts of a biosensor. The binding of the target molecules, which often results in a chemical reaction or change and generates a biological, chemical, or physical signal, is the responsibility of the recognized components [30]. The signals generated by the recognizing components will be identified and received by the detection components. Using signal processors, these

Table 9.1. Comparison between the three generations of biosensors.

Generation	First generation	Second generation	Third generation
Mechanism	Product dispersal reaction.	Involvement of mediators.	Direct response without mediators.
Description	An electrical response is produced by the reaction product spreading to the sensor.	Introducing specific mediators between the sensor and the response will improve and strengthen the response.	There is no direct intermediary between the emotion and the response.

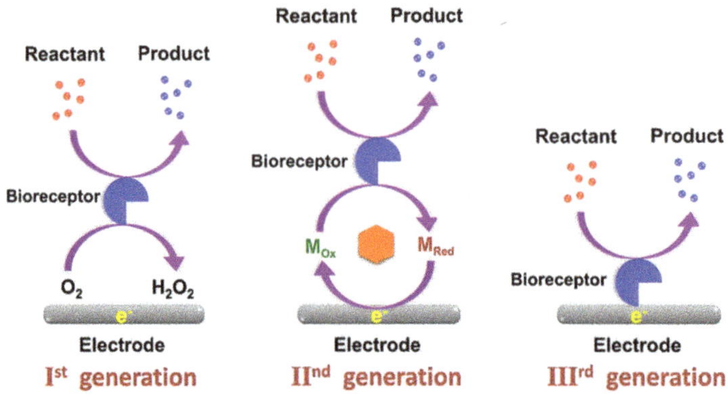

Figure 9.2. Pictorial representation of the three generations of biosensor. Reproduced from [32]. CC BY 4.0.

signals will be converted into digital signals that the researcher may read and view on a screen. Different biosensors have different detecting components, so they may be categorized into cultural, immunological, metabolic technology, nucleic acid-based, biosensor, optical, piezoelectric sensors, chromatography, and mass-based biosensors [34]. Every approach has a set of corresponding procedures. For instance, PCR is used for nucleic acid-based procedures, while ELISA is used for immunological tests. These techniques can recognize various chemical, physical, and biological pollutants. Every approach has specific benefits and drawbacks (see table 9.2). Traditional methods, for example, are simple but require much time and are not very sensitive. The electrochemical biosensors will be the primary focus of this chapter because the relative simplicity of electrochemical biosensors is one of their main advantages. Cost-effective electrodes and basic electronics may be used to create compact, user-friendly portable devices that can conduct quick measurements [35]. For monitoring current circumstances and variables associated with the environment, having the ability to identify the concentration of an analyte within a complicated sample at the point of care and in almost real time is highly appealing [25].

Since the concept of carbon-based biosensors first emerged, carbon-based detection systems have been applied in various industries, including food safety, environmental protection, and medicine. The benefit of miniaturization with high-throughput analysis and changed nanostructure characteristics compared to bulk qualities may be obtained through carbon-based functional materials. Because carbon-based nanomaterials have special biochemical and physical features (e.g., optical, mechanical, structural, and thermal capabilities), the scientific community has focused on exploring them for biosensing applications [36]. Because of the characteristics given above, various materials have been thoroughly studied, including graphene oxide, carbon nanotubes, graphite, nitrogen-vacancy center diamonds, ultra-nanocrystalline diamonds, glassy carbon electrodes, and graphene quantum dots [37]. The physicochemical properties of the materials used to construct the transducer and the matrices used to immobilize the enzymes, stabilizers, and mediators affect how well the biosensor performs [32]. In the development of biosensors, carbon-based materials such as graphite paste, carbon

Table 9.2. Comparing the methods used in biosensor-based techniques to find agricultural contaminants [10].

Technique type	Method	Detected analyte	Advantages	Disadvantages
Biosensor based	Electrochemical	Biological pollutants	• Simple • Good repeatability • A large number of samples can be used • Automated • Label-free detection	• Low specificity • High sample volume is required • Analysis may interfere with detection matrices • Many washings • A homogenous sample is required
	Optical	Biological, chemical, and physical pollutants	• High sensitivity • Fast • Real-time detection • Label-free detection	• Complex equipment required • High cost
	Piezoelectric biosensors	Biological, chemical, and physical pollutants	• Automated • High sensitivity	• Complex equipment required
	Mass-based biosensors	Biological, chemical, and physical pollutants	• Cost-effective • Easy to operate • Label-free detection • Real-time detection	• Low specificity • Low sensitivity • Long incubation time with the analyte • Many washing and drying steps

nanotubes (CNTs), and graphene oxide (GO) are commonly used because of their low background current, surface regeneration ability, and ease of production. These materials have desirable physical properties and predictable electrochemical behavior, providing simple surface biomolecular interaction. Certain carbon materials have excellent porosity and conductivity, which makes them perfect for adsorbing big molecules (e.g., polyelectrolyte/enzyme complexes) and electrochemical signal transmission without requiring the enzyme to be chemically manipulated. For a biosensor to be effective in a particular application, it has to have a few specific qualities. A biosensor's response time, throughput, stability, specificity, selectivity, and sensitivity are among its performance requirements. When developing a new biosensor, analytical parameters such as dynamic range, linearity, detection limits, limit of quantitation, and response time should be considered [32]. These variables are sometimes referred to as a biosensor's analytical figures of merit. In this chapter, we have presented several carbon-based biosensors by evaluating these criteria.

9.2 Need to develop electrochemical biosensors to determine agricultural pollutants

Recent developments in material science and nanotechnology have made it possible to create ultrasensitive sensors that can take advantage of the structural and functional characteristics of metallic and carbon nanomaterials and composites made of conducting polymers. This has dramatically improved sensor performance and the overall stability of biosensors. The advances in electrochemical biosensors will help sectors such as agriculture, medicine, and many growing sectors. Many existing functional electrochemical biosensors have shown good repeatability and near-to-ideal results. This should be discussed and compared to better understand how biosensors work, which will help in the upcoming advances in this field (figure 9.3).

An electrical component and a biological ingredient, such as an enzyme or antibody, are combined in a biosensor to produce a detectable signal. The electronic component detects, records, and transmits information about a physiological change or the presence of various chemical or biological components in the environment. Biosensors can identify and quantify even minute quantities of certain diseases, hazardous substances, and pH values. They are available in a variety of sizes and forms [38]. The components of a standard biosensor are an analyte, a transducer, a bioreceptor, electronics, and a display. The substance being examined, such as

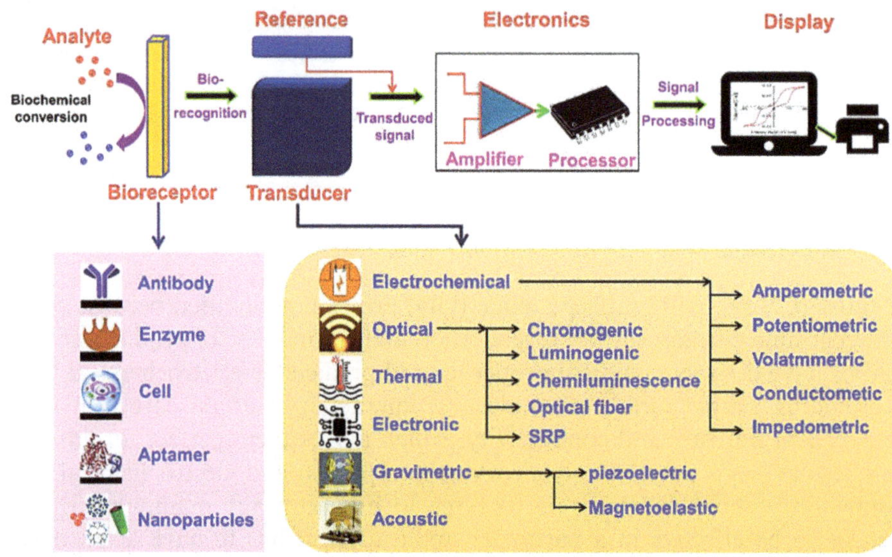

Figure 9.3. A biosensor's schematic design shows the many types of bioreceptors and transducers that are used in biosensors in addition to the electrical system (processor, amplifier), display (PC or printer), and other components. Reproduced from [32]. CC BY 4.0.

glucose or ammonia, is the analyte. An enzyme, cell, aptamer, DNA, RNA, or antibody is an example of a bioreceptor in the biosensing domain. It identifies and interacts with the target analyte to produce signals such as light, heat, pH changes, or mass modifications [39]. We call this process biorecognition. Transducers, which function as devices that change the form of energy, are essential. Most importantly, they convert the biorecognition event into a quantifiable electrical signal for use in biosensors. Many different kinds of transducers work on other principles. These include electrochemical, optical, thermal, electronic, and gravimetric transducers. After transduction, electronics produce the electrical impulses, amplifying them and converting them into a digital representation. In doing so, the signals are ready for presentation. The display device incorporates a user interpretation system, such as a computer or printer, and generates an output for user comprehension. The output can be tabular, graphical, or numerical, depending on the user's requirements. The complex route of biosensing, an essential technology in disciplines ranging from environmental monitoring to medical diagnostics, comprises an all-encompassing process from analyte identification to user-readable output. Following specific guidelines is critical to producing an effective biosensor for use in industry. Essential considerations include selectivity in the selection of bioreceptors, sensitivity for precise detection at low concentrations, and linearity for reliable results [32]. Response speed is essential for real-time applications, and repeatability guarantees consistent outcomes. For continuous monitoring, stability, which is determined by the degradation and affinity of the bioreceptor, is crucial. The listed characteristics are essential for maximizing the dependability and performance of biosensors.

Based on the electrochemical characteristics of the analyte and transducer, electrochemical biosensors are the most extensively studied and utilized biosensors. Electrochemical biosensors are characterized by their high sensitivity, selectivity, and detection capabilities [31]. This biosensor uses an electrochemical interaction between the analyte and bioreceptor on the transducer's surface to provide observable electrochemical signals regarding capacitance, voltage, current, and impedance. Electrochemical biosensors fall into five categories: conductometric, voltammetric, impedimetric, potentiometric, and amperometric, all based on the transduction principle. Concerning the reference electrode at zero current, potentiometric biosensors measure the charge from the interaction between the analyte and bioreceptor at the working electrode. Ion-sensitive field-effect transistors and ion-selective electrodes convert biological processes into potential signals [40]. In two- or three-electrode setups, amperometric biosensors measure current from electrochemical oxidation or reduction of electroactive species at the working electrode at a constant voltage. This technique is suitable for mass manufacturing because it provides sensitive, quick, accurate, and linear responses [41]. Conductometric biosensors, which are frequently used to track metabolic processes, assess the change in conductance brought on by electrochemical reactions [31]. Impedimetric biosensors use low-amplitude AC voltage to measure electrical impedance at the electrode/electrolyte contact [32]. Voltammetric biosensors can simultaneously detect several analytes and give very sensitive readings due to their ability to monitor current under-regulated potential change (figure 9.4) [32].

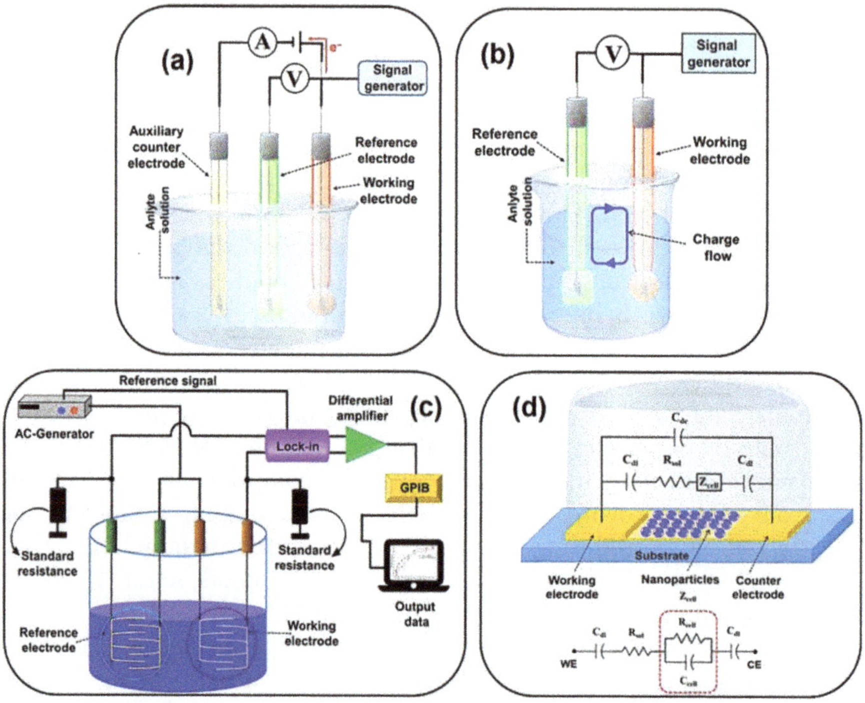

Figure 9.4. Schematics of the (a) amperometric/voltammetric, (b) potentiometric, and (c) conductometric biosensors. (d) Diagram showing the equivalent circuit of the impedimetric biosensor (C_{dl} = double-layer capacitance of the electrodes, R_{sol} = resistance of the solution, C_{de} = capacitance of the electrode, Z_{cell} = impedance introduced by the bound nanoparticles, and R_{cell} and C_{cell} = resistance and capacitance in parallel). Reproduced from [32]. CC BY 4.0.

In contrast, sample analysis has often been neglected because reporting a sensor's sensitivity and specificity usually depends on its optimization and interrogation using buffered solutions. However, the method's detection limit acquired when a produced sensor is tested with actual samples might differ significantly from the instrumental limit of detection obtained using 'laboratory' solutions. The actual matrix of the intended use, which is far more complex than a buffered solution, must be measured to ascertain the latter. The impact of this measurement can be seen in several ways, including the analyte's interaction with matrix molecules and its detrimental effects on the sensor's detection limit. Depending on the sample's characteristics and the biorecognition molecule, several solutions have been developed to address matrix interference and actual sample analysis, two common issues that all biosensors face [32]. Consequently, a real or extracted sample's matrix interference with the sensor's performance might be disproportionately great, leading to significant departures from the expected behavior. Therefore, comparing the generated carbon-based biosensors in matrices pertinent to the actual sensor application is crucial. This makes it possible to determine and explain the cause of measurement aberrations, which could be anything from matrix effects and the presence of interferents to low analyte recovery after sample pretreatment or even a combination of these. Ultimately, this makes it possible to understand truly robust assays and carbon-based biosensors that can obtain accurate readings [42].

9.3 Electrochemical biosensors for pesticides

The Food and Agriculture Organization of the United Nations defines pesticides as any substance or combination of substances used to control, prevent, or destroy any pests that pose a risk to humans or animals, as well as any unwanted plants or animal species that may have an impact on the production, management, sale, storage, or transportation of food. Agrochemicals such as pesticides destroy weeds, fungi, rodents, and insects. They consist of plant growth regulators, fungicides, molluscicides, herbicides, nematicides, and other substances. In commercial and food-based industrial processes, such as aquaculture, agriculture, food processing, and storage, they play essential roles in crop protection, food preservation, and the general prevention of diseases carried by vectors. Pests are any living organisms, whether plants or animals, that pose a risk to humans or other creatures—pesticides are used to destroy pests or stop them from growing [10]. When pesticides are applied to plants, the desired result may be that the plants absorb the pesticide and produce fruit, vegetables, and other consumable plant products. Some of the examples are mentioned in table 9.3, where the electrochemical carbon-based biosensors are used for the detection of pesticides or pesticide classes such as malathion, paraoxon, methyl parathion, chlorpyrifos, diazinon, organophosphate, chlorpyrifos-methyl, acetamiprid, phosmet, triazophos, carbamate, and organophosphorus.

Pesticides can be categorized into two groups according to their chemical and physical characteristics [67]. They are categorized based on the type of pest they target and their nature (i.e., natural or synthetic). The bulk of synthetic pesticides are organic compounds divided into four categories: pyrethroids, carbamates, organochlorines, and organophosphates. Biopesticides, naturally occurring pesticides, are made of living things such as fungi, bacteria, and plants (figure 9.5) [10].

Pesticides behave and have different biological activities in soil depending on their molecular weight, ionizability, lipophilicity, polarizability, and volatility, among other physical and chemical qualities. Pesticides translocate in soil and water as a result of various agricultural practices, and depending on several factors, such as temperature, moisture, pH, texture of the soil, and the content of organic and mineral compounds, their persistence in that environment can last for a few weeks, months, or even years [68]. The dosage and exposure duration are the main variables determining a pesticide's acute and chronic toxicity. Only acute toxicity is recognized by the World Health Organization for pesticide categorization based on lethal dosage (LD50), divided into two types: acute cutaneous toxicity and acute oral toxicity. Acute cutaneous toxicity is defined as follows: significantly: less than 50 mg kg^{-1} body weight of rat; highly: 50–200 mg kg^{-1} body weight of rat; moderately: 200–2000 mg kg^{-1} body weight of rat; etc [10].

Pesticide/insecticide detection using biosensors uses analytical methods that use biological recognition components and transducers to identify and measure

Table 9.3. Examples of carbon-based biosensors used to detect pesticides in the food matrix.

Nanomaterial	Biorecognition material	Pesticide or pesticide class	LOD	Food matrix	References
PEDOT-MWCNTs	Antibody	Malathion	1.0×10^{-6} nM	Lettuce	[43]
AgNPs-GQDs	AChE	Paraoxon	1.7 ng ml^{-1}	Apple and carrot	[44]
f/MWCNTs	AChE	Chlorpyrifos-methyl	1.0×10^{-3} μg l^{-1}	Lettuce	[45]
CS@TiO_2-CS/rGO	AChE	Dichlorvos	29.0 nM	Cabbage juice	[46]
ZnS/Mn-QDs and MWCNTs	Aptamer	Acetamiprid	7.0×10^{-10} M	Cabbage leaves	[47]
MWCNTs	AChE	Chlorpyrifos	5.0×10^{-8} g l^{-1}	Cabbage, rape, and lettuce	[48]
	AChE	Malathion	$1.0 \times 10^{-9.}$ μg l^{-1}	Lettuce	[49]
	ds-DNA	Diazinon	3.0×10^{-10} mol l^{-1}	Lettuce and tomato juice	[50]
	AChE	Paraoxon	1.0×10^{-10} M	Potato	[51]
	AChE	Organophosphate	4.0×10^{-6} μM	Spinach and cabbage	[52]
r-GO	Aptamer	Acetamiprid	7.12×10^{-2} pM	Tea	[53]
CdTe-QD's	AChE and CHOx	Malathion, Triazophos, Paraoxon, and Dichlorvos	Malathion: 2.3×10^{-2} μM Triazophos: 1.06×10^{-5} μM Paraoxon: 1.62×10^{-9} μM Dichlorvos: 7.53×10^{-8} μM	Tomato juice and apple	[54]
MHCS and Fe_3O_4@MHCS	AChE	Malathion	MHCS: 14.8 ng l^{-1} Fe_3O_4@MHCS: 18.2 ng l^{-1}	Pear	[55]
AuNPs and VNSWCNTs	AChE	Malathion, Chlorpyrifos, and Methyl parathion	Malathion: 1.96×10^{-6} μg l^{-1} Chlorpyrifos: 2.06×10^{-6} μg l^{-1} Methyl parathion: 3.04×10^{-6} μg l^{-1}	Cabbage juice	[40]
CNT	M Cell	Paraoxon	3.0×10^{-9} μmol l^{-1}	Spinach juice	[56]
Fe_3O_4 and graphene	AChE	Chlorpyrifos	2.0×10^{-8} g l^{-1}	Spinach and cabbage	[57]

AuNSs/QDs	Antibodies	Malathion, Diazinon, and Chlorpyrifos	Malathion: 7.4×10^{-7} g l^{-1} Diazinon: 6.9×10^{-7} g l^{-1} Chlorpyrifos: 7.3×10^{-7} g l^{-1}	Apple, blueberry, cabbage, cauliflower, eggplant, lettuce, Long bean, maize, orange, oyster, shiitake mushroom, spinach, and tomato	[58]
WO_3@g-C_3N_4	Tc-AChE	Phosmet	3.6×10^{-3} μM	Wheat flour	[59]
AuNPs/rGO	AChE	Methyl parathion and Malathion	Methyl parathion: 2.17×10^{-5} μg l^{-1} Malathion: 2.78×10^{-3} μg l^{-1}	Chinese cabbage	[60]
r-GO	AChE	Carbamate	19.0×10^{-8} mol l^{-1}	Tomato	[61]
CuNW/rGO/TEPA	AChE	Malathion	0.39 ng ml^{-1}	Cabbage and carrot	[62]
Ir NRs@CdS QDs	AChE and ChOx biocomposite	Organophosphorus	1.67×10^{-6} μM	Cabbage, lettuce, and pakchoi	[63]
PB/SWCNTs	AChE	Methyl parathion and Malathion	Methyl parathion: 1.88×10^{-7} μg l^{-1} Malathion: 3.11×10^{-3} μg l^{-1}	Chinese cabbage	[64]
CdTe-QD	AChE	Organophosphorus and Carbamate	Pirimicarb: 0.05 ppm Dichlorvos: 0.01 ppm Carbaryl: 0.01 ppm	Lettuce, choy, and rice	[65]
CuO NFs and C-SWCNTs	Oligonucleotides	Chlorpyrifos	7.0×10^{-10} g l^{-1}	Cabbage and apple	[66]

Abbreviations: PEDOT-MWCNTs = Poly(3,4-ethylene dioxythiophene)-MWCNTs; AgNPs-GQDs = Graphene quantum dots-Silver nanoparticles; AuNPs-VNSWCNTs = Gold nanoparticles-vertical nitrogen-doped single-walled carbon nanotubes; QDs-AuNSs = Quantum dots gold nanostars; MWCNTs = Multi-walled carbon nanotubes; ZnS: Mn-QDs = Zinc Sulphide: Manganese-quantum dots, CNT = Carbon nanotube, PB-SWCNTs = Prussian blue-SWCNTs; WO_3/g-C_3N_4 = Tungsten oxide/Graphitic carbon nitride; CdTe-QD = Cadmium telluride-quantum dots; rGO/AuNPs = Reduced graphene oxide/gold nanoparticles; rGO-TEPA-CuNW = Reduced graphene oxide-Tetraethylenepentamine-copper nanowire; CuO NFs and C-SWCNTs = Copper oxides nanoflowers and carboxyl-functionalized SWCNTs; f-MWCNTs = Functionalized MWCNTs; CS@TiO2-CS/rGO = Chitosan integrated Titanium oxide-Chitosan/Reduced graphene oxide, Ir NRs@CdS QDs = Iridium nanorods integrated cadmium sulphide quantum dots; MHCS and Fe_3O_4@MHCS = Mesoporous hollow carbon spheres and Iron oxide integrated mesoporous hollow carbon spheres.

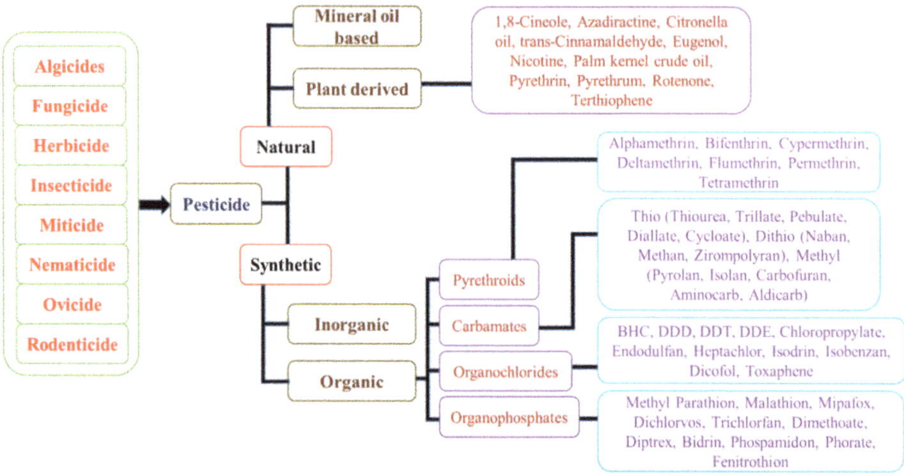

Figure 9.5. Classification of pesticides.

pesticides in various samples. These biosensors are essential for monitoring the environment, guaranteeing food safety, and adhering to regulations. Biosensors have helped us obtain the data for multiple pesticide/insecticide contamination regulated around agricultural applications. Specific systems are used for electrochemical or colorimetric detection based on the characteristics of the nanomaterial. For instance, SWCNTs and MWCNTs have outstanding thermal conductivities, but graphene has a larger surface area than CNTs. The lower electrical conductivity of GO and carbon-based quantum dots and their exceptional photoluminescence qualities, biocompatibility, and low toxicity make them excellent materials for various applications [69].

9.4 Electrochemical biosensors for heavy metal ions

The four central systems of the world are the hydrosphere, biosphere, atmosphere, and geosphere. These spheres are nutrient- and mineral-rich. In the form of ores, more than 35 metals have been detected. Of these, 23 metals have an atomic weight of more than 40.04 and a high specific density greater than 5 g cm^{-3}, indicating that they are environmentally hazardous and five times denser than water [70]. The soil environment is frequently contaminated by heavy metals, which include lead (Pb), copper (Cu), zinc (Zn), nickel (Ni), arsenic (As), cadmium (Cd), chromium (Cr), mercury (Hg), and zinc. This pollution is widespread, long-lasting, and physiologically harmful to the soil ecosystem. A range of heavy metal-contaminated soils pose a hazard to the environment and human health due to the economy's and society's fast development. There are three categories for soil replacement: spading, importing fresh soil, and replacing soil. Replacing contaminated soil with fresh soil involves taking the old soil out. This technique works well for small areas of polluted soil. However, the replacement soil must be managed practically to avoid secondary contamination. To achieve the goal of dilution and natural degradation, soil spading involves extensively excavating the contaminated soil, allowing the pollutant to penetrate the deep places. To lower the pollutant concentration, new soil importation consists of adding a large amount of clean soil to the contaminated soil, covering it on the surface or mixing it [71]. To understand the level of contamination and act upon it, we need efficient detection techniques that can correctly calibrate the amount of contamination caused by the pollutants. Below are some examples that show the electrochemical sensing platform for heavy metal sensing (see table 9.4).

Heavy metal ion detection electrochemical biosensors have become indispensable environmental surveillance and public health defense instruments. Ecosystems and human health are seriously threatened by heavy metal pollution, which makes

Table 9.4. Examples of carbon-based electrochemical sensors for detecting heavy metal contamination.

Electrochemical sensing platform	Target analyte	Linear dynamic range	Limit of detection	References
Tl/MWCNT/IP/CPE	Tl^{+}	3.0–240 × 10^{-9} g ml^{-1}	0.76 × 10^{-9} g ml^{-1}	[72]
Ag/MWCNTs/IIP	Ag^{+}	0.5 nM–0.28 μM	0.12 nM	[73]
MWCNTs/IIP/GCE	Pb^{2+}	5.0–10.0 μg l^{-1}	0.16 μg l^{-1}	[74]
GCE–IIP–MWCNTs	Hg^{2+}	0.1 nM–7.0 × 10^{-4}M	0.5 × 10^{-10} M	[75]
Ce-IIP-MWCNTs	Ce^{3+}	1.0 μM–25.0 pM	10.0 pM	[76]
CPE-IIP-MWCNTs	Cr^{3+}	1.0 μM–1.0 M	5.9 × 10^{-7} M	[77]
CS/GR-IIP	Cr^{6+}	1.0 × 10^{-9}–1.0 × 10^{-5} M	6.4 × 10^{-10} M	[78]
g-C_3N_4/IIP	Hg^{2+}	0.06–25.0 nM	18.0 pM	[79]
IIP-MWCNT-CS-IL/GCE	Mn^{2+}	2.0–9.0 μM	0.15 μM	[80]
MWCNTs/CPE/IIP	Pb^{2+}	0.1 pM–0.8 nM	3.8 × 10^{-3} nM	[81]
MWCNT/CH=CH_2/IIP	Zn^{2+}	1.0–5.0 ppm	13.2 nM	[82]
	Cr^{3+}		51 nM	[83]
	Pb^{2+}		2 × 10^{-2} μM	[84]
MWCNT/CH=CH_2-IIP/PE	Co^{2+}		1.01 × 10^{-5} μM	[85]
MWCNT/CH=CH_2=/IIP/Pt	Ni^{2+}		0.028 μM	[86]
	Cd^{2+}		0.03 μM	[87]
	Mn^{2+}		0.0138 μM	[88]
GR/IIM/GCE	Pd^{2+}	2.0 × 10^{-8}–2.0 × 10^{-4} M	6.4 × 10^{-9} M	[89]
CS-AuNPs-GR/GCE	Cd^{2+}	0.1–0.9 μM	1.62 × 10^{-4} μM	[90]
Ag/GR/IIP-CPE	Zn^{2+}	2.62 × 10^{-1}–6.54 × 10^{-5} μg l^{-1}	1.93 × 10^{-1} μg l^{-1}	[91]
GO-IIP-GCE	Cd^{2+}	4.2 pM–5.6 mM	7 × 10^{-5} nM	[92]
GQDTU-IIP	Hg^{2+}	0.5 nM–0.23 μM	23.5 ×10^{-9} M	[93]
rGO/IIP	Hg^{2+}	0.07–80.0 μg l^{-1}	0.02 μg l^{-1}	[94]
PPy-rGO-IIP	Cd^{2+}	1.0–100.0 μg l^{-1}	0.26 μg l^{-1}	[95]
CS-GO/IIP	Cu^{2+}	0.5 × 10^{-6}–1.0 × 10^{-4} M	0.15 × 10^{-6} M	[96]
GO-MWCNT-IIP	Cu^{2+}	1.0 μM–1.0 × 10^{-1} M	4.0 × 10^{-7} M	[97]
PoPD-ERGO-IIP/GCE	Cd^{2+}	1.0–50.0 ng ml^{-1}	0.13 ng ml^{-1}	[98]
Al_2O_3/rGO/IIP	Hg^{2+}	4.00 nM–1.30 × 10^{-3} M	1.95 nM	[99]
N-CS-rGO-IIP	Cd^{2+}	0.01–0.1 μM	3.51 × 10^{-9} M	[100]

Abbreviations: IIPs = Ion-imprinted polymers, IIMs = Ion-imprinted membranes, IL = Ionic liquid, GCE = Glassy carbon electrode, SWCNTs = Single-walled carbon nanotubes, MMWCNTs = Magnetic multi-walled carbon nanotubes, GR = Graphene, rGO = Reduced graphene oxide, CS = Chitosan, PPy = Polypyrrole, PoPD = Poly (o-phenylenediamine), g-C_3N_4 = Graphitic carbon nitride, GQDTU = Thiourea derivative-functionalized graphene quantum dots.

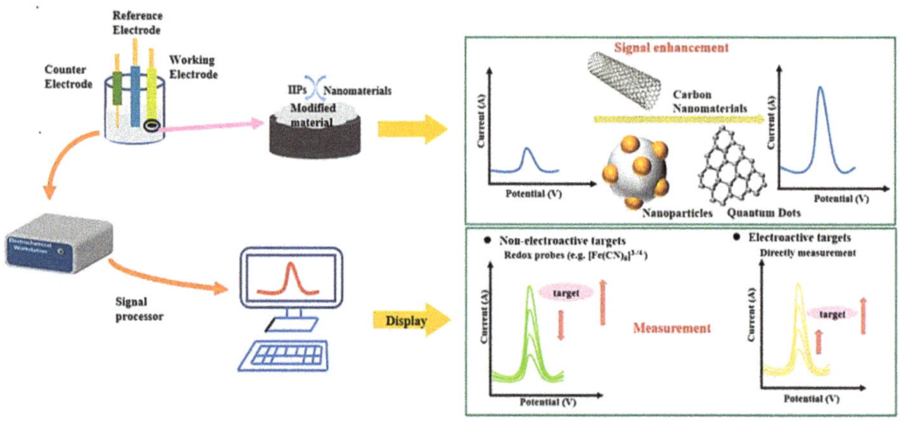

Figure 9.6. Construction and detection principle of heavy metal ions electrochemical sensors. Reproduced from [101]. CC BY 4.0.

effective and trustworthy analytical methods for detection and quantification necessary. Utilizing the concepts of electrochemistry, electrochemical biosensors provide a strong response to these problems. Figure 9.6 shows a instance of carbon-based electrochemical sensors for heavy metal ion detection. Electrochemistry is necessary to accomplish the biosensing process in different biomarker tests. As a result of its many benefits, electrochemical biosensing has garnered interest in a wide range of applications. An electrical signal proportional to the analyte concentration is produced by electrochemical biosensors when they react with the target analyte or compounds. An electrolyte separates the reference and the detecting electrodes, or working electrodes, in a traditional electrochemical biosensor. The reference electrode of an electrochemical biosensor is usually connected to a potentiostat in a three-electrode configuration. It may be finished by adding a counter electrode to allow current to flow across the circuit [102]. The remarkable sensitivity of electrochemical biosensors is one of their main advantages. These tools enable the early detection of environmental contamination because they can identify traces of heavy metal ions. Given the detrimental effects of heavy metals on biological systems and the environment, sensitivity is essential. In summary, electrochemical biosensors for heavy metal ions represent an advanced and effective method of environmental surveillance. Together, their sensitivity, selectivity, mobility, cost-effectiveness, and real-time monitoring capabilities make them invaluable instruments for preventing the harmful effects of heavy metal contamination on ecosystems and public health.

9.5 Conclusion

Electrochemical biosensors for pesticides and heavy metal ions embody a sophisticated and efficient approach to environmental monitoring. Their sensitivity, selectivity, real-time monitoring capabilities, portability, and cost-effectiveness collectively position them as indispensable tools in safeguarding ecosystems and human health from the perils of both pesticides and heavy metal pollution.

Biosensors, particularly those utilizing carbon-based materials, are widely employed for this purpose, employing diverse compositions to achieve optimal sensitivity, selectivity, and detection limits. Electrochemical techniques serve as critical components, converting signals for further analysis. Among these biosensors, electrochemical carbon-based biosensors stand out because of their effectiveness, boasting portability, user-friendliness, and affordability, making them ideal for detecting environmental pollutants. Although conventional analytical techniques such as GC/LC–MS and AAS provide sensitivity and accuracy, their disadvantages, such as expensive cost and time-consuming procedures, make them impractical for on-site monitoring. Furthermore, these techniques frequently lack the essential toxicity information that is required to evaluate the effects of different contaminants in aquatic and agricultural environments. This chapter explored the most recent developments in electrochemical biosensors to identify environmental pollutants, such as heavy metals and pesticides.

References

[1] Fu H, Tan P, Wang R, Li S, Liu H, Yang Y and Wu Z 2022 Advances in organophosphorus pesticides pollution: current status and challenges in ecotoxicological, sustainable agriculture, and degradation strategies *J. Hazard. Mater.* **424** 127494

[2] Khan N, Ray R L, Sargani G R, Ihtisham M, Khayyam M and Ismail S 2021 Current progress and future prospects of agriculture technology: gateway to sustainable agriculture *Sustainability* **13** 4883

[3] Monteiro A, Santos S and Gonçalves P 2021 Precision agriculture for crop and livestock farming—brief review *Animals* **11** 2345

[4] Adhikari P *et al* 2018 System of crop intensification for more productive, resource-conserving, climate-resilient, and sustainable agriculture: experience with diverse crops in varying agroecologies *Int. J. Agric. Sustain.* **16** 1–28

[5] Smith S R 2009 Organic contaminants in sewage sludge (biosolids) and their significance for agricultural recycling *Philos. Trans. R. Soc. A: Math. Phys. Eng. Sci.* **367** 4005–41

[6] Zahoor I and Mushtaq A 2023 Water pollution from agricultural activities: A critical global review *Int. J. Chem. Biochem. Sci.* **23** 1664–76

[7] Chel A and Kaushik G 2011 Renewable energy for sustainable agriculture *Agron. Sust. Developm.* **31** 91–118

[8] Muzari W, Gatsi W and Muvhunzi S 2012 The impacts of technology adoption on smallholder agricultural productivity in sub-saharan Africa: a review *J. Sustain. Dev.* **5** 69–77

[9] Tiwari A K and Pal D B 2022 Nutrients contamination and eutrophication in the river ecosystem *Ecological Significance of River Ecosystems* ed S Madhav, S Kanhaiya, A Srivastav, V Singh and P Singh (Amsterdam: Elsevier) ch 11 pp 203–16

[10] Pathak V M *et al* 2022 Current status of pesticide effects on environment, human health and it's eco-friendly management as bioremediation: a comprehensive review *Front. Microbiol.* **13** 962619

[11] Alengebawy A, Abdelkhalek S T, Qureshi S R and Wang M-Q 2021 Heavy metals and pesticides toxicity in agricultural soil and plants: ecological risks and human health implications *Toxics* **9** 42

[12] Kirchman D L 2021 *Dead Zones: The Loss of Oxygen from Rivers, Lakes, Seas, and the Ocean* (Oxford: Oxford University Press)

[13] Khan N and Rehman S 2022 *Reclamation of deteriorated soils utilizing green approaches* (Nova Science) (book ref) Nova Science Publishers, Inc. 978-1-68507-614-6

[14] Tudi M, Daniel Ruan H, Wang L, Lyu J, Sadler R, Connell D, Chu C and Phung D T 2021 Agriculture development, pesticide application and its impact on the environment *Int. J. Environ. Res. Public Health* **18** 1112

[15] Ansari I, El-Kady M M, Arora C, Sundararajan M, Maiti D and Khan A 2021 A review on the fatal impact of pesticide toxicity on environment and human health *Global Climate Change* ed S Singh, P Singh, S Rangabhashiyam and K K Srivastava (Amsterdam: Elsevier) ch 16 pp 361–91

[16] Kumar V, Kumar R, Singh J and Kumar P 2019 *Contaminants in Agriculture and Environment: Health Risks and Remediation* (Agro Environ Media, Publication Cell of AESA, Agriculture and Environmental Science Academy)

[17] Karthick Rajan D, Mohan K, Rajarajeswaran J, Divya D, Thanigaivel S and Zhang S 2024 Toxic effects of organophosphate pesticide monocrotophos in aquatic organisms: a review of challenges, regulations and future perspectives *Environ. Res.* **244** 117947

[18] Vats S 2015 Herbicides: history, classification and genetic manipulation of plants for herbicide resistance *Sustainable Agriculture Reviews* **Vol. 15** Sustainable Agriculture Reviews E Lichtfouse (Cham: Springer International Publishing) pp 153–92

[19] Schütte G, Eckerstorfer M, Rastelli V, Reichenbecher W, Restrepo-Vassalli S, Ruohonen-Lehto M, Saucy A-G W and Mertens M 2017 Herbicide resistance and biodiversity: agronomic and environmental aspects of genetically modified herbicide-resistant plants *Environ. Sci. Eur.* **29** 5

[20] Rajmohan K S, Chandrasekaran R and Varjani S 2020 A review on occurrence of pesticides in environment and current technologies for their remediation and management *Indian J. Microbiol.* **60** 125–38

[21] Khan B A *et al* 2023 Pesticides: impacts on agriculture productivity, environment, and management strategies *Emerging Contaminants and Plants: Interactions, Adaptations and Remediation Technologies* Emerging Contaminants and Associated Treatment Technologies T Aftab (Cham: Springer International Publishing) pp 109–34

[22] El-Shahawi M S, Hamza A, Bashammakh A S and Al-Saggaf W T 2010 An overview on the accumulation, distribution, transformations, toxicity and analytical methods for the monitoring of persistent organic pollutants *Talanta* **80** 1587–97

[23] Huang C-W, Lin C, Nguyen M K, Hussain A, Bui X-T and Ngo H H 2023 A review of biosensor for environmental monitoring: principle, application, and corresponding achievement of sustainable development goals *Bioengineered* **14** 58–80

[24] Manjakkal L, Mitra S, Petillot Y R, Shutler J, Scott E M, Willander M and Dahiya R 2021 Connected sensors, innovative sensor deployment, and intelligent data analysis for online water quality monitoring *IEEE Internet Things J.* **8** 13805–24

[25] Dagar M, Yadav S, Sai V V R, Satija J and Bhatia H 2022 Emerging trends in point-of-care sensors for illicit drugs analysis *Talanta* **238** 123048

[26] Vogiazi V, de la Cruz A, Mishra S, Shanov V, Heineman W R and Dionysiou D D 2019 A comprehensive review: development of electrochemical biosensors for detection of cyanotoxins in freshwater *ACS Sens.* **4** 1151–73

[27] Lopes L C, Santos A and Bueno P R 2022 An outlook on electrochemical approaches for molecular diagnostics assays and discussions on the limitations of miniaturized technologies for point-of-care devices *Sensors Actuators Rep.* **4** 100087

[28] Zulkifli S N, Rahim H A and Lau W-J 2018 Detection of contaminants in water supply: a review on state-of-the-art monitoring technologies and their applications *Sensors Actuators* B **255** 2657–89

[29] Singh J S, Pandey V C and Singh D P 2011 Efficient soil microorganisms: a new dimension for sustainable agriculture and environmental development *Agric. Ecosyst. Environ.* **140** 339–53

[30] Singh S, Kumar V, Dhanjal D S, Datta S, Prasad R and Singh J 2020 Biological biosensors for monitoring and diagnosis *Microbial Biotechnology: Basic Research and Applications* Environmental and Microbial Biotechnology J Singh, A Vyas, S Wang and R Prasad (Singapore: Springer) pp 317–35

[31] Mehrvar M and Abdi M 2004 Recent developments, characteristics, and potential applications of electrochemical biosensors *Anal. Sci.* **20** 1113–26

[32] Naresh V and Lee N 2021 A review on biosensors and recent development of nano-structured materials-enabled biosensors *Sensors* **21** 1109

[33] Rapp B E, Gruhl F J and Länge K 2010 Biosensors with label-free detection designed for diagnostic applications *Anal. Bioanal. Chem.* **398** 2403–12

[34] Aggarwal S, Sehgal S and Tandon A W 2021 Biosensors—types and application in food processing industry *J. Postharvest Technol.* **9** 1–19

[35] Hernandez-Vargas G, Sosa-Hernández J E, Saldarriaga-Hernandez S, Villalba-Rodríguez A M, Parra-Saldivar R and Iqbal H M N 2018 Electrochemical biosensors: a solution to pollution detection with reference to environmental contaminants *Biosensors* **8** 29

[36] Liang X, Li N, Zhang R, Yin P, Zhang C, Yang N, Liang K and Kong B 2021 Carbon-based SERS biosensor: from substrate design to sensing and bioapplication *NPG Asia Mater.* **13** 36

[37] Dandu N K, Chandaluri C G, Ramesh K, Saritha D, Mahender Reddy N and Ramesh G V 2022 Carbon nanomaterials: application as sensors for diagnostics *Advanced Nanomaterials for Point of Care Diagnosis and Therapy* ed S Dave, J Das and S Ghosh (Amsterdam: Elsevier) ch 11 pp 211–48

[38] Chadha U *et al* 2022 Recent progress and growth in biosensors technology: a critical review *J. Ind. Eng. Chem.* **109** 21–51

[39] Karunakaran C, Rajkumar R and Bhargava K 2015 Introduction to biosensors *Biosenssors and Bioelectronics* ed C Karunakaran, K Bhargava and R Benjamin (Amsterdam: Elsevier) ch 1 pp 1–68

[40] Ma X, Peng R, Mao W, Lin Y and Yu H 2023 Recent advances in ion-sensitive field-effect transistors for biosensing applications *Electrochem. Sci. Adv.* **3** e2100163

[41] Ronkainen N J, Halsall H B and Heineman W R 2010 Electrochemical biosensors *Chem. Soc. Rev.* **39** 1747–63

[42] Fahmy H M, Abu Serea E S, Salah-Eldin R E, Al-Hafiry S A, Ali M K, Shalan A E and Lanceros-Méndez S 2022 Recent progress in graphene- and related carbon-nanomaterial-based electrochemical biosensors for early disease detection *ACS Biomater. Sci. Eng.* **8** 964–1000

[43] Kaur N, Bhatnagar A, Bhalla A and Prabhakar N 2021 Determination of an organo-phosphate pesticide using antibody immobilised hybrid nanocomposites *Int. J. Environ. Anal. Chem.* **101** 1485–98

[44] Li X, Gao X, Gai P, Liu X and Li F 2020 Degradable metal–organic framework/methylene blue composites-based homogeneous electrochemical strategy for pesticide assay *Sensors Actuators* B **323** 128701

[45] Kaur N, Thakur H, Kumar R and Prabhakar N 2016 An electrochemical sensor modified with poly(3,4-ethylenedioxythiophene)-wrapped multi-walled carbon nanotubes for enzyme inhibition-based determination of organophosphates *Microchim. Acta* **183** 2307–15

[46] Cui H-F, Wu W-W, Li M-M, Song X, Lv Y and Zhang T-T 2018 A highly stable acetylcholinesterase biosensor based on chitosan–TiO_2–graphene nanocomposites for detection of organophosphate pesticides *Biosens. Bioelectron.* **99** 223–9

[47] Lin B, Yu Y, Li R, Cao Y and Guo M 2016 Turn-on sensor for quantification and imaging of acetamiprid residues based on quantum dots functionalized with aptamer *Sensors Actuators* B **229** 100–9

[48] Chen D, Fu J, Liu Z, Guo Y, Sun X, Wang X and Wang Z 2017 A simple acetylcholinesterase biosensor based on ionic liquid/multiwalled carbon nanotubes-modified screen-printed electrode for rapid detecting chlorpyrifos *Int. J. Electrochem. Sci.* **12** 9465–77

[49] Kaur N, Thakur H and Prabhakar N 2016 Conducting polymer and multi-walled carbon nanotubes nanocomposites based amperometric biosensor for detection of organophosphate *J. Electroanal. Chem.* **775** 121–8

[50] Zare A R, Ensafi A A and Rezaei B 2019 An impedimetric biosensor based on poly(l-lysine)-decorated multiwall carbon nanotubes for the determination of diazinon in water and fruits *J. Iran. Chem. Soc.* **16** 2777–85

[51] Thakkar J B, Gupta S and Prabha C R 2019 Acetylcholine esterase enzyme doped multiwalled carbon nanotubes for the detection of organophosphorus pesticide using cyclic voltammetry *Int. J. Biol. Macromol.* **137** 895–903

[52] Mahmoudi E, Fakhri H, Hajian A, Afkhami A and Bagheri H 2019 High-performance electrochemical enzyme sensor for organophosphate pesticide detection using modified metal–organic framework sensing platforms *Bioelectrochemistry* **130** 107348

[53] Yi J, Liu Z, Liu J, Liu H, Xia F, Tian D and Zhou C 2020 A label-free electrochemical aptasensor based on 3D porous CS/rGO/GCE for acetamiprid residue detection *Biosens. Bioelectron.* **148** 111827

[54] Korram J *et al* 2020 CdTe QD-based inhibition and reactivation assay of acetylcholinesterase for the detection of organophosphorus pesticides *RSC Adv.* **10** 24190–202

[55] Luo R, Feng Z, Shen G, Xiu Y, Zhou Y, Niu X and Wang H 2018 Acetylcholinesterase biosensor based on mesoporous hollow carbon spheres/core–shell magnetic nanoparticles-modified electrode for the detection of organophosphorus pesticides *Sensors* **18** 4429

[56] Han L, Chen D and Li F 2018 Rational Integration of biomineralization, microbial surface display, and carbon nanocomposites: ultrasensitive and selective biosensor for traces of pesticides *Adv. Mater. Interfaces* **5** 1801332

[57] Wang H, Zhao G, Chen D, Wang Z and Liu G 2016 A sensitive acetylcholinesterase biosensor based on screen printed electrode modified with Fe_3O_4 nanoparticle and graphene for chlorpyrifos determination *Int. J. Electrochem. Sci.* **11** 10906–18

[58] Cheng N, Song Y, Fu Q, Du D, Luo Y, Wang Y, Xu W and Lin Y 2018 Aptasensor based on fluorophore-quencher nano-pair and smartphone spectrum reader for on-site quantification of multi-pesticides *Biosens. Bioelectron.* **117** 75–83

[59] Bilal S, Mudassir Hassan M, Fayyaz ur Rehman M, Nasir M, Jamil Sami A and Hayat A 2021 An insect acetylcholinesterase biosensor utilizing WO_3/g-C_3N_4 nanocomposite modified pencil graphite electrode for phosmet detection in stored grains *Food Chem.* **346** 128894

[60] Dong P, Jiang B and Zheng J 2019 A novel acetylcholinesterase biosensor based on gold nanoparticles obtained by electroless plating on three-dimensional graphene for detecting organophosphorus pesticides in water and vegetable samples *Anal. Methods* **11** 2428–34

[61] da Silva M K L, Vanzela H C, Defavari L M and Cesarino I 2018 Determination of carbamate pesticide in food using a biosensor based on reduced graphene oxide and acetylcholinesterase enzyme *Sensors Actuators* B **277** 555–61

[62] Li S, Qu L M, Wang J F, Ran X Q and Niu X 2020 Acetylcholinesterase based rGO-TEPA-copper nanowires biosensor for detecting malathion *Int. J. Electrochem. Sci.* **15** 505–14

[63] Yang G, He Y, Zhao J, Chen S and Yuan R 2021 Ratiometric electrochemiluminescence biosensor based on Ir nanorods and CdS quantum dots for the detection of organophosphorus pesticides *Sensors Actuators* B **341** 130008

[64] Jiang B, Lu M and Xu M 2019 Amperometric sensing of organophosphorus pesticides based on covalently attached multilayer assemblies of diazo-resin, prussian blue single-walled carbon nanotubes, and acetylcholinesterase *Rev. Roum. Chim.* **64** 763–74

[65] Apilux A, Siangproh W, Insin N, Chailapakul O and Prachayasittikul V 2017 Paper-based thioglycolic acid (TGA)-capped CdTe QD device for rapid screening of organophosphorus and carbamate insecticides *Anal. Methods* **9** 519–27

[66] Xu G, Huo D, Hou C, Zhao Y, Bao J, Yang M and Fa H 2018 A regenerative and selective electrochemical aptasensor based on copper oxide nanoflowers-single walled carbon nanotubes nanocomposite for chlorpyrifos detection *Talanta* **178** 1046–52

[67] Kamalesh C P C, Senthil Kumar T, Rangasamy P and G 2023 An insights of organochlorine pesticides categories, properties, eco-toxicity and new developments in bioremediation process *Environ. Pollut.* **333** 122114

[68] Rasool S, Rasool T and Gani K M 2022 A review of interactions of pesticides within various interfaces of intrinsic and organic residue amended soil environment *Chem. Eng. J. Adv.* **11** 100301

[69] Eivazzadeh-Keihan R *et al* 2022 Applications of carbon-based conductive nanomaterials in biosensors *Chem. Eng. J.* **442** 136183

[70] Velusamy K, Periyasamy S, Kumar P S, Rangasamy G, Nisha Pauline J M, Ramaraju P, Mohanasundaram S and Nguyen Vo D-V 2022 Biosensor for heavy metals detection in wastewater: a review *Food Chem. Toxicol.* **168** 113307

[71] Priya A K, Muruganandam M, Ali S S and Kornaros M 2023 Clean-up of heavy metals from contaminated soil by phytoremediation: a multidisciplinary and eco-friendly approach *Toxics* **11** 422

[72] Nasiri-Majd M, Taher M A and Fazelirad H 2015 Synthesis and application of nano-sized ionic imprinted polymer for the selective voltammetric determination of thallium *Talanta* **144** 204–9

[73] Zhiani R, Ghanei-Motlag M and Razavipanah I 2016 Selective voltammetric sensor for nanomolar detection of silver ions using carbon paste electrode modified with novel nanosized Ag(I)-imprinted polymer *J. Mol. Liq.* **219** 554–60

[74] Tarley C R T, Basaglia A M, Segatelli M G, Prete M C, Suquila F A C and de Oliveira L L G 2017 Preparation and application of nanocomposite based on imprinted poly(methacrylic acid)-PAN/MWCNT as a new electrochemical selective sensing platform of Pb^{2+} in water samples *J. Electroanal. Chem.* **801** 114–21

[75] Rajabi H R, Roushani M and Shamsipur M 2013 Development of a highly selective voltammetric sensor for nanomolar detection of mercury ions using glassy carbon electrode modified with a novel ion imprinted polymeric nanobeads and multi-wall carbon nanotubes *J. Electroanal. Chem.* **693** 16–22

[76] Alizadeh T, Ganjali M R, Akhoundian M and Norouzi P 2016 Voltammetric determination of ultratrace levels of cerium(III) using a carbon paste electrode modified with nano-sized cerium-imprinted polymer and multiwalled carbon nanotubes *Microchim. Acta* **183** 1123–30

[77] Alizadeh T, Mirzaee S and Rafiei F 2017 All-solid-state Cr(III)-selective potentiometric sensor based on Cr(III)-imprinted polymer nanomaterial/MWCNTs/carbon nanocomposite electrode *Int. J. Environ. Anal. Chem.* **97** 1283–97

[78] Wu S, Dai X, Cheng T and Li S 2018 Highly sensitive and selective ion-imprinted polymers based on one-step electrodeposition of chitosan-graphene nanocomposites for the determination of Cr(VI) *Carbohydrate Polym.* **195** 199–206

[79] Ganjali M R, Rahmani A R, Shokoohi R, Farmany A and Khazaei M 2019 A highly sensitive and selective electrochemical mercury(II) sensor based on nanoparticles of Hg(II)-imprinted polymer and graphitic carbon nitride (g-C_3N_4) *Int. J. Electrochem. Sci.* **14** 6420–30

[80] Roushani M, Saedi Z, Hamdi F and Dizajdizi B Z 2017 Preparation an electrochemical sensor for detection of manganese (II) ions using glassy carbon electrode modified with multi walled carbon nanotube-chitosan-ionic liquid nanocomposite decorated with ion imprinted polymer *J. Electroanal. Chem.* **804** 1–6

[81] Alizadeh T, Hamidi N, Ganjali M R and Rafiei F 2017 An extraordinarily sensitive voltammetric sensor with picomolar detection limit for Pb^{2+} determination based on carbon paste electrode impregnated with nano-sized imprinted polymer and multi-walled carbon nanotubes *J. Environ. Chem. Eng.* **5** 4327–36

[82] Sebastian M and Mathew B 2018 Carbon nanotube-based ion imprinted polymer as electrochemical sensor and sorbent for Zn(II) ion from paint industry wastewater *Int. J. Polym. Anal. Charact.* **23** 18–28

[83] Aravind A and Mathew B 2018 Electrochemical sensor based on nanostructured ion imprinted polymer for the sensing and extraction of Cr(III) ions from industrial wastewater *Polym. Int.* **67** 1595–604

[84] Sebastian M and Mathew B 2018 Ion imprinting approach for the fabrication of an electrochemical sensor and sorbent for lead ions in real samples using modified multiwalled carbon nanotubes *J. Mater. Sci.* **53** 3557–72

[85] Sebastian M and Mathew B 2018 Multiwalled carbon nanotube based ion imprinted polymer as sensor and sorbent for environmental hazardous cobalt ion *J. Macromol. Sci., Part* A **55** 455–65

[86] Aravind A and Mathew B 2018 An electrochemical sensor and sorbent based on mutiwalled carbon nanotube supported ion imprinting technique for Ni(II) ion from electroplating and steel industries *SN Appl. Sci.* **1** 23

[87] Aravind A and Mathew B 2018 Tailoring of nanostructured material as an electrochemical sensor and sorbent for toxic Cd(II) ions from various real samples *J. Anal. Sci. Technol.* **9** 22

[88] Aravind A and Mathew B 2020 Nano layered ion imprinted polymer based electrochemical sensor and sorbent for Mn (II) ions from real samples *J. Macromol. Sci., Part* A **57** 256–65

[89] Bai H, Wang S, Liu P, Xiong C, Zhang K and Cao Q 2016 Electrochemical sensor based on *in situ* polymerized ion-imprinted membranes at graphene modified electrode for palladium determination *J. Electroanal. Chem.* **771** 29–36
[90] Wu S, Li K, Dai X, Zhang Z, Ding F and Li S 2020 An ultrasensitive electrochemical platform based on imprinted chitosan/gold nanoparticles/graphene nanocomposite for sensing cadmium (II) ions *Microchem. J.* **155** 104710
[91] Shirzadmehr A, Rezaei M, Bagheri H and Khoshsafar H 2016 Novel potentiometric sensor for the trace-level determination of Zn2+ based on a new nanographene/ion imprinted polymer composite *Int. J. Environ. Anal. Chem.* **96** 929–44
[92] Abdallah A B, El-kholany M R, Molouk A F S, Ali T A, El-Shafei A A and Khalifa M E 2021 Selective and sensitive electrochemical sensors based on an ion imprinting polymer and graphene oxide for the detection of ultra-trace Cd(II) in biological samples *RSC Adv.* **11** 30771–80
[93] Soman S, Aswathy P V and Ramakrishnan K 2021 Covalently modified graphene quantum dot using a thiourea based imprinted polymer for the selective electrochemical sensing of Hg(II) ions *J. Polym. Res.* **28** 359
[94] Ghanei-Motlagh M, Taher M A, Heydari A, Ghanei-Motlagh R and Gupta V K 2016 A novel voltammetric sensor for sensitive detection of mercury(II) ions using glassy carbon electrode modified with graphene-based ion imprinted polymer *Mater. Sci. Eng.* C **63** 367–75
[95] Hu S, Gao G, Liu Y, Hu J, Song Y and Zou X 2019 An electrochemical sensor based on ion imprinted PPy/rGO composite for Cd(II) determination in water *Int. J. Electrochem. Sci.* **14** 10714–30
[96] Wei P, Zhu Z, Song R, Li Z and Chen C 2019 An ion imprinted sensor based on chitosan graphene oxide composite polymer modified glassy carbon electrode for environmental sensing application *Electrochim. Acta* **317** 93–101
[97] Topcu C, Lacin G, Yilmaz V, Coldur F, Caglar B, Cubuk O and Isildak I 2018 Electrochemical determination of copper(II) in water samples using a novel ion-selective electrode based on a graphite oxide–imprinted polymer composite *Anal. Lett.* **51** 1890–910
[98] Wang J, Hu J, Hu S, Gao G and Song Y 2020 A novel electrochemical sensor based on electropolymerized ion imprinted PoPD/ERGO composite for trace Cd(II) determination in water *Sensors (Basel)* **20** 1004
[99] Shirzadmehr A, Afkhami A and Madrakian T 2015 A new nano-composite potentiometric sensor containing an Hg^{2+}-ion imprinted polymer for the trace determination of mercury ions in different matrices *J. Mol. Liq.* **204** 227–35
[100] Chen J, Chen Y and Liang Y 2021 Application of chitosan-N-doped graphene oxide ion-imprinted sensor in Cd (II) ions detection *Diam. Relat. Mater.* **119** 108591
[101] Yu L, Sun L, Zhang Q, Zhou Y, Zhang J, Yang B, Xu B and Xu Q 2022 Nanomaterials-based ion-imprinted electrochemical sensors for heavy metal ions detection: a review *Biosensors* **12** 1096
[102] Hui Y, Huang Z, Alahi M E E, Nag A, Feng S and Mukhopadhyay S C 2022 Recent advancements in electrochemical biosensors for monitoring the water quality *Biosensors* **12** 551

Chapter 10

Application of carbon nanomaterial-modified FET and impedance-based sensors for agricultural pollutant detection

G Manasa and Chandra Sekhar Rout

Agricultural pollutants can have a considerable influence on both the environment and human health. Therefore, it is crucial to detect these pollutants to ensure that agricultural practices are sustainable and safe. Researchers have been exploring alternative sensing technologies that are rapid, sensitive, and cost-effective to tackle this challenge. One promising approach involves using field-effect transistors (FETs) and sensors based on impedance, both modified with carbon nanomaterials. The sensing of agro-pollutants using a potentiometric ion-selective mechanism is discussed in this chapter. The principles underlying these sensing mechanisms will be explained, along with their advantages. Additionally, various methods to enhance sensor performance through the functionalization of carbon nanomaterials will be discussed in this chapter. Farmers and environmental regulators can quickly and accurately identify and address potential pollution issues by utilizing these innovative sensing technologies, ensuring that agricultural practices are safe and sustainable.

10.1 Introduction

Over the past few years, the agricultural sector has encountered an increasing challenge of soil and water contamination with harmful pollutants such as heavy metals, agrochemical residues, herbicides, and pesticides. These pollutants pose a grave threat to human health and the environment, which calls for the prompt and accurate detection of these substances through efficient sensing technologies. Detecting these pollutants promptly and accurately is critical for ensuring food safety, environmental protection, and human health [1]. Unfortunately, traditional

doi:10.1088/978-0-7503-5879-8ch10

analytical methods often involve time-consuming sample preparation and expensive equipment, making them unsuitable for on-site monitoring in agricultural settings. Therefore, there is an imperative need to develop rapid, sensitive, and economical sensing technologies that can detect agricultural pollutants in real time. However, analyzing agricultural pollutants using traditional methods is time-consuming and requires expensive equipment and sample preparation procedures [2]. Such methods are unsuitable for on-site monitoring of farming settings where rapid detection is necessary. To address this issue, there is a need for alternative sensing technologies that are sensitive, rapid, and cost-effective. The promising approach involves using carbon nanomaterial-modified FETs and electrochemical impedance spectroscopy (EIS)-based sensors.

However, several limitations may arise when using bare or pristine working electrodes in sensing applications. These limitations include low sensitivity, lack of selectivity, poor stability, limited dynamic range, and susceptibility to electrode fouling. These electrodes may not provide enough sensitivity toward the target analyte, and they may interact with interfering species in a nonspecific manner. They are also vulnerable to fouling or degradation over time, compromising sensor performance [3]. Therefore, modifying or functionalizing the electrode surface is typically necessary to enhance sensitivity, improve selectivity by introducing specific binding sites, increase stability, expand the dynamic range, and mitigate electrode fouling. This modification enables more reliable and accurate detection of target analytes in complex sample matrices [4, 5]. Carbon nanomaterial-modified sensors are emerging as a promising solution to surpass the limitations of traditional sensing methods [6]. Carbon nanomaterials, such as graphene, carbon nanotubes, and carbon nanofibers, exhibit exceptional properties such as high surface area, excellent electrical conductivity, and chemical stability, which make them the most suitable candidates for sensor development. By integrating these nanomaterials into sensing platforms, we can achieve enhanced sensitivity, selectivity, and response time for detecting target analytes. The remarkable properties of these carbon nanomaterials have opened up new horizons in sensor technology, offering significant advantages over traditional sensing methods [7–9].

FET and impedance-based sensors are promising candidates for next-generation biosensors. Researchers are exploring the benefits of these sensors, which offer label-free detection, easy operation, cost-effectiveness, and the ability to directly detect target analytes in liquid environments. With the rapid advances in nanotechnology and biotechnology, efforts are being made to reinforce the sensitivity of these sensors and expand their potential applications. The objective of this chapter is to provide a review of the latest developments in using carbon nanomaterial-modified sensors (FET and EIS) to detect agricultural pollutants. This will involve examining FET-based and impedance-based sensing mechanisms, and their sensitivity, selectivity, and miniaturization benefits. Additionally, this chapter will cover various approaches to functionalizing carbon nanomaterials to enhance their performance in detecting pollutants. Focusing on the technical details described below is essential to help researchers understand and utilize FET/EIS biosensors more effectively.

10.2 Fundamentals of FET-based sensors and their application for agro-pollutant analysis

The FET is a device that controls the conductivity of charge carriers (electrons or holes) in the channel material using an electric field. The FET sensor is composed of three different parts: the source, drain, and gate. In a regular FET, the source and drain are two p-n junctions that supply and receive electrons or holes. The gate electrode is created on a thin insulating layer that is applied to the semiconductor between the source and drain [10, 11]. The voltage applied to the gate controls the conductivity between the source and drain terminals (figure 10.1(a)). Thus, the device becomes active only when the gate voltage reaches a certain threshold, known as the 'threshold voltage' (V_{th}), after which carriers start flowing alongside the channel between the drain and the source. The device can either be in an 'on' or 'off' state, and this is determined by the relative magnitude of the gate bias voltage (V_g) applied to the FET and V_{th}. Four basic structures of FET are determined by the electrode's relative position and the semiconductor layer. These structures are shown in figure 10.1(b). The FET can have two geometries: bottom-gate and top-gate.

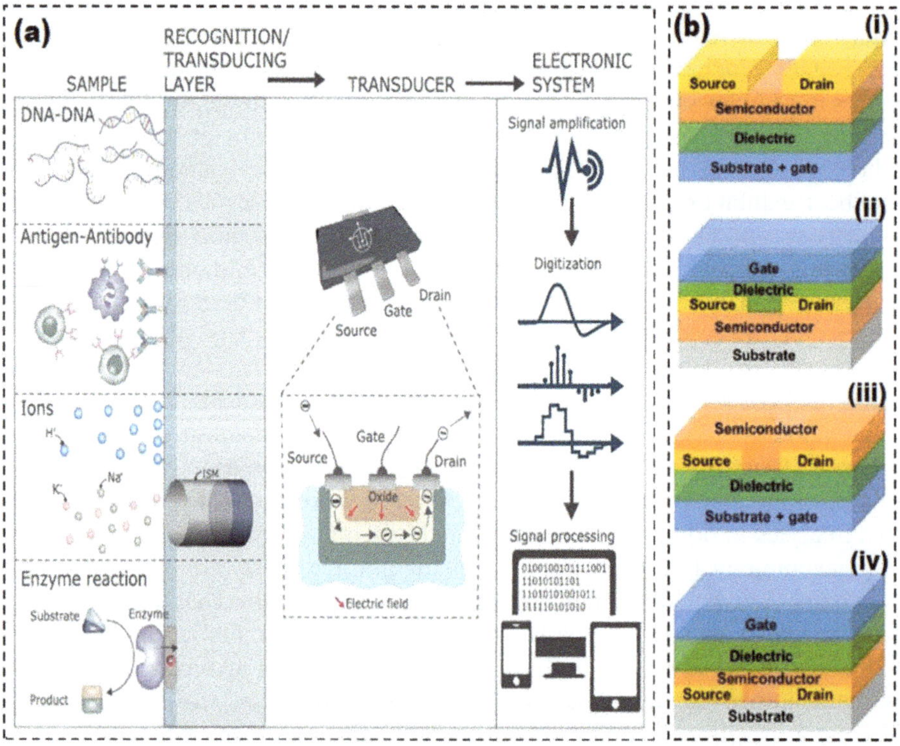

Figure 10.1. (a) Illustration of chemical and biological FET sensor construction. Reprinted from [10], Copyright (2017), with permission from Elsevier. (b) Scheme of FET configurations: (i) bottom-gate top contact, (ii) bottom-gate bottom contact, (iii) top-gate top contact, and (iv) top-gate bottom contact. Reproduced from [12]. CC BY 4.0.

These geometries depend on the position of the source-drain and gate electrodes. The top-gate geometry is also known as top contact, while the bottom-gate geometry is either back channel-etch or coplanar. Another variation of the bottom-gate geometry is known as an etch stopper [12]. In recent years, advances have been made in FET configurations. An example is thin-film transistors (TFTs), which use non-silicon semiconductors as substrates. There are several types of TFT configurations, including ion-sensitive field-effect transistor (ISFET), top-gate TFT, electrolyte-gate FET (EG-FET), electrochemical transistor (ECT), and chemically sensitive FETs (ChemFETs) [13].

Over the last decade, numerous sensing mechanisms have been proposed for FET biosensing. Despite this, many proposed mechanisms only account for some experimental findings, leaving a universal mechanism elusive. Existing sensing mechanisms include: (i) the electrostatic gating effect can be used for sensing, (ii) another sensing mechanism involves the charge transfer effect, (iii) the Donnan potential effect is also used for sensing, and (iv) the charge scattering effect is also currently in use. Meanwhile, FET biosensing has seen numerous response signals proposed to aid researchers' comprehension of the relationship and the existing response signals for the sensing mechanisms, including [14]: (i) Driac response, (ii) threshold voltage response, (iii) current response, and (iv) capacitance response. There are two primary mechanisms of FET sensing, which are the gating effect and electron transfer between the semiconductor channel material and analyte. When the platform is exposed to charged ions, they contribute to electron transfer with the channel material, which changes the concentration of carriers (holes or electrons) in the channel film. Consequently, there is a corresponding change in the current between the source and drain electrodes. Additionally, the charged ions on the sensor surface generate an electric field that attracts or repels carriers in the channel material. This phenomenon also leads to a change in the current between the source and drain electrodes.

The conductivity of the channel in a FET is determined by the voltage applied to the gate and source terminals. With its specialized semiconductor layer, FET technology is well-suited for electronic sensing and chemical and electronic process monitoring. These sensors rely on nanomaterials such as nanowires, nanotubes, and nanoparticles, offering performance comparable to or better than traditional methods like ELISA [15]. FET sensors can detect heavy metal ions (HMIs) using the interaction between the analyte and the semiconductor, with semiconducting nanomaterials such as single-walled carbon nanotubes (SWCNTs) and graphene being particularly attractive due to their high surface-to-volume ratios and charge mobility [11]. However, these nanomaterials' surface modification/functionalization is often necessary for the specific detection of chemicals, and thus devoid of degrading properties and device instability. In recent years, there has been a lot of research interest in developing FET biosensors using different types of nanomaterials, such as silicon nanowires (SiNWs), carbon nanotubes (CNTs), graphene, metal oxide, and transition metal dichalcogenide-based (TMDs). From 2010 to July 2019, a search for literature on ISI Web of Science revealed that carbon (graphene) was utilized as the primary material (52%), followed by other nanomaterials [16].

Carbon nanomaterials have unique physical and chemical properties that suit biosensing applications. Among different types of CNTs, graphene has particularly attractive features, such as atomic thickness, excellent electrical properties and stability, and good biocompatibility. These properties endow carbon-based FETs with inherent advantages in biosensing applications. Let us take a look at the latest developments in carbon-based FET sensors that are used to detect agro-pollutants.

Zhu *et al* [17] developed a flexible enzymatic acetylcholinesterase graphene-based FET biosensor for detecting organophosphorus compounds. This sensor fixes the enzyme to the gold electrode with a molecule called 3-mercapto propionic acid (MPA). The fabrication and functionalization are presented in figure 10.2(a) (i) and (ii), respectively. The sensor has excellent detection indexes for isocarbophos, a common organophosphorus pesticide. The pesticide residue attached to the sensor caused an increase in holes with a positive charge, which increased the FET's bias current. The enzymatic biosensor demonstrated a significant detection limit index for isocarbophos (100.0 μg mL^{-1}) in water samples. Jimenez *et al* [18] developed a sensing platform to selectively detect HMI lead(II). The sensor employs self-assembled polyethyleneimine-functionalized carbon nanotubes (PEI-CNTs) and graphene oxide (GO) films that are deposited onto gold-interdigitated electrodes (figure 10.2(b)). The nanostructure made of graphene has a resistive characteristic.

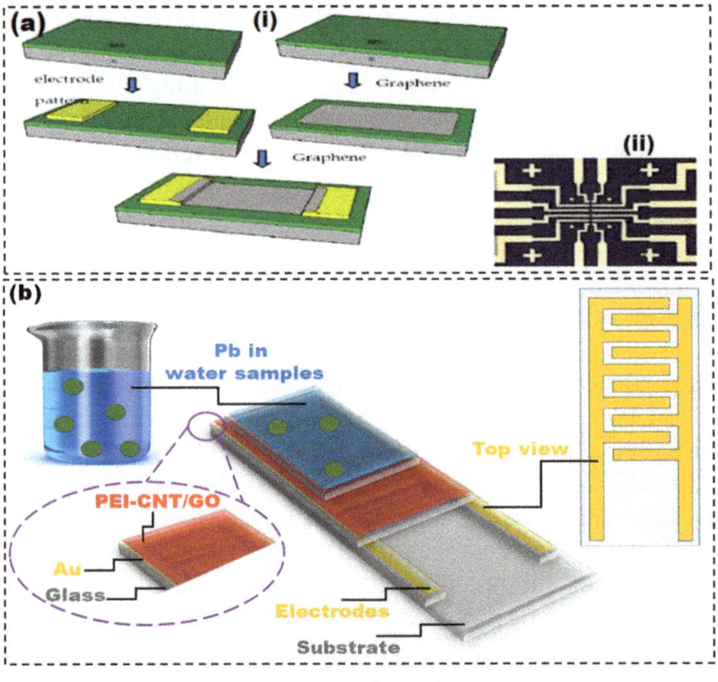

Figure 10.2. (a) Schematic illustration of biosensor fabrication. (i) Photolithography process of sensor fabrication, (ii) patterns of gold electrodes: source and drain electrode pairs. Reproduced from [17]. CC BY 4.0. (b) Lead is detected by constructing a sensor that utilizes self-assembled PEI-CNTs and GO films deposited onto gold-interdigitated electrodes.

The scientists tested a film made layer by layer to detect Pb(II) acetate in a solution by comparing three electrochemical techniques: amperometry, impedance spectroscopy, and potentiometry stripping analysis. The calculated detection limit stood at 36.0 pmol L^{-1}, while the sensitivity was as high as 4.3 μAL μmol^{-1}. The strong affinity of HMIs with the functional groups present in the PEI-CNTs and GO was the reason for the detection mechanism. These results show promise for developing integrated monitoring and sensing platforms for detecting Pb(II) contamination in drinking water. Furthermore, Deng *et al* [13] and Falina *et al* [19] recently published a detailed review of carbon-based FET sensors for detecting various HMIs. Yao *et al* [20] describe CNT-FETs for gas sensing, particularly the agro-pollutant gas ammonia. Graphene possesses a vast delocalized π-electron system and has a theoretically specific surface area that makes it a perfect material for the adsorption of organic compounds. The review by Zafar *et al* [21] highlights successful pesticide detection using graphene-based sensors applied for the detection of pesticides: carbofuran, isocarbophos, dimethoate, chlorpyrifos, paraquat, methamidophos, methyl parathion, and diuron. These sensors, designed with three electrodes and FET principles, offered notable sensitivity and selectivity. The sensors that were fabricated have consistently exhibited sensitivity that is considered acceptable. Additionally, the detection ranges of these sensors have been wide and linear. However, the setbacks are cost constraints and portability.

Estimating soil nutrient availability and pH is vital for improving soil fertility, crop growth, and yield. ISFET sensors are a promising technology that can accomplish this. Electrochemical-based sensors can estimate the pH and available nutrients present in soils. ISFETs are electronic devices that measure ions in an electrolyte solution. These sensors need a recognition element, such as an ion-sensitive membrane integrated with a reference electrode. This integration converts a chemical response, such as ion concentration, into a potential electrical signal. The fundamentals of the device are: (i) the ISFET device can adjust the threshold voltage by controlling the potential at the interface of the oxide and solution; and (ii) it includes a gate connection that is separate from the chip and a reference electrode (usually Ag/AgCl) immersed in an aqueous solution, which is in contact with the gate membrane (figure 10.3(a)) [22]. Thus, Vyacheslav *et al* [23] demonstrated that a multienzyme membrane ISFET-based biosensor could monitor various environmentally hazardous pollutants due to its versatile enzyme activities. A recent review by Archbold *et al* [22] gave an up-to-date evaluation of ISFET sensors and their application in soil nutrients and pH analysis. This review highlighted the technical potential and limitations of implementation, including essential concepts such as basic operation principles, algorithms, sensor representations, behavioral models, and simulation examples. The review's authors analyzed the performance characteristics of ISFET sensors in precision agriculture, including relevant electronic instrumentation, nonidealities, variables, application examples, and implementation perspectives. They aimed to raise awareness of ISFET sensors in the agriculture community and offer a resource for those considering adopting ISFET sensors in precision agriculture. Overall, it provides valuable insights into the potential of

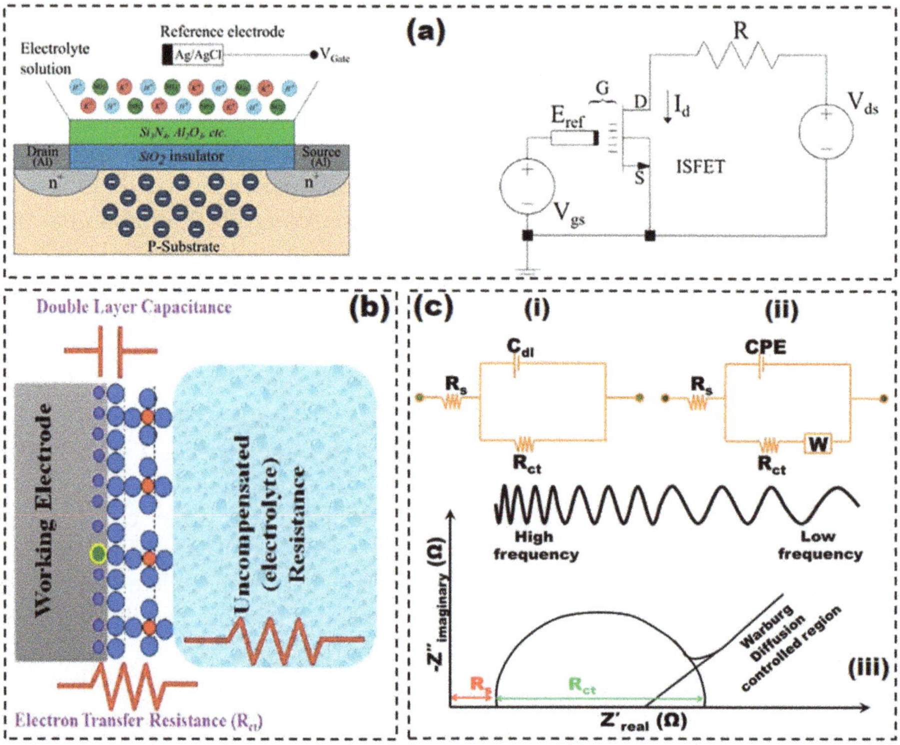

Figure 10.3. (a) ISFET device: D = drain, S = source, G = gate, V_{ds} = drain-source voltage, E_{ref} = reference electrode, I_d = current drain, and V_{gs} = gate voltage. Reprinted from [22], Copyright (2023), with permission from Elsevier. (b) A simplified EIS cell (three-electrode system) and the redox reaction occur at the interface of the working electrode and the electrolyte solution: (c) Randle's circuit: (i) simplified circuit, and (ii) circuit with constant phase element and Warburg impedance. Reproduced from [24]. CC BY 4.0.

ISFET sensors for soil nutrient and pH analysis, which can help improve crop yield and sustainability in agriculture.

10.3 Principle of impedance-based sensors and their application for agro-pollutant analysis

EIS is a powerful technique for investigating the properties of surfaces modified for biorecognition events. One of the benefits of EIS is that it employs small amplitude perturbations from a steady state, making it a nondestructive method (figure 10.3(b)) [24]. Interactions between matter, redox species, and electrodes occur in an electrochemical cell and involve different factors such as electron transfer, the concentration of electroactive species, mass transfer from the bulk solution to the electrode surface, and electrolyte resistance [25]. An electrical circuit can represent these features, consisting of resistances (electrolyte resistance (R_s), charge transfer resistance (R_{ct})), and capacitors (C_{dl}), (and constant phase elements and or Warburg impedance (W)) in series or parallel connections to create an equivalent circuit, as illustrated in figure 10.3(c) (i) and (ii). EIS can investigate mass, charge transfer, and diffusion processes and evaluate intrinsic material properties or specific processes that may affect an electrochemical system's resistance, conductance, or capacitance. It is essential to recognize that impedance and resistance are different because resistance in DC circuits follows Ohm's Law without exception. A small signal excitation is used to measure the impedance response. The electrochemical cell response is approximately pseudo-linear but with a phase shift. On the other hand, the current response to a sinusoidal potential is sinusoidal at the frequency of the applied potential [26].

Information about electron-transfer kinetics and diffusional characteristics can be derived from the impedance spectrum of an electrochemical system. The impedance versus frequency graph, known as the Nyquist plot, usually exhibits a semicircular segment at higher frequencies and a linear segment at lower frequencies. The semicircle section corresponds to the electron-transfer-limited process, while the linear segment represents the diffusion-limited process, as seen in figure 10.3(c) (iii). In swift electron-transfer processes, the impedance spectrum shows only the linear portion, while in prolonged electron-transfer processes, a large semicircular region is present. The electron-transfer resistance is equal to the diameter of the semicircle. The impedance spectrum can also be represented using the Bode plot, which displays the logarithm of impedance's absolute value and phase against the logarithm of frequency. This is an alternative method to showcase the impedance spectrum [24].

It is possible to measure impedance in the presence or absence of a redox couple. This kind of measurement is referred to as faradaic impedance measurement when the redox couple is present, and non-faradaic impedance measurement when it is absent. Faradaic biosensors detect biomolecular interactions by measuring the change in the faradaic current (interfacial electron-transfer resistance) due to steric hindrance caused by the biomolecular interaction or electrostatic repulsion between the free charges of the target molecules and the electroactive species in the supporting electrolyte. The choice of a redox indicator is influenced by different factors, including the charge, hydrophobicity/hydrophilicity, size of the redox pair, and the chemical and physical attributes of the modified electrodes [25].

A key aspect of formulated fertilization is determining soil nutrient levels, followed by specific site fertilization recommendations. This reduces the excessive application of nutrients and promotes sustainable farming. Eldeeb and researchers [27] have constructed an ion-selective electrode (ISE) electrochemical soil nutrient-nitrate sensor that uses EIS to measure soil nitrate in real time without soil pretreatment. The working electrode was modified by drop casting, which was then subjected to testing on three distinct soil textures—clay, loamy clay, and sandy loam (covering the soil texture triangle) (figures 10.4(a)–(c)). They used the non-linear regression models to analyze the nitrate-dependent response of the sensor, resulting in an R^2 value greater than 0.97 for the nitrate range of 5.0–512.0 ppm. The sensor's accuracy was verified, and an error rate of less than 20% was found when measuring nitrate levels in various soil textures. During a week-long study in the soil, the sensor performed well and measured nitrate levels dynamically over time with an error rate of less than 20%. In another study, Akhter *et al* [28] proposed an interdigital phosphate sensor using MWCNTs and PDMS for the electrodes and

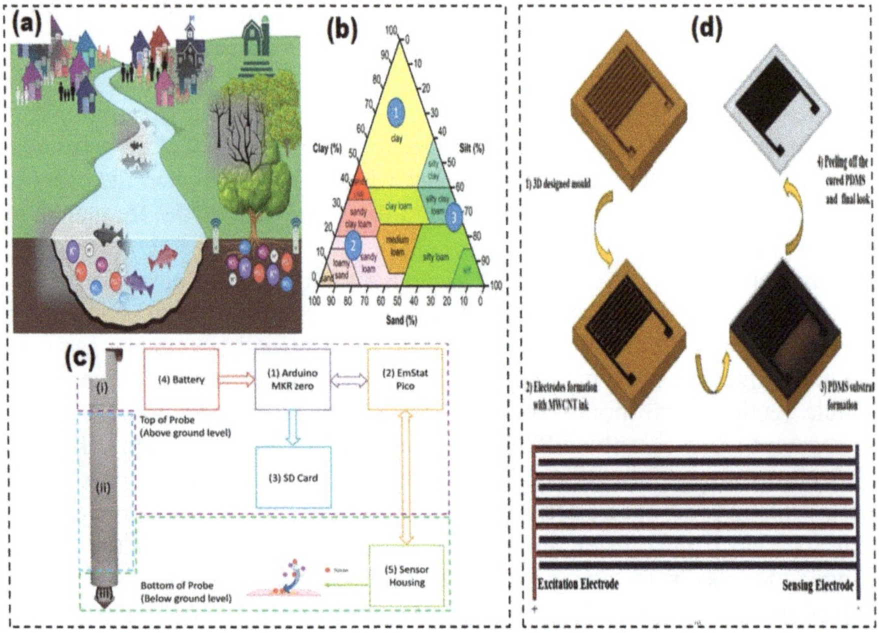

Figure 10.4. (a) Illustration of nitrate sensing, which shows how the absence of real-time monitoring of soil nitrate can have a negative impact on humanity. (b) A detailed classification of various soil types through the soil texture triangle. (c) This study is illustrated through a block diagram showcasing the hardware and probe employed. Reproduced from [27]. CC BY 4.0. (d) Sensor fabrication for phosphate sensing using PDMS and MWCNTs for the substrate and electrodes, respectively, and a 3D-printed mold. Reprinted from [28], Copyright (2021), with permission from Elsevier.

substrate, respectively, and a 3D-printed mold was used for sensor fabrication (figure 10.4(d)). This sensor was characterized using EIS for various temperatures and phosphate detection. The results show that the sensor can differentiate between 0.01 ppm and 40.0 ppm of phosphate concentration levels. Furthermore, an Internet of Things (IoT)-enabled portable innovative phosphate detection system was also developed using an Arduino-based system. This system enables continuous water quality monitoring and allows experts to provide their opinions remotely. Overall, the portable phosphate detection system has the potential to impact smart agriculture significantly. Furthermore, agro-pollutants also include various pesticides. This issue is addressed by Dhamu *et al* [29], who present detailed case studies that are explored to understand better current electrochemical biosensors for pesticide screening and environmental monitoring.

Bacterial infections significantly contribute to various diseases globally, resulting in extensive economic damage, particularly in the agriculture and food sectors. Detecting pathogens is critical in safeguarding the agricultural industry from potential outbreaks that could have devastating consequences. Patel and researchers [30] have constructed a sensor for detecting pathogenic cells in real potato samples. A rapid and straightforward method to identify the existence of gram-negative *Escherichia coli* bacteria has been developed using a gold-interdigitated microelectrode-based impedance biosensor. The metabolic activity of the organisms was monitored by measuring the change in impedance as they were incubated in a growth medium. After analyzing real potato samples using a standardized measurement protocol, this preliminary study presents potential benefits for detecting food pathogens. Furthermore, Rose *et al* [31] show the utilization of amine-functionalized graphene oxide (fGO) nanomaterial to attach *E. coli* to its surface. The nanosensors based on GO were utilized to measure the changes in impedance resulting from varying concentrations of *E. coli.* The resultant potential difference was recorded. The nanosensor's impedance changes were found to be inversely proportional to bacterial concentrations and were fed to the Arduino microcontroller. The detection of *E. coli* in aquatic environments was confirmed through real-time analysis. The efficiency of the developed nanosensor was validated in complex water matrices by conducting experiments.

10.4 Other sensors for agricultural pollutant determination

ISE and potentiometric detection are two techniques that involve measuring potential differences. However, ISEs are sensors designed to detect specific ions selectively. At the same time, potentiometric detection has a broader range of applications beyond ion measurement, such as redox reactions and pH measurement [32]. The key differences between the two can be found elsewhere [33–35]. Potentiometry is a static (zero-current) technique in which the potential generated across an electrochemical cell measures the target species value. To measure the concentration of a substance in a sample, one can determine the voltage difference between an indicator electrode and a reference electrode. This measurement uses two electrodes: the indicator and the reference electrodes. The voltage difference between these electrodes is used to determine the concentration of the substance in the sample. The reference electrode maintains a constant voltage, usually silver–silver chloride or calomel. The indicator electrode can be a traditional metallic or ISE with a liquid or solid inner solution. Potentiometric cells can also use ISFETs as indicators. The equation gives the ISE response [36]:

$$E = E^{\circ} + \frac{RT}{nF} \ln \frac{a_{\text{ox}}}{a_{\text{red}}}$$

where E = measured potential, E° = characteristic constant for ISE (the summation of the potential differences at all interfaces, excluding the interface between the membrane and the analyte solution, is what makes the analyte unique), R = gas constant, T = absolute temperature, n = number of electrons involved in the reaction (ionic charge of the analyte), F = Faraday constant, and α = activity of the analyte. This Nernst equation for ISEs is a well-known formula that characterizes their distinct response properties, i.e., Nernstian response, where the sensor signal is proportional to the logarithm of the analyte activity rather than the activity itself. At the same time, the slope of an E versus ln α plot is utilized to determine the target analyte based on charge. Due to the logarithmic relationship between the potential and the analyte activity, a broad spectrum of analyte activity can be measured.

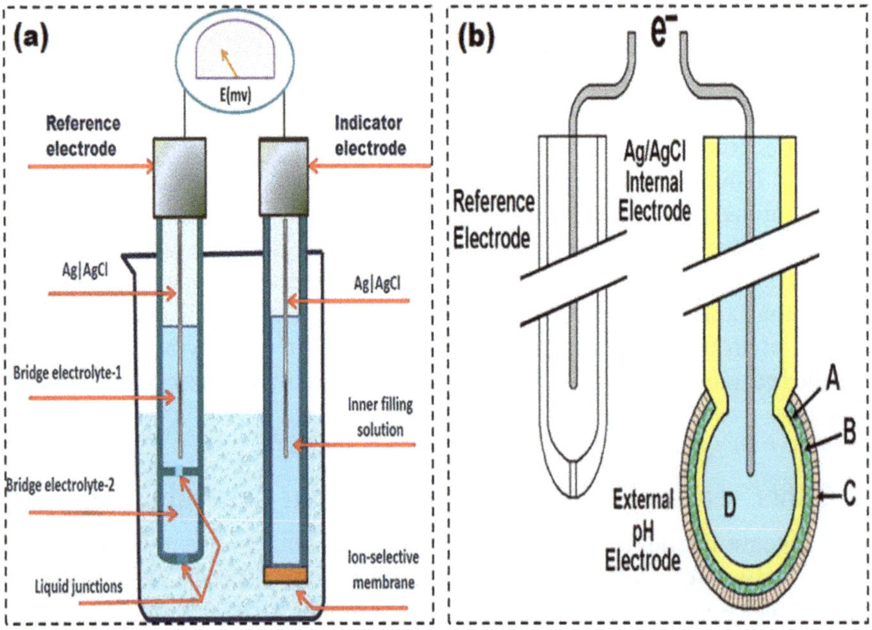

Figure 10.5. (a) In a potentiometric cell assembly, an ion-selective membrane electrode is used as an indicator electrode. In contrast, a reference electrode with a double junction is utilized. Reprinted from [38], Copyright (2018), with permission from Elsevier. (b) A typical potentiometric biosensor. An active glass membrane (A) is enclosed by a biocatalyst (B), held in position by a semi-permeable membrane (C). A difference in electric potential occurs between the internal electrode, which is immersed in dilute HCl (D), and the exterior pH electrode. Reproduced from [42]. CC BY-ND 4.0.

In order to identify low analyte activity, the potential difference must be measured rather than relying on detecting a very small signal. For instance, a glass membrane pH electrode is an example of this [37]. Thus, potentiometric selectivity is magnified by incorporating the ISEs with a polymeric membrane (figure 10.5(a)) [38].

Another type of indicator electrode is the ISE, in which the response of the ions in the sample is a complex phenomenon that depends on the properties of the membrane, including its composition, thermodynamics, and kinetics. The selectivity of the electrode to a target analyte (*I*) can be affected by the presence of interfering chemical species (*J*) in a complex matrix. The Nikolsky–Eisenman equation typically provides an estimate of the potential of an ISE [39]:

$$E = E^{\circ} + \frac{2.303RT}{z_I F}\log\left(a_I + \sum_{n=1}^{x} K_{I,J}^{\mathrm{pot}}(a_J)^{z_I/z_J}\right)$$

where a_I and a_J = primary and interfering ion activity, z_I and z_J = charges of the ions (responses coming from either a cation or an anion are subjected to plus or minus signs for their representation), and $K_{I,J}^{\mathrm{pot}}$ = potentiometric selectivity coefficient (a numerical measurement of the membrane electrode's capability to discriminate the primary ion '*I*' in the presence of an interfering ion '*J*').

There are four types of ISE based on the membrane material that they use:

(a) The pH glass electrode is widely used, and is one of the most commonly used glass membrane electrodes. Its fragile glass membrane, shaped like a bulb, detects hydrogen ions in a solution.

(b) Solid-state membrane electrodes are composed of crystalline substances or insoluble precipitates. An instance of a solid-state membrane sensor recently emerged for the detection of Zn(II) using ZnS nanoparticles [40].

(c) Sensors called liquid membrane electrodes use an organic ion exchanger dissolved in a suitable solvent and enclosed in an inert polymer matrix. For example, tantalum was determined with a hexafluorotantalate(V) extract in nitrobenzene, which was utilized as electroactive material in fabricating a hexafluorotantalate(V)-selective membrane. A PVC support was used to fabricate this liquid membrane electrode [41].

(d) Gas-sensing electrodes and biosensors are referred to as compound electrodes. In this category, a membrane that is highly hydrophobic facilitates gas diffusion, resulting in a pH change in the solution layer, which is detected by a glass electrode. In the second type of compound electrode, target analytes are detected by enzymes or other bio-catalytic species [38].

Furthermore, an electrical potential is generated as an analytical signal by potentiometric biosensors, which connect a biological sensing element to a physicochemical transducer. Figure 10.5(b) depicts the typical architecture of a potentiometric biosensor [42]. Several factors characterize these biosensors—the components of a sensor usually include a recognition element, a transducer, a method to immobilize the sensing element, and specific performance parameters such as sensitivity range, selectivity, accuracy, response time, lifetime, and reversibility. The applications of potentiometric biosensors span a wide range of fields, including public health, environmental monitoring, and industrial process control.

10.4.1 Determination of nutrients and fertilizers

10.4.1.1 Potentiometric nitrate sensors

Jiang *et al* [43] have reviewed the electrochemical determination of nitrates in the environment and food matrices up to 2020. However, the latest report was by Baumbauer and team [44], who developed a printed sensor that measures nitrate levels using potentiometry created by an ISE modified with polymeric membranes. Their sensor is capable of detecting nitrate concentrations ranging from 0.62 to 6200.0 ppm in solution, with a sensitivity of −48.0 mV/decade. In peat soil, the sensor has a sensitivity of −47 mV/decade. Passive sensors require very little power to be read. Integrating them into wireless sensor nodes becomes beneficial (figures 10.6(a)–(e)). Nitrate sensors can be used to map the movement of nitrate through a landscape. This information is essential for informing the efficient application of fertilizer and alerting residents to elevated nitrate levels in drinking water. Nitrate sensors can be widely distributed throughout a watershed to gather data on the movement of nitrate.

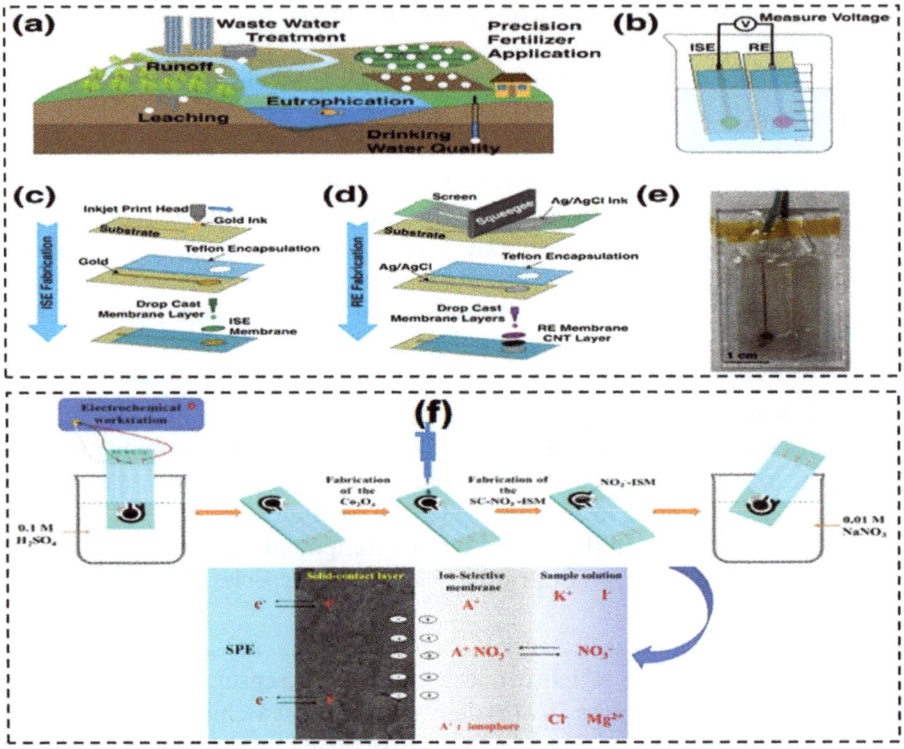

Figure 10.6. (a) Printed sensors are used to map nitrate distribution effectively, which results from applying fertilizers to runoff. (b) The output of the sensor is obtained by reading the potential difference between the printed ion-selective and printed reference electrodes, which is determined by the nitrate concentration in the solution. (c) Gold is printed onto a substrate using inkjet to create ISEs. The trace is encapsulated using Teflon tape. The electrode's area is exposed by drop casting a membrane solution onto it. (d) Ag/AgCl ink is screen-printed onto the substrate to create reference electrodes. The Teflon coating is used to encapsulate the trace. The CNT transducing layer is made by first drop casting it. Next, the PVB/salt membrane is then applied. (e) An acrylic-backed, entirely printed sensor with attached wires is available for soil testing. Reproduced from [44]. CC BY 4.0.(f) Schematic illustration of NO_3^--ISM/Co_3O_4 NPs/SPE sensor fabrication. Reproduced from [45]. CC BY 4.0.

Thuy and researchers [45] developed NO_3^--ISM/Co_3O_4 NPs/SPEs to detect NO_3^- in aquaponic water. Aquaponics is a modern type of circulating technology combining two agricultural engineering methods: aquaculture and hydroponics. In traditional aquaculture systems, the ammonia nitrogen concentration in the water gradually increases due to fish excreta accumulation, which increases the water's toxicity. This ammonia nitrogen in water decomposes into nitrite and then into nitrate. This might be a threat to aquatic life and the biosphere as a whole. The surface of the carbon ink electrode was modified using Co_3O_4 NPs to prevent the formation of an aqueous layer at the interface between the membrane and the inner electrode (figure 10.6(f)). Results indicate orders of magnitude increased the electrode capacitance by introducing Co_3O_4 NPs required for stable output. The sensors also exhibited an excellent sensitivity of −56.78 mV/decade. The results obtained from analyzing actual water samples taken from an aquaponic system indicated that the NO_3^--ISM/Co_3O_4 NPs/SPE are efficient sensors.

Signal-to-noise drift and short lifespans are common problems that ISEs encounter, which can be attributed to water uptake and the formation of aqueous layers. Hjort and team [46] introduced a nitrate ISE with hydrophobic laser-induced graphene (LIG) coated with a PVC-based nitrate selective membrane to overcome these challenges. The polyimide substrate was used to create the LIG through a double-lasing process conducted in ambient conditions. This resulted in a static water contact angle of 135.5° ± 0.7° when subjected to wettability testing. The Nernstian response of LIG-ISE was found to be −58.17 ± 4.21 mV/decade, with a limit of detection (LOD) of 6.01 ± 1.44 μM. The portable potentiostat analyzing water samples from two lakes showed that the sensor produced results comparable ($p > 0.05$) to those obtained through a US EPA-accepted analytical method. These promising results make developing hydrophobic LIG-ISEs attractive for long-term in situ surface water quality applications. Kim *et al* [47] have developed a solid-contact ISE (SC-ISE) for the detection of NO_3^- and Ca^{2+} ions using a rGO aerogel (rGOA) as the solid-contact material. Carbon-based materials are not water-attracting, which makes them a suitable choice for ion-to-electron converters in SC ISEs. Among carbon materials, rGO stands out due to its high chemical stability, mechanical strength, and excellent electrical conductivity. The atomic structure of rGO is a sp^2 nanostructure, which provides a hybrid bond arrangement. Furthermore, rGO has a high electrical double-layer capacitance, which makes it a promising material for improving the performance of SC-ISEs. However, the aggregation of rGO occurs when GO is reduced to rGO, leading to a decreased surface area. To tackle this issue, researchers proposed the use of aerogels, which have a 3D porous structure with a large surface area, to provide a more stable potential signal. The rGOA was synthesized by self-assembling GO via heat treatment (figure 10.7(a)). The durability of the electrode was confirmed by water layer tests and potentiometry experiments, which showed that it remained stable over a long period of time. This improvement in stability was attributed to the hydrophobic properties of rGOA. The sensor comprising rGOA exhibited excellent Nernstian responses with 59.1 mV $\log^{-1}$ [NO_3^-] and 28.4 mV $\log^{-1}$ [Ca^{2+}] and ion detection limits of 759.0 nM for NO_3^- and 186 nM for Ca^{2+}. The exceptional electrical conductivity and vast surface area of rGOA were responsible for this accomplishment. Furthermore, the sensor exhibited long-term potential stability and strong immunity to interference. Thus, the developed sensor, being compact, could detect ions in actual leaf sap, potentially enabling real-time detection. The findings indicate that rGOA may serve as a fresh ion-to-electron transducer for SC-ISEs. Additionally, it is a disposable device that can be used immediately in crop cultivation, particularly in hydroponic systems and environmental monitoring.

10.4.1.2 Potentiometric urea biosensors

Potentiometric urea biosensors are simple devices that are constructed using components like an ISE, a pH-selective electrode, or an ISFET. These devices

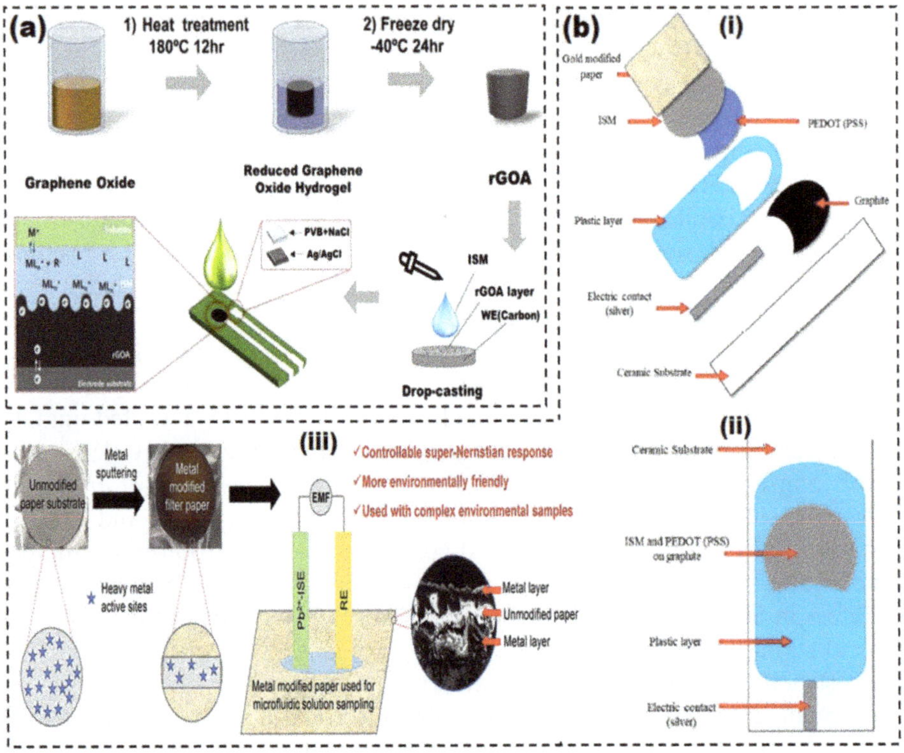

Figure 10.7. (a) Nitrate sensor. The fabrication procedures for rGO-aerogel-based SC-ISE are schematically represented. Reprinted from [47], Copyright (2021), with permission from Elsevier. (b) Lead detection. Construction of SPE Pb^{2+}-ISE: (i) detailed components description, (ii) assembled model screen-printed electrode used as Pb^{2+}-ISE-carbon working electrode, (iii) measurement of Pb^{2+}-ISE through potentiometry was carried out in simulated environmental samples that were prepared beforehand. Reprinted from [61], Copyright (2022), with permission from Elsevier.

utilize enzyme immobilization via matrices (e.g., PVC and carboxylated PVC) or polymers (e.g., polyaniline and polypyrrole) to measure urea concentration in various experimental settings. For a biosensor to be efficient, the immobilized enzyme should have excellent repeatability and stability during storage. These potentiometry-based urea biosensors provide real-time urea quantification in various experimental settings, as reviewed by Ozbek *et al* [48] who discussed the proposed urea potentiometric biosensors from the literature. These biosensors have been classified based on (i) the type of nanoparticles utilized in fabricating the sensor, (ii) urease enzyme immobilized potentiometric biosensors, and (iii) electrodeposited conducting polymer film-based potentiometric biosensors. They discussed the structure and performance parameters of each methodology to facilitate a better understanding of the advances. More recently, Urbanowicz constructed a potentiometric established on a glassy carbon/polyazulene/NH^{4+}-selective membrane and used it for urea detection [49].

10.4.1.3 Potentiometric phosphate detection

A common way of supplying plants with nutrient phosphorus is by adding it externally as fertilizers. However, the unregulated use of such fertilizers has caused an excess buildup of phosphorus in agricultural watersheds, leading to eutrophication and water pollution on a global scale. Since most of these nutrients come from current farming practices, it is highly recommended to apply phosphorus to soil only as needed. This has led to the development of new laboratory and in-field measurements for phosphorus. Another issue is regulating the concentration of phosphate in drinking water. Maintaining acceptable phosphate concentration levels is vital to ensure good water quality and preserve natural water sources. The WHO has set international standards for acceptable phosphate levels. Hence, Zeitoun and their team [50] have reviewed the various phosphate electrochemical sensors and recommended enhancing the functionality of their software in order to ensure better and consistent performance of phosphate sensors that are proven to be reliable and widely accepted. These sensors can be used widely in agricultural and water treatment systems. They have discussed the current and upcoming technologies for phosphate ISE sensing that use cobalt (Co) and their successful implementation in determining soil and wastewater. The measurement principle, detection limit, analysis range, lifetime, and response time are all fundamental principles that are emphasized for each approach. The various methods that have been researched can be categorized into the following groups: (i) Co-metal-phosphate ISE, (ii) Co-alloy-phosphate ISE, (iii) Co-needle-type-phosphate ISE, (iv) Co-nanosensors-phosphate ISE, (v) on-chip, and screen-printed-Co-phosphate ISE. Co phosphate electrode research has predominantly concentrated on Co's stability and detection limit. The operational aspects of dissolved oxygen and solution pH require careful consideration in the context of Co frameworks for phosphate measurement. Since significant fluctuations in dissolved oxygen and pH levels can substantially impact the accuracy of phosphate quantification, it is imperative to integrate dissolved oxygen and pH sensing with cobalt phosphate testing. Such integration could result in a three-in-one sensor that provides the necessary data to refine sensing electrode measurements.

10.4.2 Potentiometric pesticide detection

Kamel *et al* [51] validated the potentiometric transduction constructed to evaluate bispyribac herbicide. The sensors utilized tridodecyl methyl ammonium chloride (TDMAC) as the recognition material, made with a PVC matrix plasticized with TDMAC. The sensing device exhibited a Nernstian anionic slope of −63.6 mV/decade within a linear range of 9.1×10^{-6} to 1.0×10^{-2} M. The detection limit for the sensors was 6.0×10^{-6} M. The test method has been meticulously validated for accuracy, trueness, bias, between-day variability, and within-day variability and has been found to perform well. The sensor has successfully determined bispyribac in complex commercial bispyribac sodium, rice samples, and agricultural wastewater matrices. Mashuni *et al's* [52] research aimed to improve the performance of the catalytic biosensors by optimizing surface conditions using nanocomposite-based Ag-rGO and chitosan to immobilize acetylcholinesterase (AChE) enzyme. The Ag/rGO/CS nanocomposite membrane was used with a potentiometer transducer to detect carbaryl pesticide (1-naphthyl methylcarbamate). The biosensor for AChE showed a high attraction to acetylthiocholine chloride (ATCl). It catalyzed the hydrolysis of ATCl and turned it into an oxidized form, which could be detected. The biosensor was able to detect concentrations of carbaryl pesticide within a linear range under ideal conditions of 1.0×10^{-8} to 1.0×10^{-1} $\mu g\ mL^{-1}$, with a LOD of 1.0×10^{-9} $\mu g\ mL^{-1}$. The fabricated biosensor demonstrated straightforward fabrication processes, good sensitivity, acceptable stability, and reproducibility, which make it a very promising approach for analyzing pesticide residues. Khaled and team [53] developed a potentiometric biosensor that detected the presence of specific anticholinesterase pesticides. By measuring the degree of inhibition of the cholinesterase enzyme, the biosensor could identify three commonly used pesticides, i.e., methomyl, chlorpyrifos, and prothiofos, as well as their degradation products. The sensitivity level to each pesticide varied based on the extent of enzyme inhibition it causes. The results indicated that methomyl has the highest sensitivity, followed by chlorpyrifos and prothiofos. This highlights the significance of monitoring pesticide degradation products. The proposed sensor has the potential to be cost-effective and a straightforward screening tool for monitoring detoxification processes.

10.4.3 Potentiometric heavy metal ion detection

Malon *et al* [54] reported that direct potentiometry could achieve sub-femtomole LODs for Pb^{2+}, Ca^{2+}, and Ag^{2+}. However, applying this method to real samples with unknown composition remains challenging due to the difficulty in predicting the required optimal applied current [55]. Frag and researchers [56] have developed a carbon paste electrode (CPE) that uses 1,8-dihydroxyanthraquinone (DHAQ) as an ionophore in CP matrices to detect Cu^{2+} ions. By incorporating nanomaterials such as graphene nanoplatelets and multi-walled carbon nanotubes, the researchers significantly improved the response properties of the potentiometric sensor. They successfully detected Cu^{2+} in natural water samples with reasonable accuracy. Additionally, they proved CPE-DHAQ to be an effective indicator electrode in potentiometric titration of Cu^{2+} against EDTA. Recently, You *et al* [57] addressed the issue of traditional ISE devices that are limited in detecting HMI (Hg^{2+}, Cd^{2+}, Pb^{2+}, and AsO_2^-), with detection being limited to ppm levels. Nonetheless, a micro-ISE (μISE) array has been developed that enables the multiplex detection of HMIs on a single chip. They report the detection limit for Pb^{2+}, Cd^{2+}, AsO_2^-, and Hg^{2+} using the array to be 1.0, 3.0, 10.0, and 1.0 ppb, respectively, which adheres to the permissible limits for drinking water. The uniformity, sensitivity, and response time of the μ-meter-scale device arrays are enhanced through the microfabrication process, in comparison to traditional ISE devices. Furthermore, they have demonstrated exceptional selectivity and investigated their performance dependence on temperature and pH values.

Sun *et al* [58] proposed ionophores in ionophore-based polymeric membrane HMI ion-selective electrodes (IBPMHM) ISEs to detect HMIs, including Hg^{2+}, Ag^{2+}, Cd^{2+}, Zn^{2+}, Pb^{2+}, Cu^{2+}. They discussed a protocol that utilizes screening parameters to determine the best ionophores for ISEs. The parameters are based on the selectivity coefficients of five major interfering ions, and the molecular categories of preferred ionophores vary based on the metal ion being detected. Their approach follows the complex soft acids and bases rule for efficient screening of ionophores. New ionophores for other types of ionophore-based ISEs and potentiometric sensors for HMIs can be investigated using them. Ozbek and team [59] proposed the development of a novel all-solid-state Cd^{2+}-selective sensor based on a poly(vinyl chloride) (PVC) membrane. The linear concentration range of this innovative sensor is operational at 1.0×10^{-5} to 1.0×10^{-1} mol L^{-1}. The sensing device has specific traits such as a low detection limit (1.77×10^{-1} mol L^{-1}), wide pH working range, short response time, selectivity, and good reusability. Various environmental samples and a waste battery sample were analyzed using the sensor, and it was successfully applied to detect cadmium ions. The recovery rates were reasonable and within acceptable limits. It is understood from these studies that the potentiometric sensor's membrane is a crucial component that can be made of polymeric, polycrystalline, or glass materials [60]. The sensor's selectivity and performance depend on the chosen membrane's properties. However, these membranes are prone to interference ions and potential drift over time, requiring subtle handling and prior measurement calibrations.

Silva *et al* [61] demonstrated metal-modified paper-based substrates for microfluidic paper-based solution sampling along with Pb^{2+}-ISEs to control the super-Nernstian response that typically occurs with unmodified paper substrates. Substrates made of paper that have been coated with 38 nm gold layers on both sides were found to be the optimal choice for regulating the super-Nernstian response of ISEs during nonequilibrium conditions (figure 10.7(b) (i) and (ii)). Furthermore, using paper-based substrates with Pb^{2+}-ISEs in complex environmental samples with high solid-to-liquid content doubled the sensors' lifetime. The inductively coupled plasma optical emission spectrometry confirmed the determination of lead in actual samples by using paper substrates that were modified with metal and coupled with Pb^{2+}-ISEs. (figure 10.7(b) (iii)).

Reviews from several researchers, including Gupta *et al*, Bansod *et al*, Ferrari *et al*, and Lisak *et al*, demonstrate the advances in potentiometric sensors for HMI determinations [62–65]. In some cases, ISEs for analyzing complex environmental samples are impossible due to their selectivity limitations. This requires pretreatment of the sample, such as acidification and selective ion masking/removal. HMIs especially require highly acidic conditions to be ionized. HMIs can form hydroxyl species in an aquatic environment without strongly complexing agents, making it impossible to quantify them using ISEs. Therefore, analyzing heavy metals in $pH < 4$ is essential to ensure that most heavy metals are in their ionized forms. As a result, adjusting the pH in the sample is usually necessary. For online analysis, pH changes would be impractical, and measuring HMIs in environmental conditions typically requires pH measurements to estimate free and bound forms of HMIs.

10.4.4 Conclusion

The development of practical applications using FET transduction still faces some critical challenges. One of the main issues is the unstable electrical performance of the FET over time. Another challenge is the fluctuation of the sensing performance due to slight variations in the surroundings, such as buffer conditions. The achievement of portable and miniaturized systems using FET and EIS transduction is obstructed by these problems. To overcome these challenges, it is critical to lower the manufacturing cost of FET and EIS-based sensors significantly. Further investigation is required to examine the feasibility of ISFET sensors for mobile platform integration and to establish comprehensive macronutrient mapping systems in vast agricultural areas, considering factors such as robustness, repeatability, durability, and accuracy. Establishing IoT-based systems could be highly viable due to the portability and adaptability of FET and EIS-based sensors to custom-made electronic systems. Addressing these technical and research questions is crucial to successfully implement ISFET sensors in agricultural practices.

The ISEs are highly sensitive to ion activity. However, they can only detect ionized species present in a solution. Although ISEs offer rapid response, low energy consumption, and cost-effectiveness, their LODs and multielement determination remain challenging. Unfortunately, when exposed to the environmental sample matrices, none of the potentiometric electrodes were operational outside of laboratory conditions. The design of sensors that can accurately measure low concentrations of analytes in different matrices of environmental samples and conditions presents a significant challenge. Before the measurement protocols and sensor modifications can be addressed to enhance sensitivity at low analyte concentrations, fundamental issues in sensor design must be resolved. The most critical challenge in achieving on-site and online ISEs is the selectivity of the ISM. The ISM must respond to concentration changes over interfering ions, which becomes even more crucial when measuring at trace levels where the concentration of the analyte of interest usually is much lower than that of the background electrolyte in the sample. In addition to selectivity, the electrode's ability to resist parallel processes, such as the presence of gases in solution, water ingress to the ISM, temperature change, light sensitivity, and pH, followed by being resistant to fouling, including mechano-, physical-, chemo-, and bio-fouling, is crucial. Although the stability of the sensor, potential reproducibility, resistance to the formation of the water layer, and any fouling are already extensively explored, the search for new ionophores that could provide better selectivity to the ISM appears to be relatively stagnant. Therefore, the field of potentiometric sensors requires new and more selective ionophores to improve the accuracy and reliability of measurements.

References

[1] Versatile MXenes as electrochemical sensors for heavy metal ions and phenolic moiety-containing industrial chemicals: recent development and prospects *Mater. Adv.*

[2] Shanbhag M M, Manasa G, Mascarenhas R J, Mondal K and Shetti N P 2023 Fundamentals of bio-electrochemical sensing *Chem. Eng. J. Adv.* **16** 100516

[3] Manasa G, Bhakta A K, Bafna J, Mascarenhas R J, Malode S J and Shetti N P 2022 An amperometric sensor composed of carbon hybrid-structure for the degradation of amino-triazole herbicide *Environ. Res.* **212** 113541

[4] Manasa G, Mascarenhas R J, Satpati A K, D'Souza O J and Dhason A 2017 Facile preparation of poly(methylene blue) modified carbon paste electrode for the detection and quantification of catechin *Mater. Sci. Eng.* C **73** 552–61

[5] Manasa G, Mascarenhas R J, Satpati A K, Basavaraja B M and Kumar S 2018 An electrochemical bisphenol F sensor based on ZnO/G nano composite and CTAB surface modified carbon paste electrode architecture *Colloids Surf.* B **170** 144–51

[6] Manasa G 2020 MWCNT/nileblue heterostructured composite electrode for flavanone naringenin quantification in fruit juices *Electroanalysis* **32** 939–48

[7] Manasa G, Mascarenhas R J and Basavaraja B M 2019 Sensitively-selective determination of Propyl Paraben preservative based on synergistic effects of polyaniline-zinc-oxide nano-composite incorporated into graphite paste electrode *Colloids Surf.* B **184** 110529

[8] Manasa G, Bhakta A K, Mekhalif Z and Mascarenhas R J 2019 Voltammetric study and rapid quantification of resorcinol in hair dye and biological samples using ultrasensitive maghemite/MWCNT modified carbon paste electrode *Electroanalysis* **31** 1363–72

[9] Manasa G, Mascarenhas R J, Bhakta A K and Mekhalif Z 2021 Nano-graphene-platelet/brilliant-green composite coated carbon paste electrode interface for electrocatalytic oxidation of Flavanone Hesperidin *Microchem. J.* **160** 105768

[10] Kaisti M 2017 Detection principles of biological and chemical FET sensors *Biosens. Bioelectron.* **98** 437–48

[11] Shkodra B, Petrelli M, Costa Angeli M A, Garoli D, Nakatsuka N, Lugli P and Petti L 2021 Electrolyte-gated carbon nanotube field-effect transistor-based biosensors: principles and applications *Appl. Phys. Rev.* **8** 041325

[12] Hao R, Liu L, Yuan J, Wu L and Lei S 2023 Recent advances in field effect transistor biosensors: designing strategies and applications for sensitive assay *Biosensors* **13** 426

[13] Deng Y, Liu L, Li J and Gao L 2022 Sensors based on the carbon nanotube field-effect transistors for chemical and biological analyses *Biosensors* **12** 776

[14] Chen S, Sun Y, Fan X, Xu Y, Chen S, Zhang X, Man B, Yang C and Du J 2023 Review on two-dimensional material-based field-effect transistor biosensors: accomplishments, mechanisms, and perspectives *J. Nanobiotechnology* **21** 144

[15] Gao X P A, Zheng G and Lieber C M 2009 Subthreshold regime has the optimal sensitivity for nanowire FET biosensors *Nano Lett.* **10** 547–52

[16] Syedmoradi L *et al* 2019 A review on nanomaterial-based field effect transistor technology for biomarker detection *Microchim. Acta.* **186** 739

[17] Zhu J, Feng M and Lian G 2022 Graphene based FET biosensor for organic-phosphorous sample detection and the enzymatic analysis *Crystals* **12** 1327

[18] Martinez Jimenez M J, Avila A, de Barros A, Lopez E O, Alvarez F, Riul A J and Perez-Taborda J A 2021 Polyethyleneimine-functionalized carbon nanotube/graphene oxide composite: a novel sensing platform for Pb(II) acetate in aqueous solution *ACS Omega* **6** 18190–9

[19] Falina S, Syamsul M, Rhaffor N A, Sal Hamid S, Mohamed Zain K A, Abd Manaf A and Kawarada H 2021 Ten years progress of electrical detection of heavy metal ions (HMIs) using various field-effect transistor (FET) nanosensors: a review *Biosensors* **11** 478

[20] Yao X, Zhang Y, Jin W, Hu Y and Cui Y 2021 Carbon nanotube field-effect transistor-based chemical and biological sensors *Sensors* **21** 995

[21] Zafar M A, Waligo D, Varghese O K and Jacob M V 2023 Advances in graphene-based electrochemical biosensors for on-site pesticide detection *Front. Carbon* **2** 1325970

[22] Archbold G, Parra C, Carrillo H and Mouazen A M 2023 Towards the implementation of ISFET sensors for *in situ* and real-time chemical analyses in soils: a practical review *Comput. Electron. Agric.* **209** 107828

[23] Vyacheslav V and Kim N-S 2003 Ion-sensitive field effect transistor-based multienzyme sensor for alternative detection of mercury ions, cyanide, and pesticide *J. Microbiol. Biotechnol.* **13** 373–7

[24] Magar H S, Hassan R Y A and Mulchandani A 2021 Electrochemical impedance spectroscopy (EIS): principles, construction, and biosensing applications *Sensors* **21** 6578

[25] Bahadır E B and Sezgintürk M K 2016 A review on impedimetric biosensors *Artif. Cells Nanomed. Biotechnol.* **44** 248–62

[26] Radhakrishnan R, Suni I I, Bever C S and Hammock B D 2014 Impedance biosensors: applications to sustainability and remaining technical challenges *ACS Sustain. Chem. Eng.* **2** 1649–55

[27] Eldeeb M A, Dhamu V N, Paul A, Muthukumar S and Prasad S 2023 Electrochemical soil nitrate sensor for *in situ* real-time monitoring *Micromachines* **14** 1314

[28] Akhter F, Siddiquei H R, Alahi M E E and Mukhopadhyay S C 2021 Design and development of an IoT-enabled portable phosphate detection system in water for smart agriculture *Sensors Actuators* A **330** 112861

[29] Dhamu V N, Poudyal D, Samson M, Paul A, Muthukumar S and Prasad S 2023 Review—environmental biosensors for Agro-safety based on electrochemical sensing mechanism with an emphasis on pesticide screening *ECS Sens. Plus* **2** 024601

[30] Patel R, Vinchurkar M, Patkar R, Pranjale G and Baghini M S 2021 Impedance based biosensor for agricultural pathogen detection *2021 IEEE 21st Int. Conf. on Nanotechnology (NANO)* pp 385–8

[31] Rose L, Mary X A, Johnson I, Srinivasan G, Priya L and Bhagavathsingh J 2021 Polyaza functionalized graphene oxide nanomaterial based sensor for *Escherichia coli* detection in water matrices *Sci. Rep.* **11** 16872

[32] *Electrochemical Methods: Fundamentals and Applications* 2nd edn (New York: Wiley)

[33] Zdrachek E and Bakker E 2019 Potentiometric sensing *Anal. Chem.* **91** 2–26

[34] Bakker E 1999 Polymer membrane ion-selective electrodes—what are the limits? *Electroanalysis* **11** 915–33

[35] Pretsch E 2007 The new wave of ion-selective electrodes *TrAC, Trends Anal. Chem.* **26** 46–51

[36] Jin W and Maduraiveeran G 2018 Nanomaterial-based environmental sensing platforms using state-of-the-art electroanalytical strategies *J. Anal. Sci. Technol.* **9** 18

[37] Amemiya S 2007 Potentiometric ion-selective electrodes *Handbook of Electrochemistry* ed C G Zoski (Amsterdam: Elsevier) ch 7 pp 261–94

[38] Ma'mun A, Abd El-Rahman M K and Abd El-Kawy M 2018 Real-time potentiometric sensor; an innovative tool for monitoring hydrolysis of chemo/bio-degradable drugs in pharmaceutical sciences *J. Pharm. Biomed. Anal.* **154** 166–73

[39] Gil R, Amorim C G, Araújo A N and Montenegro M C B S M 2019 Process analysis—electroanalytical techniques *Encyclopedia of Analytical Science* 3rd edn ed P Worsfold, C Poole, A Townshend and M Miró (Oxford: Academic) pp 384–8

[40] Elmosallamy M A F, Hashem H A and Abdalmoez F F 2022 New solid-state membrane and coated wire potentiometric sensors for the determination of Zn(II) ions based on nanoparticles *Anal. Bioanal. Chem.* **414** 8277–87
[41] Megersa N, Chandravanshi B S and Moges G 1995 Potentiometric determination of tanatalum with a hexafluorotantalate(V)-selective liquid membrane electrode *Anal. Chim. Acta* **311** 183–92
[42] Hossain M Z, Shrestha D S and Kleve M G 2010 Biosensors for biodiesel quality sensing *J. Arkansas Acad. Sci.* **64** 17
[43] Jiang C, He Y and Liu Y 2020 Recent advances in sensors for electrochemical analysis of nitrate in food and environmental matrices *Analyst* **145** 5400–13
[44] Baumbauer C L, Goodrich P J, Payne M E, Anthony T, Beckstoffer C, Toor A, Silver W and Arias A C 2022 Printed potentiometric nitrate sensors for use in soil *Sensors* **22** 4095
[45] Thuy N T D, Wang X, Zhao G, Liang T and Zou Z 2022 A Co_3O_4 nanoparticle-modified screen-printed electrode sensor for the detection of nitrate ions in aquaponic systems *Sensors* **22** 9730
[46] Hjort R G *et al* 2022 Hydrophobic laser-induced graphene potentiometric ion-selective electrodes for nitrate sensing *Microchim. Acta* **189** 122
[47] Kim M-Y, Lee J-W, Park D J, Lee J-Y, Myung N V, Kwon S H and Lee K H 2021 Highly stable potentiometric sensor with reduced graphene oxide aerogel as a solid contact for detection of nitrate and calcium ions *J. Electroanal. Chem.* **897** 115553
[48] Özbek O, Berkel C, Isildak Ö and Isildak I 2022 Potentiometric urea biosensors *Clin. Chim. Acta* **524** 154–63
[49] Urbanowicz M, Sadowska K, Paziewska-Nowak A, Sołdatowska A and Pijanowska D G 2021 Highly stable potentiometric (bio)sensor for urea and urease activity determination *Membranes* **11** 898
[50] Zeitoun R and Biswas A 2020 Review—potentiometric determination of phosphate using cobalt: a review *J. Electrochem. Soc.* **167** 127507
[51] H. Kamel A, Almehizia A A, Galal H R, Amr A E-G E and Elsayed E A 2020 Rapid and accurate validated potentiometric method for bispyribac herbicide assessment in rice and agricultural wastewater *Water* **12** 2216
[52] Mashuni M, Ritonga H, Jahiding M, Rubak B and Hamid F H 2022 Highly sensitive detection of carbaryl pesticides using potentiometric biosensor with nanocomposite Ag/r-graphene oxide/chitosan immobilized acetylcholinesterase enzyme *Chemosensors* **10** 138
[53] Khaled E, Kamel M S, Hassan H N A, Malhat F M and Abdel-Gawad H 2015 Rapid detection of methomyl and organophosphorous pesticides with portable potentiometric biosensor *Anal. Chem. Lett.* **5** 117–26
[54] Malon A, Vigassy T, Bakker E and Pretsch E 2006 Potentiometry at trace levels in confined samples: ion-selective electrodes with subfemtomole detection limits *J. Am. Chem. Soc.* **128** 8154–5
[55] Höfler L, Bedlechowicz I, Vigassy T, Gyurcsányi R E, Bakker E and Pretsch E 2009 Limitations of current polarization for lowering the detection limit of potentiometric polymeric membrane sensors *Anal. Chem.* **81** 3592
[56] Frag E Y Z, Mohamed M E, Ali A E and Mohamed G G 2020 Potentiometric sensors selective for Cu(II) determination in real water samples and biological fluids based on graphene and multi-walled carbon nanotubes modified graphite electrodes *Indian J. Chem.* **59A** 162–73

[57] You R, Li P, Jing G and Cui T 2019 Ultrasensitive micro ion selective sensor arrays for multiplex heavy metal ions detection *Microsyst. Technol.* **25** 845–9
[58] Sun L, Sun C and Sun X 2016 Screening highly selective ionophores for heavy metal ion-selective electrodes and potentiometric sensors *Electrochim. Acta* **220** 690–8
[59] Özbek O, Isildak Ö, Gürdere M B and Berkel C 2022 Cadmium(II)-selective potentiometric sensor based on synthesised (E)-2-benzylidenehydrazinecarbothioamide for the determination of Cd^{2+} in different environmental samples *Int. J. Environ. Anal. Chem.* **102** 6819–34
[60] Tang X, Wang P-Y and Buchter G 2018 Ion-selective electrodes for detection of lead (II) in drinking water: a mini-review *Environments* **5** 95
[61] Silva R, Ahamed A, Cheong Y H, Zhao K, Ding R and Lisak G 2022 Non-equilibrium potentiometric sensors integrated with metal modified paper-based microfluidic solution sampling substrates for determination of heavy metals in complex environmental samples *Anal. Chim. Acta* **1197** 339495
[62] Gupta V K 2005 Potentiometric sensors for heavy metals—an overview *CHIMIA* **59** 209 209
[63] Bansod B, Kumar T, Thakur R, Rana S and Singh I 2017 A review on various electrochemical techniques for heavy metal ions detection with different sensing platforms *Biosens. Bioelectron.* **94** 443–55
[64] Ferrari A G-M, Carrington P, Rowley-Neale S J and Banks C E 2020 Recent advances in portable heavy metal electrochemical sensing platforms *Environ. Sci.: Water Res. Technol.* **6** 2676–90
[65] Lisak G 2021 Reliable environmental trace heavy metal analysis with potentiometric ion sensors—reality or a distant dream *Environ. Pollut.* **289** 117882

Chapter 11

Conclusion, prospects, and summary

G Manasa and Chandra Sekhar Rout

11.1 Introduction

The necessity for detecting agricultural pollutants, a topic of significant relevance, arises from the profound consequences of agricultural activities on environmental and human health. As agriculture continues to be a fundamental element of global food production, the use of fertilizers, pesticides, and other agrochemicals has significantly increased to meet escalating demands. However, these practices have introduced a wide range of pollutants into the soil, water, and air ecosystems, posing significant risks to biodiversity, water quality, and food safety. Identifying these pollutants, which can be effectively accomplished through advanced sensing technologies such as electrochemical sensors, is thus pivotal in protecting environmental integrity, ensuring sustainable agricultural practices, and mitigating adverse health effects of contaminant exposure. By implementing these sensors, we can effectively monitor pollutant levels, identify sources of contamination, and implement targeted mitigation strategies. Such efforts are indispensable for preserving the long-term viability of agricultural systems, safeguarding natural resources, and promoting a healthier and more resilient future for ecosystems and communities worldwide. Thus, the urgency and significance of this issue cannot be overstated. Technologies for monitoring and detection, including sensor networks, remote sensing, and analytical techniques, play a vital role in evaluating levels of pollutants, identifying the origin of contamination, and guiding efforts for mitigation. In addition, sustainable agricultural practices, such as nutrient management planning, integrated pest management, and precision farming, can help to reduce the amount of pollutants introduced while promoting water conservation, soil health, and biodiversity. Researchers, industry stakeholders, policymakers, and farmers must collaborate to implement effective strategies to mitigate agricultural pollution, protect the environment, and ensure the sustainability of global food systems.

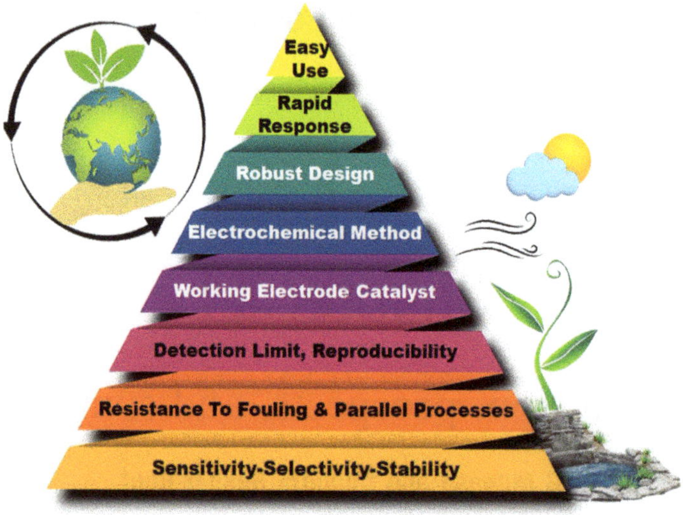

Figure 11.1. Hierarchical significant parameters for consideration during designing and fabricating electrochemical sensors to deploy on-field and online agropollutant detection, quantification, and monitoring.

Electrochemical sensors are sensitive and selective, offering precise analyte detection even at minute concentrations. Their rapid response times and wide dynamic ranges make them ideal for real-time monitoring of dynamic systems. Additionally, their portability and miniaturization make them suitable for field applications. Electrochemical sensors are cost-effective, user-friendly, and environmentally friendly, ensuring widespread accessibility and sustainability. Their stability and compatibility across various sample matrices make them indispensable solutions for multiple industries, from environmental monitoring to healthcare diagnostics. Hence, electrochemical sensors have driven scientific progress, providing efficient and precise analytical solutions (figure 11.1).

11.2 Electrochemical sensors for agricultural pollutants

The electrochemical electrodes, a key focus of this book, are crucial tools in the sensing field. They can be classified into four main measurement categories: current, potential, impedance, and field-effect transistor. Each category plays a significant role in our research, ensuring high precision in the work. For instance, voltammetric and amperometric techniques apply a potential to the working electrode versus a reference electrode and measure the current. Amperometric electrodes portray the current proportional to the concentration of the electroactive species in the sample. With their precise measurements, these sensors can guide farmers in taking necessary actions without wasting time and money, empowering them in their agricultural practices.

Meanwhile, potentiometric sensors rely on measuring the potential of an electrochemical cell while drawing negligible current. They are commonly used in pH electrodes and ion-selective electrodes. Among the various techniques, field-effect transistor (FET)-based electrochemical sensors stand out for their versatility. Leveraging field-effect transistor principles and electrochemical reactions at the sensing interface, they offer a wide range of applications. Analyte interaction alters gate electrode properties, modulating FET conductivity. This change in conductivity indicates analyte presence and concentration. With the addition of selective receptor molecules, these sensors enhance sensitivity and selectivity, making them valuable for diverse detection applications. This versatility empowers researchers to explore various research avenues, making these sensors a promising study area. The potential of carbon nanomaterial-based sensors in this field is particularly exciting, as discussed in this book, because they offer even greater sensitivity and selectivity, and pave the way for more advanced detection methods. ion-selective electrodes (ISEs) and ion-sensitive field-effect transistors (ISFETs) have both demonstrated successful applications. Integrating one or multiple sensors with an ISE/ISFET system makes it feasible to create an automated multianalyte/parameter sensor, including a sensor array on one chip. Such microsensors are designed for automatic control and can be easily operated, even by untrained users. However, the potential blocking of microchannels by small particles must be considered.

In a three-electrode cell, the working electrode is where the electrochemical reaction occurs, such as the oxidation or reduction of analytes. Its surface area, composition, and potential directly impact reaction kinetics and sensitivity. Typically made of platinum, gold, or carbon, its properties can be tailored for specific applications. Researchers can manipulate the reaction rate and direction by controlling the potential applied to the working electrode. Its importance lies in its ability to enable precise measurement and manipulation of electrochemical processes, a crucial aspect of sensor development. Carbon substrates are preferred among the various working electrode substrates because of their cost-effectiveness and good electrochemical traits. Electrochemical sensing electrodes play a crucial role in accurately detecting target species. They require specific sensitive materials to be modified onto their surface, including nanomaterials, ion-selective membranes, and biorecognition elements (enzymes, antibodies, and nucleic acids). A meticulous selection and application of these materials are critical to the success of the research.

Nanomaterials have emerged as excellent catalysts in sensing applications due to their unique properties and tailored functionalities. With an exceptionally high surface area-to-volume ratio, nanomaterials provide numerous active sites for catalytic reactions, leading to improved sensitivity. Their properties, such as size, shape, and surface chemistry, can be precisely engineered to optimize catalytic activity and selectivity for specific analytes, making them highly versatile across various sensing platforms. Additionally, nanomaterials exhibit remarkable catalytic activity at the nanoscale due to quantum size effects and surface characteristics, resulting in rapid response times and lower detection limits. Their compatibility with miniaturization techniques allows for developing portable, integrated sensor devices for real-time monitoring in diverse environments. As a result, nanomaterial-based catalysts represent a cutting-edge approach to sensing technology, providing unparalleled sensitivity, selectivity, and versatility for various applications in research and industry. This book emphasizes carbon nanomaterials, elevating their discussion above that of other nanomaterials. This is not just due to their exceptional properties but also to their potential to revolutionize the field of electrochemical sensing, a fact that we aim to underscore in this book.

Carbon nanomaterials, including carbon nanotubes, graphene, carbon nanofibers, and others, boast unique features such as high aspect ratio and surface-to-volume ratio, providing ample active sites for catalytic reactions, excellent mechanical strength, high electrical conductivity, and chemical stability. These unique characteristics and adaptability make carbon nanomaterials promising candidates for developing sensitive, selective, and reliable sensors across several real-world applications. Carbon-based sensors present advantages and challenges when applied to detect argo-pollutants such as pesticides, fertilizers, and heavy metal ions. These sensors have offered acceptable sensitivity, enabling the detection of low concentrations of pesticide residues in various matrices. Their rapid response allows for real-time monitoring, which is critical for ensuring food safety and environmental protection. However, matrix interference from complex ecological samples poses a significant challenge, affecting sensor accuracy. Furthermore, ensuring the long-term stability and reliability of carbon-based sensors remains a concern, particularly under harsh environmental conditions. Despite these challenges, ongoing research efforts are focused on addressing these limitations to fully harness the potential of carbon-based sensors for agropollutants detection, offering invaluable contributions to agricultural sustainability and public health.

11.3 Prospects

The integration of sensors in agriculture is still developing, with a long path to traverse before it becomes a ubiquitous technology worldwide. However, the indisputable benefits of electrochemical sensor-based agriculture have increased acceptance of this technology. This trend indicates that sensor technology will play a critical role in the future of sustainable agriculture. Market predictions reinforce this view, suggesting that the global agricultural sensor market will experience significant growth. The employment of sensors in agriculture has been identified as a potent tool with the potential to revolutionize the industry. Although these devices can potentially revolutionize the agricultural sector, their reliance on a wireless connection may limit their impact in developing nations. Furthermore, the high cost of acquiring these sensors and the lack of awareness among farmers in these regions about their potential benefits are significant obstacles to their widespread adoption. As the underlying technology behind sensors advances, the scalability and practicability of using these devices will improve, thereby elevating their importance to the farming industry. Here are a few prospects regarding electrochemical sensing technology that we would like to highlight for detecting, qualifying, and continuously monitoring agropollutants in real-world scenarios.

11.3.1 Modification and need for an advanced catalyst

Regrettably, the current configuration of the sensor design, specifically its working electrode and measurement protocol, cannot detect environmental trace concentration analyses with the required sensitivity without modification. In particular,

modifying the sensor design and measurement protocol is necessary to identify and measure concentrations lower than micro-molar. Several critical attributes warrant enhancement to bolster sensor performance in the domain of nanomaterial catalysts for sensing applications. Heightened sensitivity is pivotal, allowing the detection of minute concentrations of target analytes, thereby augmenting the sensor's capability to identify trace levels of agropollutants. Furthermore, elevating selectivity is crucial, ensuring precise detection and differentiation of target analytes within complex sample matrices. Recent developments in this field have focused on improving the performance of electrochemical sensors. For example, researchers have developed novel electrode materials, such as graphene and carbon nanotubes, that can enhance the sensitivity of the sensors. They have also used different types of functional groups to modify the electrode surface, improving the selectivity of the sensors. Strategies involving surface functionalization with specific receptors or recognition elements can enhance selectivity by enabling exclusive binding/interaction with target molecules. Minimizing response time is imperative for facilitating rapid detection and real-time monitoring of analyte concentrations, which can be achieved through optimization of catalytic reaction kinetics or improving mass transport properties at the sensor's interface. Stability enhancements of these nanomaterials are also indispensable to ensure reliable, long-term performance under diverse environmental conditions, necessitating refinement of nanomaterial synthesis, surface functionalization, or encapsulation techniques. Designing sensors with reusable or regenerative catalyst properties reduces operational costs and environmental footprint, advocating for robust nanomaterials or incorporating regeneration methods. By meticulously addressing these facets, nanomaterial-catalyst sensors can be optimized for diverse sensing applications, propelling advances in environmental monitoring.

11.3.2 Multitarget and simultaneous detection

This book highlights the current methods for detecting soil nutrients, which only measure one target ion at a time using conventional electrochemical measurement (with a nanocatalyst or an ion-selective membrane). However, integrating electrochemical sensors onto one chip as a sensor array allows multi-target simultaneous detection. Unfortunately, the nanocatalyst or the membranes developed for target species (including nutrients, pesticides, and heavy metal ions) detection respond to the specific ion of interest and other interfering ions in the sample. The main challenge is ensuring the reliability of the sensor array and minimizing interferences from other ions during simultaneous detection.

Thus, traditional electrochemical sensors are limited in detecting a single analyte, making them less useful for multianalyte analysis applications. Simultaneous detection of multiple analytes promises to expand the capabilities of electrochemical sensors and address complex analytical challenges. First, it enables comprehensive analysis of complex samples containing multiple analytes, providing a more holistic understanding of the sample composition. Second, simultaneous detection enhances analytical throughput and efficiency, reducing analysis time and resource requirements. But perhaps most importantly, it opens up new possibilities for real-time monitoring of dynamic processes and multiplexed analysis, thereby revolutionizing applications in environmental monitoring, food safety, and beyond. Strategies to realize simultaneous detection in electrochemical sensors include: (i) integrating multiple sensing elements, such as electrode arrays or multi-channel systems, to enable parallel measurement of different analytes; and (ii) advances in sensor materials, signal processing algorithms, and miniaturization techniques have improved sensor performance and enabled simultaneous detection with high sensitivity and selectivity.

11.3.3 Miniaturization and automation

One area of focus in electrochemical sensors and analyzers is the miniaturization of these devices to make them more practical for infield applications. Miniaturization and integration of nanomaterial-catalyst sensors into compact, portable devices foster decentralized sensing, bolstered by advances in microfabrication techniques and nanomaterial synthesis. Additionally, there is a push to implement remotely controlled automated systems for continuous contaminant detection and early pollution prevention. These advances have the potential to improve environmental monitoring and protection significantly because they offer the following benefits: (i) reduced sample (target analyte) volume, (ii) faster analysis, (iii) improved precision and accuracy, and (iv) portability and accessibility.

11.3.4 Cost-effectiveness

One potential advantage of using electrochemical sensors is their cost-effectiveness. By utilizing MEMS-based microfabrication technology and laser scribing, these sensors can be produced in batches at a fraction of the cost of other sensors. They can even be designed for one-time or multiple uses. Additionally, the use of small-sized sensors reduces costs by requiring a smaller volume of reagents and samples when testing soil, water, crops, or food.

Traditional approaches often involve using multiple specialized sensors to detect a specific species. However, this approach comes with high equipment procurement, maintenance, and operational logistics costs. We can substantially reduce these financial burdens by consolidating multiple detection capabilities into a single sensor platform. This, in turn, will enable broader access to advanced monitoring technologies and enhance the value of electrochemical sensor research. Additionally, space constraints can make it challenging to deploy sensor networks, especially in resource-limited settings. As researchers, it is crucial to recognize the importance of spatial efficiency in sensor design. Hence, sensors capable of detecting multiple species simultaneously must be engineered. This approach will allow stakeholders to maximize the utility of limited space while maintaining comprehensive monitoring coverage. This will, in turn, make them feel involved and essential in the process.

11.3.5 Disposable platforms

The development of disposable platforms and lab-on-a-chip technologies for detecting agropollutants remains elusive. However, these technologies hold immense promise in operating with minimal sample volumes and being integrated into hand-held devices. When deployed on-site, they can provide real-time analysis for various agropollutants. Incorporating such technologies represents a significant step forward in agropollutant detection, opening up new avenues for research and innovation.

Figure 11.2 illustrates the primary distinctions between conventional electrode platforms and screen-printed electrodes (SPEs). SPEs are characterized by their disposability, reproducibility, and ease of use. They eliminate the need for rigorous polishing and cleaning before each measurement, which is required for solid electrodes such as glassy carbon electrodes, edge plane and basal plane pyrolytic graphite, or highly ordered pyrolytic graphite. Moreover, solid electrodes necessitate external reference and auxiliary electrodes to function correctly. By providing a disposable, cost-effective, reproducible, and easily customizable platform, SPEs or laser scribbled electrodes represent a noteworthy advance in electrode technology.

11.3.6 Regulations and protection agencies

The limited adoption rate of agro-sensor technology by farmers can be attributed to the lack of supportive infrastructure and regulatory frameworks established by

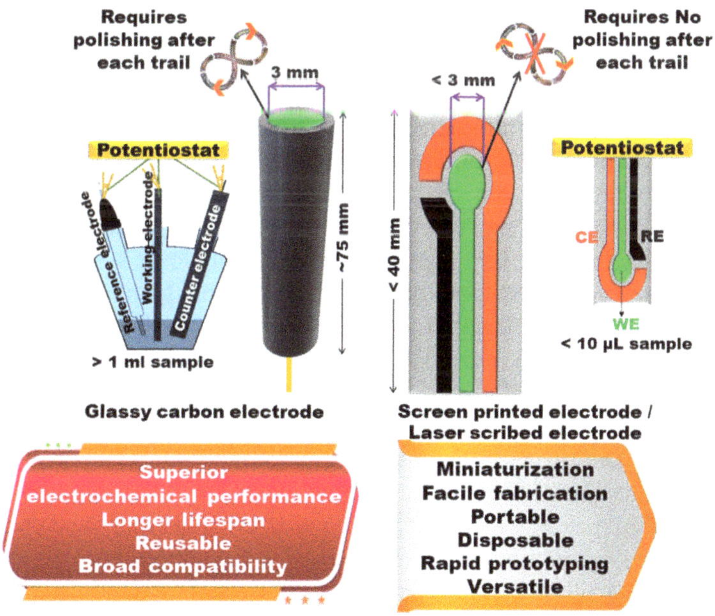

Figure 11.2. Illustration comparing a classical electrochemical cell with laser-scribed or SPE platforms that perform with just a single drop of the target species.

governmental authorities. The inadequate infrastructure, including communication networks and power supply systems, hinders the widespread deployment of agro-sensors, particularly in underdeveloped or developing nations. Moreover, the absence of clear regulations and standards creates uncertainty about data privacy, interoperability, and adherence to agricultural practices, further discouraging farmers from embracing this technology. To overcome these challenges, it is necessary to coordinate efforts to invest in infrastructure development, establish regulatory guidelines, and promote awareness initiatives. Governments can facilitate the integration of agro-sensor technology into agricultural practices, unlocking its potential to enhance productivity, sustainability, and resilience in farming communities by addressing these barriers.

11.3.7 Sustainable agricultural practices to avoid environmental contamination (use of bio-fertilizers and pesticides)

Adopting sustainable agricultural practices has gained significant traction due to their potential to promote environmentally friendly and economically feasible farming systems. One of the critical components of these practices is the utilization of bio-based inputs, including bio-fertilizers and bio-pesticides. These inputs have been demonstrated to enhance soil fertility and reduce dependence on chemical inputs, which are detrimental to the environment. However, the widespread adoption of bio-based inputs faces many challenges, such as variable efficacy and cost constraints. To overcome these obstacles, concerted research, education, and policy formulation efforts must be made to integrate bio-based inputs into conventional agricultural frameworks. By leveraging the inherent ecological benefits of microorganisms and natural compounds, agricultural stakeholders can transition towards greener, economically viable farming systems. This helps safeguard ecosystems and public health and contributes to global food security. Therefore, continuous commitment to research, innovation, and collaborative partnerships is essential to overcoming existing barriers and encouraging the widespread adoption of sustainable agricultural practices globally.

The potential of rapid, efficient electrochemical sensors in agroecosystems is vast and multidimensional. These systems are versatile, robust, and dynamic, and their capabilities should be explored further. They are intelligent diagnostic systems that assess and manage soil, water health, and food quality. They also help to achieve high production without excessive use of fertilizers and pesticides. To make these systems accessible to small-scale farmers, it is essential to foster public–private partnerships. These partnerships can help to develop, promote, and distribute these systems, making them more affordable and more accessible to adopt for small-scale farmers. To achieve sustainable agriculture further, international collaboration in policy-making, strategy, and legislation must improve, and a broad databank (on available contaminants detection) must be created to disseminate knowledge worldwide. We hypothesize that targeted efforts by governments and academia will make nanotechnology a transformational force in agriculture by focusing research and development on sustainable agriculture (figure 11.3).

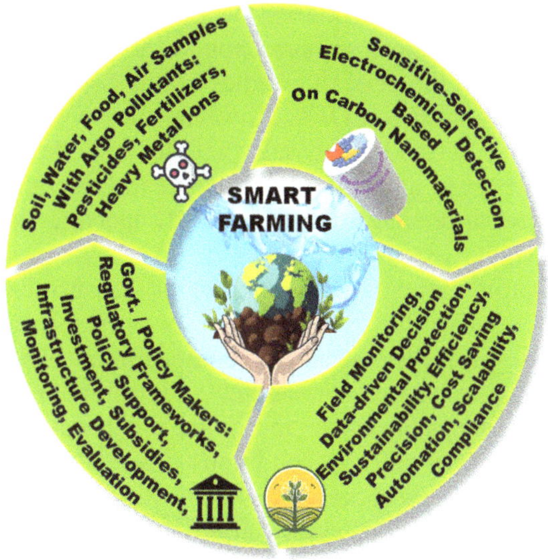

Figure 11.3. Schematic illustrating the steps to incorporate electrochemical sensors in agriculture and promote agricultural reform.

11.4 Summary

Despite the current lack of attention, electrochemical sensors for agropollutant assessment hold significant potential for farming. Their user-friendly and affordable nature can simplify farming management, a feature that farmers increasingly demand. As farmers become more aware of technological advancements, the need for advanced and updated approaches in farming becomes apparent. These sensors, with their ability to guide farmers to take necessary actions without wasting time and money, are a valuable tool in modern agriculture. Efforts are underway to develop miniaturized electrochemical sensing systems for soil quality assessment (nutrients), and to manage pesticide and fertilizer runoff. Thanks to advances in nanotechnology, these systems are becoming more innovative and more efficient, offering practical benefits to farmers and policymakers. This promising future of precision agriculture, driven by electrochemical sensors, should inspire optimism and excitement among our readers.

Our book covers the latest advances and applications of electrochemical sensors for agropollutants and provides insights into the prospects of precision agriculture. We highlight the significance of sensors in real-time monitoring, which is critical for farmers and policymakers, and emphasize the need for multi-sensing systems to detect agropollutants. Notably, we focused on detecting and quantifying pesticides, heavy metal ions, and fertilizers, which are essential for crop growth metrics. We discussed each electrochemical sensor's operating mechanism and performance, and evaluated their applicability in real-world scenarios. This emphasis on practicality and real-world applicability should instill confidence in our readers about the potential of electrochemical sensors in precision agriculture.

This book comprehensively introduces the parameters that one must consider when developing electrochemical sensors capable of meeting the newly imposed limits of detection (LODs). Most of the studies in this book offer sensing platforms that are capable of meeting these LODs. However, they typically require expensive and extensively labored electrode materials that can only be used in a laboratory, need reagents and chemicals, and suffer multi-elemental interferences. A few studies demonstrate a realistic approach to cost-effectively meeting the new international regulations committees.

It is important to note that environmental analysis cannot be approached with a 'one solution fits all' mindset due to factors such as temperature, pH, light, salinity, ionic strength, solid impurities, chemical composition, biological activity, etc. Instead of relying on idealized sensor designs and validation in simplified sample matrices, future development of on-site and online environmental sensors should be tailored to the specific environmental conditions present in that environment. This customization is crucial for successfully implementing electrochemical sensors in precision agriculture, where accurate and reliable data is essential for decision-making. This emphasis on customization that should underline our readers' need to adapt to specific environmental conditions when implementing electrochemical sensors.

Research must focus on developing cost-effective, portable detection technologies that facilitate efficient and rapid infield electrochemical detection devices. Integrating electrochemical techniques, enabled by miniaturized and portable potentiostats, with inexpensive, calibration-free, and customizable SPEs presents a promising solution to support this transition. Further work is required regarding determination methods, composition/ design of working electrodes, etc, to produce in situ sensor devices that are capable of meeting the regulation requirements and quality targets and effectively monitoring various global health parameters that affect us all. In situ monitoring of soil, water, and food quality at the source point of human consumption is vital to comply with the new lower permissible contaminant levels imposed by directives worldwide.

The present book delves into the intricacies of electrochemical sensor-based agropollutant assessment. It underscores the considerable potential of electrochemical sensors in selectively detecting multiple agropollutants, rendering them indispensable components for advancing innovative farming systems. These compact, intelligent sensing systems possess the capacity for soil, water, and food diagnostics, marking a crucial necessity for the next generation of farming practices owing to their affordability, swift detection capabilities, facile data storage and sharing, timely analysis, and decision-making prowess. Nonetheless, substantial scientific, administrative, and policy endeavors are imperative to steer future research endeavors in novel electrochemical sensing systems for the effective and efficient assessment of soil, water, and food quality, which are vital for intelligent farming. Such advances hold promise in curbing farming costs, mitigating excessive utilization of pesticides and fertilizers, managing crop growth, and ensuring high-quality food production for a healthier tomorrow.

www.ingramcontent.com/pod-product-compliance
Ingram Content Group UK Ltd.
Pitfield, Milton Keynes, MK11 3LW, UK
UKHW051859100926
8556IPUK00005B/693

9 780750 358774